EMBALMING
Principles and Legal Aspects

EMBALMING
Principles and Legal Aspects

Second Edition

Editor

ML Ajmani
BSc MBBS MD MAMS

Former Professor
Department of Anatomy
All India Institute of Medical Sciences
New Delhi, India

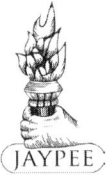

JAYPEE BROTHERS MEDICAL PUBLISHERS
The Health Sciences Publisher
New Delhi | London | Panama

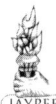

Jaypee Brothers Medical Publishers (P) Ltd

Headquarters

Jaypee Brothers Medical Publishers (P) Ltd
4838/24, Ansari Road, Daryaganj
New Delhi 110 002, India
Phone: +91-11-43574357
Fax: +91-11-43574314
E-mail: jaypee@jaypeebrothers.com

Overseas Offices

J P Medical Ltd
83 Victoria Street, London
SW1H 0HW (UK)
Phone: +44 20 3170 8910
Fax: +44 (0)20 3008 6180
E-mail: info@jpmedpub.com

Jaypee-Highlights Medical Publishers Inc
City of Knowledge, Bld. 235, 2nd Floor, Clayton
Panama City, Panama
Phone: +1 507-301-0496
Fax: +1 507-301-0499
E-mail: cservice@jphmedical.com

Jaypee Brothers Medical Publishers (P) Ltd
Bhotahity, Kathmandu, Nepal
Phone: +977-9741283608
E-mail: kathmandu@jaypeebrothers.com

Website: www.jaypeebrothers.com
Website: www.jaypeedigital.com

© 2019, Jaypee Brothers Medical Publishers

The views and opinions expressed in this book are solely those of the original contributor(s)/author(s) and do not necessarily represent those of editor(s) of the book.

All rights reserved. No part of this publication may be reproduced, stored or transmitted in any form or by any means, electronic, mechanical, photocopying, recording or otherwise, without the prior permission in writing of the publishers.

All brand names and product names used in this book are trade names, service marks, trademarks or registered trademarks of their respective owners. The publisher is not associated with any product or vendor mentioned in this book.

Medical knowledge and practice change constantly. This book is designed to provide accurate, authoritative information about the subject matter in question. However, readers are advised to check the most current information available on procedures included and check information from the manufacturer of each product to be administered, to verify the recommended dose, formula, method and duration of administration, adverse effects and contraindications. It is the responsibility of the practitioner to take all appropriate safety precautions. Neither the publisher nor the author(s)/editor(s) assume any liability for any injury and/or damage to persons or property arising from or related to use of material in this book.

This book is sold on the understanding that the publisher is not engaged in providing professional medical services. If such advice or services are required, the services of a competent medical professional should be sought.

Every effort has been made where necessary to contact holders of copyright to obtain permission to reproduce copyright material. If any have been inadvertently overlooked, the publisher will be pleased to make the necessary arrangements at the first opportunity. The **CD/DVD-ROM** (if any) provided in the sealed envelope with this book is complimentary and free of cost. **Not meant for sale**.

Inquiries for bulk sales may be solicited at: jaypee@jaypeebrothers.com

Embalming: Principles and Legal Aspects

First Edition: 1998

Reprint: 2009

Second Edition: **2019**

ISBN: 978-93-89129-74-8

Printed at Sanat Printers

Dedicated to

*My wife Kamla, son Deep,
daughter Anjali and grand-daughters Anisha and Sanya
without whose love, support and encouragement,
I could never have been able to complete this book*

Contributors

ML Ajmani
Former Professor
Department of Anatomy
All India Institute of Medical Sciences
New Delhi, India

DN Bhardwaj
Professor
Department of Forensic Medicine and Toxicology
All India Institute of Medical Sciences
New Delhi, India

Reenu Dhingra
Professor
Department of Anatomy
All India Institute of Medical Sciences
New Delhi, India

TD Dogra
Former Professor
Department of Forensic Medicine and Toxicology
All India Institute of Medical Sciences
New Delhi, India

T Jayavelu
Retd Professor of Anatomy
Stanley Medical College
Chennai, Tamil Nadu, India

Edward C Johnson
Funeral Director
Instructor of Clinical Embalming
City Wide College
Chicago, Illinois, USA

Gail R Johnson
Funeral Director
Instructor of Clinical Embalming
City Wide College
Chicago, Illinois, USA

Edward J Kerfoot PhD
Faculty of Allied Health Professions
Department of Occupational and Environmental Health
Detroit, Michigan, USA

Sanjeev Lalwani
Professor
Department of Forensic Medicine and Toxicology
All India Institute of Medical Sciences
New Delhi, India

Robert G Mayer
Licensed Embalmer and
Funeral Director
Pittsburgh, Pennsylvania, USA

BS Mikhell
Senior Lecturer and
Licensed Teacher (Anatomy)
Anglo European College of Chiropractic
13-15 Parkwood Road
Bournemouth, BH52DF, UK

Thomas F Mooney
Department of Occupational and Environmental Health
Detroit, Michigan, USA

Leandro Rendon
Director
Research and Educational Programs
The Champion Chemical Company
Williamsburg, Virginia, USA

A Sinha
Former Research Fellow
Department of Forensic Medicine and Toxicology
All India Institute of Medical Sciences
New Delhi, India

EO' Sullivan
Senior Technician
Department of Human Morphology
University of Southampton
Biomedical Science Building
Southampton, UK

Melina J Williams
Funeral Director
Chicago, Illinois, USA

KW Frolich
Institute of Anatomy
University of Bergen
5000 Bergen, Norway

LM Andersen
Institute of Anatomy
University of Bergen
5000 Bergen, Norway

Arne Knutsen
Institute of Anatomy
University of Bergen
5000 Bergen, Norway

Per R Flood
Institute of Anatomy
University of Bergen
5000 Bergen, Norway

Andre Bisaillon
Département d'Anatomie et Physiologie Animales, Faculté de Médecine Vétérinaire, Université de Montréal
Saint-Hyacinthe, Québec
Canada J2S 7C6

Reinhard Pabst
Center of Anatomy
Medical School of Hannover
PF 610180, D-3000 Hannover 61
Federal Republic of Germany

RP Clark
From the Laboratory for Aerobiology
Clinical Research Centre
Watford Road
Harrow, Middlesex HAI 3UJ

Richard Baurassa
Département d'Anatomie et Physiologie Animales, Faculté de Médecine Vétérinaire, Université de Montréal
Saint-Hyacinthe, Québec, Canada J2S 7C6

Preface to the Second Edition

The 2nd edition of *Embalming: Principles and Legal Aspects* adheres to the tradition established by the original publication; it provides a concise but thorough description of embalming and its clinical significance, an awareness of which is essential in the learning resource material in training surgeons for various operative skills that is not possible on an actual patient. The pedagogical features and updates in the 2nd edition help to facilitate embalmer learning.

The book deals with the art of embalming. It contains a brief historical review of the history of embalming, starting with ancient cultures such as the Egyptians and the lesser known Chinchorro culture, then going down the centuries and describing the anatomical techniques developed over the last two centuries. It also deals in detail with the chemicals used for embalming purposes. This edition includes the several approaches to evaluating embalming methods, their suitability for biomechanical testing, anatomical properties, and usability. Care has been taken in the text to provide all the necessary information conforming to the Indian environment and availability of resources in any medical school in the country.

The editor acknowledges his debt to other authors and works listed in the bibliography for the source material. He is equally indebted to the authors whose illustrations have been used in modified form.

In an effort of writing this kind of book, it is inevitable that some errors of omission are to be found, and these are the total responsibility of the editor.

The editor wishes to thanks M/s Jaypee Brothers Medical Publishers (P) Ltd, New Delhi, India, for helpful suggestions to get this work in print.

ML Ajmani

Preface to the First Edition

Books on embalming are few because the subject is seldom discussed in public or thought about until there is an urgent need to do the procedure. Recently, a National Symposium on embalming and AIDS was organized at the All India Institute of Medical Sciences (AIIMS), New Delhi, India, to disperse information about the modern practice of embalming to the professional from various disciplines, viz. Anatomy, Pathology, Forensic Medicine, Hospital Administration, etc. During the symposium, need for detailed information on embalming was realized. This book has been written with the object of presenting procedures of practical value in the embalming practice. It is not unusual to presume that the modern embalming is revival of the art practiced in ancient civilizations, but much is to be added to the old information in modern times. This book is not a formal treatise on embalming, but aims to give the background knowledge which would assist the practitioner in the legal aspects, methods and fundamentals of embalming. Care has been taken in the text to provide all the necessary information conforming the Indian environment and availability of resources in any medical school in the country. Chapters on the antiquity of embalming, the process of decomposition and disposal of dead and chemistry embalming materials are dealt with the some length. There is a chapter added on the therapeutic use of cadaver tissue with the legislature measures that it invites urgently because of the rapid advancement in tissue transplant surgery.

In the preparation of this book, I have had the great advantage of the meticulous professional assistance of Professor G Gopinath (Head, Department of Anatomy, AIIMS, New Delhi) without which this publication would not have been possible. She has always impressed and guided me in the true spirit in the preparation of this book.

I gratefully acknowledge the contribution made by Professor TD Dogra (Head, Department of Forensic Medicine and Toxicology, AIIMS, New Delhi). I am thankful to Dr Edward J Kerfoot, Department of Occupational and Environmental Health, Detroit, Michigan, Appleton and Lange, Connecticut, USA; The Champion Chemical Company, Springfield, Ohio; US Department of Health and Human Services, Centers for Disease Control, Atlanta; and BMJ Publishing Group, London, for allowing their material to be incorporated in this book. I have endeavored throughout to mention the authorities whose work I have made use of in the text.

The editor acknowledges his debt to other authors and works listed in the bibliography for the source material. He is equally indebted to the authors whose illustrations have been used in modified form.

In an effort of writing his kind of book, it is inevitable that some errors of omission are to be found, and these are the total responsibility of the editor.

I wish to express my sincere thanks to Mr HK Sharma, for the preparation of the art work, which is presented in this book. Special appreciation goes to Ms Savita Kumari, for typing the manuscript.

The editor wishes to thank National Book Trust, India and M/s Jaypee Brothers Medical Publishers (P) Ltd, New Delhi, India, for publishing this work. My special thanks are due to Mr KB Kapoor (Assistant Director), National Book Trust, India and Shri Jitendar P Vij (Managing Director), M/s Jaypee Brothers Medical Publishers, for their helpful suggestions to get this work in print.

ML Ajmani

Acknowledgments

The author expresses his gratitude to:
- Christine Dembski, Appleton and Lange, 25 Van Zant Street, East Norwalk, Connecticut, USA
- Christopher Sheridan, John Wiley and Sons, Inc., 605 Third Venue, New York, USA
- Mrs Carol Torselli, BMJ Publishing Group, BMA House, Tavistock Square, London WC1H9JR
- Barry Mitchell, Anglo European College of Chiropractic, 13-15 Parkwood Road, Bournemouth, BH5 2DF, UK
- US Centers for Disease Control, US Department of Health and Human Services, 1600 Clifton Road NE, Atlanta GA, USA
- Service and Research Department, The Champion Chemical Company, Springfield, Ohio, USA
- BI Churchill Livingstone Pvt Ltd, New Delhi, India.

We greatly appreciate the staff of M/s Jaypee Brothers Medical Publishers (P) Ltd, New Delhi, India, for their assistance, thoroughness, patience and professional work.

We are very grateful to our families for their tremendous support and understanding.

We are thankful to Shri Jitendar P Vij (Group Chairman), Mr Ankit Vij (Managing Director), Ms Chetna Malhotra Vohra (Associate Director—Content Strategy), and Dr Savleen Kaur (Development Editor) of M/s Jaypee Brothers Medical Publishers (P) Ltd, New Delhi, India, for giving a go-ahead at the very beginning and helping us in every way possible to bring out this book.

Contents

1. **The Origin and History of Embalming** 1
   Edward C Johnson, Gail R Johnson, Melissa J Williams

2. **Environment and Personal Health Considerations** 39
   Robert G Mayer

3. **Death and Postmortem Changes** 53
   TD Dogra, A Sinha, ML Ajmani

4. **Mummification** 59
   ML Ajmani

5. **Anatomical Considerations** 63
   ML Ajmani

6. **Surface Anatomy and Exposure of Blood Vessels** 75
   ML Ajmani

7. **Embalming Chemicals and Fluids** 81
   ML Ajmani

8. **Embalming Fluids and the Safe Levels of Formaldehyde** 88
   BS Mitchell, E O'Sullivan

9. **Practical Embalming** 92
   ML Ajmani

10. **Injection Technique** 97
    ML Ajmani

11. **Cavity Embalming** 101
    ML Ajmani

12. **Embalming the Unautopsied Adult Bodies** 105
    ML Ajmani

13. **Preparation of Autopsied Bodies** 109
    ML Ajmani

14. **Embalming the Infant** 112
    ML Ajmani

15. **Delayed Embalming** 114
    ML Ajmani

16. **Selected Conditions** 116
    ML Ajmani

17. **Effect of Drugs on the Embalming Process** 120
    Robert G Mayer

18. **Guidelines for Embalming an Acquired Immunodeficiency Syndrome Body** 128
    ML Ajmani

19. **Cosmetics and Presentation** 133
    ML Ajmani

20. **Embalmer's Legal Responsibility** 134
    TD Dogra, DN Bhardwaj

21. **Soft Embalming** 137
    Renu Dhingra, Sanjeev Lalwani

22. **The Law and the Dead** 141
    T Jayavelu

23. **Establishment of the Embalming Facilities** 146
    ML Ajmani

24. **Formaldehyde and Paraformaldehyde Study in Funeral Homes** 151
    Edward J Kerfoot, Thomas F Mooney

25. **Formaldehyde Vapor Emission Study in Embalming Rooms** 156
    Edward J Kerfoot

26. **Formaldehyde Study in Preparation Rooms** 158
    Edward J Kerfoot

27. **Reported Studies on Effects of Formaldehyde Exposure** 162
    Leandro Rendon

28. **Recommendations for Prevention of HIV Transmission in Healthcare Settings** 165

29. **Mobile Embalming Unit for the Preparation of Specimens for Anatomical Studies** 177
    Andre Bisaillon, Richard Baurassa

30. **Exposure to Formaldehyde in Anatomy: An Occupational Health Hazard** 179
    Reinhard Pabst

31. **Phenoxyethanol as a Nontoxic Substitute for Formaldehyde in Long-term Preservation of Human Anatomical Specimens for Dissection and Demonstration Purposes** 185
    KW Frolich, LM Andersen, Arne Knutsen, Per R Flood

32. **Formaldehyde in Pathology Departments** 193
    RP Clark

33. **Danger of Infection** 200
    Leandro Rendon

Index 203

Introduction

Embalming is an inescapable necessity of the modern society. Since ancient times, embalming has been in practice. The specimens preserved more than thousand years back are still lying in a perfect form in British museum in London.

The early chapters of this book give a background of the history of embalming. Ancient Egyptians used tents for doing embalming and they were called as precursors of modem anatomist. It used to take 70 days in ancient times to do the embalming, which has now been reduced to 1–2 hours to complete the process.

Everybody is made up of complex system of mechanics, and that of man is rather more complex. It is essential that the embalmer possesses a sound understanding of the internal anatomy of the body. A portion of this book is devoted to the fundamentals of the angiology and surface anatomy of the important vessels used for embalming. A thorough knowledge of surface anatomy permits the embalmer to make appropriate skin incisions and anticipate the structures, which will appear when the incision is made. Chapters on the stages of decomposition, the chemistry of embalming fluids and the process by which fluid comes into contact with the body proteins to preserve and sanitize the dead human remains are dealt with at length.

There are chapters to explain the various methods of arterial injection and drainage and embalming of the autopsied and infant bodies. As a result of the disease process, embalmer sees more and more bodies with advanced arteriosclerosis, edema, secondary infection, etc. Embalming under such conditions has also been described in detail. Because of the widespread use of drugs, many strains of the bacteria and viruses have become drug resistant and might be present in the body brought for embalming. Stress has been given for the embalmer to take extraordinary precautions in the handling and embalming of such human bodies.

A few topics are repeated to make each chapter a complete entity and to save the embalmer's time in consulting the reference item.

The latter chapters of the text deal with the specific conditions of the dead human cadaver, which generally an embalmer has to deal from time to time. There is a chapter on the legal responsibilities involved in the process of embalming, which is not only important but, at times, mandatory to safeguard the interest of society and embalmer.

Attempt has also been made to present guidelines for establishing an ideal embalming facility complex.

Finally, detailed study has been presented on some of the current embalming problems. These articles focus on environmental health hazards that exist in handling the chemicals, preservatives, and the body dead from both communicable and infectious diseases.

Chapter 1

The Origin and History of Embalming

Edward C Johnson, Gail R Johnson, Melissa J Williams

INTRODUCTION

A statement in 1875 by the New York State Supreme Court is still relevant, concise, and conceptually complete.

The decent burial of the dead is a matter in which the public have concern. It is against the Public Health if it does not take place at all and against a proper public sentiment should it not take place with decency.

Winston Churchill stated in his gifted style: "Without a sense of history, no man can understand the problems of our time, the longer you can look back, the further you can look forward—the wider the span, the longer the continuity, the greater is the sense of duty in individual men and women, each contributing their brief life's work to the preservation and progress of the land in which they live, the society of which they are the servants." *Prom Robert G Mayer. Embalming—History, Theory, and Practice. Appleton and Longe, Connecticut; 1990, with permission.

Esmond R Long, a Medical Historian wrote: "Nothing gives a better perspective of the subject than an appreciation of the steps by which it has reached its present state." So it is with the subject of embalming. The authors of this chapter trust that this brief exposition of the origin and history of embalming will impart to the reader a sense of the tradition and technical advances achieved over the nearly 5,000 years that the art and science of embalming have been practiced. There is a clear indication that both tradition and new technical advances will continue to be maintained in the future.

Embalming, one of humankind's longest practiced arts, is a means of artificially preserving the dead human body.

Natural Means of Preservation

Embalming has been in vogue since time immemorial without the deliberate intervention of humans.

- *Freezing*: By this method, bodies are preserved for centuries in the ice and snow of glaciers or snowcapped mountains.
- *Dry cold*: A morgue located on the top of St Bernard Mountain in Switzerland was so constructed to permit free admission of the elements. True mummies were produced as a result of the passage of the cold, dry air current over the corpses.
- *Dry heat*: Natural mummies are produced in the extremely dry, warm areas of Egypt, Southwestern America, and Peru.
- *Nature of the soil at the place of interment*: There are recorded instances of the discovery of bodies in a good state of preservation after long-term burial in a peat bog, which had a high-tannin content, or in soils strongly impregnated with salts aluminum or copper.

Artificial Means of Preservation

The undermentioned means have been secured by the deliberate action of humans:

- *Simple heat*: Simple heat is the means employed to preserve bodies in the Capuchin Monastery near Palermo, on the island of Sicily. The Monastery is connected to a catacomb or underground burial vault composed of four separate chambers. Treatment of the bodies consists of slow drying in an oven that is heated by a mixture of slacked lime. The desiccated bodies, quite shrunken, and light in weight are placed in upright positions along the walls of the catacombs.

- *Powders*: In powder methods, the body is placed on a bed of sawdust mixed with zinc sulfate or other preserving powder.
- *Evisceration and immersion*: It was used by the Egyptians and others.
- *Evisceration and drying*: It is also known as the Guanche method.
- *Evisceration, local incision, and immersion*: It was employed in Europe, particularly in France, during the period AD 650–1830.
- *Simple immersion*: In this method, body is immersed in alcohol, brine, or other liquid preservatives).
- *Arterial injection and evisceration*: It has been used by the Hunter brothers and others.
- *Cavity injection and immersion*: It is also known as method of Gabriel Clauderus.
- *Arterial injection*: It is mode of treatment of Gannal, Sucquet, and many others.
- *Arterial injection and cavity treatment*: This method is in daily use by all present day embalmers; generally taught in schools and colleges of embalming today.
- *Artificial cold*: Here by a system of refrigeration, the body temperature inhibits bacterial activity. It is in use in· most hospitals and morgues today).

PERIODS OF EMBALMING HISTORY

Embalming originated in Egypt during the period of the first dynasty. It is estimated to have begun about 3200 BC and continued on until AD 650. The motive of Egyptian embalming was religious. According to their belief, the preservation of the human body (intact) was a necessary requirement for resurrection. During this nearly 4000 year period of embalming practice, there obviously existed a number of variations of technique. Egyptian embalming began to decline with the advent of Christianity, as the early Christians rejected the practice, associating embalming with various "Pagan religious rites". When the Arabs conquered Egypt, they, too, rejected the practice of embalming.

The second period of embalming history extends from AD 650 to AD 1861 and its principal geographical area of practice and growth was Europe. This era is termed as the period of the Anatomists, as the motive was to advance the development of embalming techniques—for the preservation of the dead to permit detailed anatomical dissection and study.

The third or modem period of embalming history extends from 1861 to the present day. It is during this period that embalming knowledge, which had been transferring from Europe to America during the previous period, finally reverted to its original use principally for funeral purposes. Embalming again became available to all who requested it. Motives in this period are diverse, with sentiment probably predominant, as the average person desires to view the decedent free of evidence of the ravages of disease or injury. Public transportation is another reason to embalm, as the procedure prevents a dead body from becoming offensive during a protracted period of travel and is required by many public transport agencies.

While the value of embalming to the public health is disputed and debated, it is most apparent that a decaying, unembalmed body is surely a health menace to those exposed to its effluvia. From earliest Egyptian times, embalmers have been closely associated with the medical profession. In fact, most embalmers in the United States were doctors of medicine until the later portion of the 19th century.

ESTABLISHMENT OF EMBALMING SCHOOLS

The incentive for embalming in the period AD 650–1861 was the preservation of anatomical material to further the study of and research in anatomy. Those who made the early strides in embalming were the anatomists, but about the time of JN Gannal (early 19th century, France) and Thomas H Holmes (late-19th century, United States), general public interest was aroused in the preservation of the dead. This interest and the later demand for preservation for funeral purposes of all human dead grew far beyond the means and desires of the few trained embalmers in the medical profession—during the late-19th century in the United States, schools of embalming instruction were established by experienced embalmers. Many funeral directors who had no knowledge of embalming attended these schools to acquire the art. Others who were neither funeral directors nor doctors attended the schools to study embalming and to seek employment. By the beginning of the 20th century in the United States, separation of the fields of embalming and medicine was complete—this brought about the advancement of both professions, particularly that of embalming, as it placed a complex art in the hands of specialists who are still striving to acquire more knowledge and skill in preserving the human dead.

How, then, and why did the practice of embalming develop?

EGYPTIAN PERIOD

During the early predynastic period, well before 3200 BC, the Egyptians had a very simple culture. When death occurred, the unembalmed body was placed in the fetal position (arms and legs folded), wrapped in cloth or straw mats, and placed in a shallow grave scooped out of the desert sand west of the Nile River. A few pieces of pottery and other artifacts were placed in the grave with the body, which was positioned on its side. The body was then covered with the sand and the grave filled. The body was preserved by drying from the contact with the arid, porous sand, and the total absence of rainfall or other moisture. From time to time, desert winds uncovered the bodies in their shallow graves, and cemetery guards or relatives saw that the bodies were indeed preserved (Fig. 1.1).

As Egyptian civilization grew, towns and villages sprang up and commerce and industry created a substantial middle and upper class of landlords and other well-to-do persons, as well as a supreme class of tribal and area rulers. When members of this group died, the old practice of simple burial in the desert sands no longer sufficed. Graves were dug deeper and were lined with wooden boards or with stone slabs, so that the body still in the fetal position, remained untouched by the sand. With these, more prosperous or noble individuals were buried more valuable artifacts such as jewelry and furniture.

Then, as now, there existed members of society who were criminals, and some devoted themselves to grave robbing. When the cemetery custodians or family survivors of such elaborate burials noted the opening and desecration of burials, they also noted and were appalled that the corpse was no longer preserved, but had begun to decay. One attempt to forestall decomposition was the enclosure of the body within a solid stone coffin cut from a single mass of stone. The body of the coffin was without seams and the cover fit tightly. These burials were subsequently plundered and again the custodians or relatives contemplated the remains which, to their horror, had on many occasion completely decomposed to a skeletal status. Without a scientific knowledge of the process of putrefaction, they expressed the belief that the stone coffins are the soft tissues. To this day, massive bronze and copper caskets are termed Sarcophagi from the Greek "sarco" (flesh) and "phagus" (eater). The Egyptians, not wishing to revert to their simple burial in the stands method, found it necessary to devise some system of preserving the human body embalming.

It is not too difficult to understand that how Egyptian embalming was first developed with it is kept in mind that Egypt has a basically warm climate. The culture was such that hunting and fishing provided some of the food requirements. Thus, a hunter or fisherman might have a successful catch and secure more birds, fish, or game than he or his family could consume immediately. Such animals, fish, or birds could like the human body, quickly decay, and become worthless for food. The hunter, however, knew how to prepare his catch and to preserve it. He eviscerated and bled his catch and by one or another method such as salting, sun drying, smoking, or cooking preserved it for future consumption. (*This procedure for the preservation of food was common knowledge and it requires little imagination to recognize the ease with which the basic food preservation process could be adapted with refinements to the preservation of the dead human body*).

Variation in Embalming Methods

The actual methods of embalming employed by the Egyptians varied from dynasty to dynasty according to custom and to the technique of the individual embalmer. History provides views of four contemporary writers on the subject who have frequently been quoted.

The earliest account is that of the Greek historian Herodotus, who lived about 484 BC.

There are certain individuals appointed for the purpose (the embalming), and who profess the art; these persons, when anybody is brought to them, show the bearers some wooden models of corpses; the most perfect they assert to

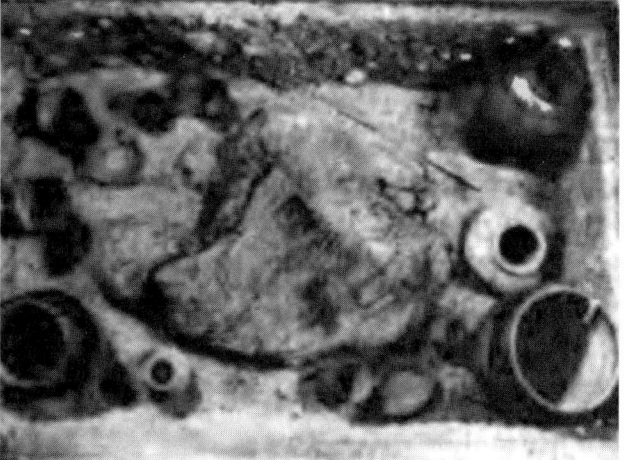

Fig. 1.1: Predynastic (3200 BC) Egyptian burial site, west of the Nile. The unembalmed corpse is in the fetal position, wrapped in straw matting.
Courtesy: The Royal Ontario Museum.

be the representation of him whose name I take it impious to mention in this matter; they show a second, which is inferior to the first and cheaper; and a third, which is cheapest of all. They then ask according to which of the models they will have the deceased prepared; having settled upon the price, the relations immediately depart, and the embalmers, remaining at home, thus proceed to perform the embalming in the most costly manner.

In the first place, with a crooked piece of iron, they pull out the brain by the nostrils; a part of it they extract in this manner, the rest by means of pouring in certain drugs; in the next place, after making an incision in the flank with a sharp Ethiopian stone, they empty the whole of the inside; and after cleaning the cavity, and rinsing it wilt) palm wine, scour it out with pounded· aromatics. Then, having filled the belly with pure myrrh pounded, and cinnamon, and all other perfumes, frankincense excepted, they sew it up again; having so done, they "steep" the body in natrum, keeping·it covered for 70 days, for it is not lawful to leave the body any longer.

When the 70 days are gone by, they first wash the corpse and then wrap up the whole body in bandages cut out of cotton cloth, which they smear with gum, a substance the Egyptians use instead of paste. The relations, having then received back the body, get a wooden case in the shape of a man to be made; and when completed, they place the body in the inside and then, shutting it up, keep it in a sepulchral repository where they stand it upright against the wall. The above is the most costly manner in which they prepare the dead.

For such who choose the middle mode, from a desire of avoiding expense, they prepare the body as follows; they first fill syringes with oil of *Cedar* to inject into the belly of the deceased, without making any incision, or emptying the inside, but by sending it in by the anus. This they then cork, to hinder the injection from it, wing backwards and lay the body in salt for the specified number of days, on the last of which they release what they had previously injected, and such is the strength it possesses that it brings away with it the bowels and insides in a state of dissolution; on the other hand, the natrum dissolves the flesh so that, in fact, there remains nothing but the skin and bones. When they have done this, they give the body back without any further operation upon it.

The third mode of embalming, which is used for such as have but scanty means, is as follows; after washing the insides with syrmas, they salt the body for the 70 days and return it to be taken back.

The second writer is Diodorus Siculus who lived about 45 BC.

When anyone·among the Egyptians dies, all his relations and friends putting dirt upon their heads, go lamenting about the city, till such time as the body shall be buried. In the mean time, they abstain from baths and wine, and all kinds of delicate meats, neither do they during that time wear any costly apparel. The manner of their burials is threefold—one very costly, a second sort less chargeable, and a third very mean. In the first,·they say, there is spent a talent of silver ($1,200); in the second 20 minae ($300); but in the last third is very little expense ($75). Those who have the care of ordering the body are such as have been taught that art by their ancestors. These, showing to the kindred of the deceased a bill of each kind of burial, ask them after which manner they will have the body prepared. When they have agreed upon the matter, they deliver the body to such as are usually appointed for this office. First, he who has the name scribe marks about the flank of the left side how much is to be cut away. Then he who is called the cutter or dissector, with an Ethiopian stone, cuts away as much of the flesh as the law commands, and presently runs away as fast as he can. Those who are present pursue him, cast stones at him, curse him, and thereby turning all the execrations, which they imagine due to his office upon him.

For whosoever offers violence, wounds, or does any kind of·injury to a body of the same nature with himself, they think him worthy of hatred;·but those who are called embalmers are worthy of honor and respect; for they are familiar with their priests and go into the temples, as holy men without any prohibition. So soon as they come to embalm the dissected body, one of them thrusts his hand through the wound into the abdomen and draws out all the viscera but the heart and kidneys, which another washes and cleanses with wine made of palms and aromatic odors.

Lastly having washed the body, they anoint it with oil of *Cedar* and other things for 30 days, and afterwards with myrrh, cinnamon, and other such like matters, which have not only a powder to preserve it for a long time, but also give it a sweet smell; afterwards, they deliver it·to the kindred in such manner that every member remains whole and tire, and no part of it changed. The beauty and shape of the face seems just as it was before, and may be known, even the hairs of the eyebrows and eyelids remaining as they were at first. By this method, many of the Egyptians, keeping the dead bodies' of their ancestors in magnificent houses, so perfectly see the true visage and countenance of those that died many ages before they themselves were born that in viewing the proportions of every one of them, and the lineaments of their faces, they take as much delight as if they were still living among them.

The third account is given by Plutarch who lived between AD 50 and 100.

The belly being opened, the bowels were removed and cast into the River Nile and the body exposed to the sun. The cavities of the chest and belly were then filled with the unguents and odorous substances.

The fourth description is by Perphry who lived about AD 230 to 300.

When those who have care of the dead proceed to embalm the body of any person of respectable· rank, they first take out the contents of the belly and place them in a separate vessel, addressing the sun, and utter on behalf of the deceased the following prayer, which Euphantus has translated from the original language into Greek—"O thou sun, our lord, and all ye gods who are the givers of life to men, accept me, and receive me into the mansions of the eternal gods; for I have worshipped piously, while I have lived in this world, those divinities whom my parents taught me to adore. I have ever honored those parents who gave origin to my body; and of other men I have neither killed any, nor robbed them of their treasure, nor inflicted upon them any grievous evil; but if I have done anything injurious to my soul either by· eating or drinking anything unlawfully, this offense has not been committed by me, but by what is contained in this chest." This refers to the intestines in the vessel, which is then cast into the River Nile. The body is afterwards regarded as pure, this apology having been made for its offenses, and the embalmer prepares it according to the appointed rites.

Differences in Translations

As may be observed, there were differences in embalming methods as described by the foregoing writers. This may be, in part, due to inaccuracies in copying and translating of the original manuscripts. Egyptologists generally dismiss the accounts of Plutarch and Porphyry as unreliable because the intestines either were removed or placed in containers that were kept near the body or were replaced in the body. As to the accounts of Herodotus and Diodorus, they were given the seal of approval for their general verity. However, scientific proof is lacking with regard to the corrosiveness of oil of *Cedar*, and it is believed that the covering of the corpse with natron took place before the filling of the trunk cavities with the spices and other substances.

Present-day translations of the Book of the Dead, a textbook guide for the Egyptian embalmer, do not agree on the 70-day period for the covering with natron. One of the chronologies of the most costly method states that the 1st–16th days were occupied with evisceration, washing, and cleansing of the body; from the 16th to the 36th days, the body was kept under natron; from the 36th to the 68th days, the spicing and bandaging took place; and from the 68th to the 70th days, the body was coffined.

Steps in Egyptian Preparation

Step 1: Removal of the Brain

The brain was generally removed by introducing a metal hook or spoon into the nostril and by forcing it through the ethmoid bone to the brain. As much as possible was scooped out in this way. In some mummies, the brain was not removed. A few craniums had the rain removed through the eye socket. There is one case on record in which the evacuation of the cranium was accomplished through the foramen magnum, after excision of the atlas vertebra. After the body was removed from under natron, the cranium was usually repacked with linen bandages soaked in resin or bitumen. One writer tells of removing 27 feet of 3-inch linen bandage from the cranium of a mummy. Sometimes, the cranium was filled with resin believed to have been introduced while molten with the aid of a funnel.

Step 2: Evisceration

Many bodies were not eviscerated. The earliest incision was made vertically in the left side, extending from the lower margin of the ribs to the anterior superior spine (crest) of the ilium. This incision would measure between 5 inches and 6 inches in length. At a later period, the incision became oblique, extending from a point near the left anterior spine (crest) of the ilium toward the pubes. A variant incision extended vertically from the symphysis pubis toward the umbilicus. In the very late 26th dynasty (665–527 BC), some bodies were eviscerated through the anus. The incision was usually made with a flint knife called Ethiopian stone because of its black color. All the viscera, with the exception of the kidneys and usually the heart, was removed, washed, and immersed in palm wine or packed in natron. ("Their disposition will be referred to later.")

Step 3: Covering with Natron

Natron is a salt obtained from the dry lakes of the desert and is composed of the chloride carbonate, and sulfate of sodium and the nitrate of potassium and sodium. Because of the corrosive action on the body, the embalmers had to affix the toe and fingernails to the body during the macerating period. This was accomplished by tying the nails on with thread or copper or gold wire. Alternatively, metal thimbles were fit over the ends of the fingers and toes for the same purpose. The body was then ready for the natron treatment. Early Egyptologists believed that the bodies were placed in a solution composed of natron dissolved in water, as described by Herodotus. Present-day authorities, in studying the original writing of Herodotus and other prime sources, detect a flaw in the translation of the text that is responsible for the misrepresentation. Present-day research, where the embalming process was recreated, indicates conclusively that only application of the concentrated dry salt over the body to some depth could dehydrate and preserve it. Experiments with different, concentrations of the natron solution, and immersion of specimens therein were largely unsuccessful in preventing decay.

Step 4: Removal from Natron

At the end of the 20th day of immersion in natron, the body was washed with water and dried in the sun.

Step 5: Wrapping and Spicing

The body was coated within and without by resin or a mixture of resin and fat. The skull was treated as in Step 1. The viscera, when removed from the body and not returned to the body, were placed in four canopic jars, the tops of which were surmounted by the images of the four children of Horus. Each jar held a specific portion of the. The jar topped with the human head represented Imset, and this jar contained the liver. The jar covered with the jackal's head represented Duamutef and contained the stomach. The jar topped with the ape's head represented Hapy and held the lungs. The fourth jar, surmounted by a hawk's head, represented Qebeh-Snewef and contained the intestines. No mention is made of the disposition of the spleen, pancreas, or pelvic organs (Fig. 1.2).

The canopic jars varied in size and material. They were from about 9 inches to 18 inches in height, and 4 inches in diameter, and were made of alabaster, limestone, basalt,

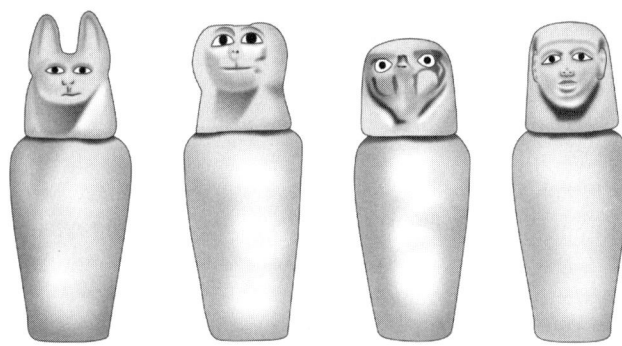

Fig. 1.2: Canopic urns—containers of the viscera removed during embalming preparation and not returned to trunk of body. From left to right are the Jackal's head. Duamutef (contained stomach), the human head, Imset (contained liver), the ape's head, Happy (contained lungs), and the hawk's head, Qebeh-Snewef (contained intestines).
Courtesy: Paula Johnson De Smet.

clay, and other materials. The Canopic jars were usually placed in a wooden box and kept near the body. When the vera were placed in these jars, images in miniature of the jars were returned to the cavity, which was padded in straw, resin-soaked linen bandages, or lichen moss. Upon return to the body cavity, the viscera were usually wrapped in four separate parcels to which were attached specific images, as mentioned above. Originally, the incision was not sewn but merely had the edges drawn together. Sometimes, the edges were stuck together by resin or wax; however, there are recorded instances in the 18th, 20th, and 21st dynasties (1700 BC, 1250 BC, and 1000 BC) of closure affected by sewing that closely resembles the familiar embalmer's stitch of today. The incision was covered, whether sewn or not, by a plate of wax or metal upon which was engraved the eye of Osiris (Egyptian god of the dead).

Ancient Restorative Art

It was during this part of the preparation in the 20th dynasty (1288–1100 BC) that a little known process was performed. Most present clay embalmers feel that the restoration to normal of emaciated facial features of corpse is of comparatively recent origin. On the contrary, the Egyptian embalmers performed this operation, but on a much more extensive scale. Not only were the facial features restored, but the entire bodily contours were subcutaneously padded to regain their normal shape. The methods and materials used varied.

The mouth was usually internally packed with sawdust to pad out the cheeks, while the eyelids were stuffed with linen pads. Then working from the original abdominal incision by burrowing under the skin of the trunk in all directions, the packing material was forced into these channels. In places, such as the back and arms, that could not be reached from the original incision, additional local incisions were made through which to pass the padding material. In later periods, the cheeks and temples were padded with resin introduced through openings in front of the ears. This material, introduced while warm, could be molded to conform to the desired contour. The packing materials most commonly used were resin, linen bandages, mud, sand, sawdust, and butter mixed with soda. It was also during this stage of preparation that repair of bodily injuries took place. Broken limbs were splinted, and bed sores were packed with resin-soaked linen bandages and covered with thin strips of antelope hide.

There is a case of a crooked spine having been straightened. Eyes were sometimes replaced with ones of stone or as in one instance, with small onions. The bodies that were to be gilded (covered with gold leaf) were then treated. Some were completely covered with a gold leaf; on others, only the face, fingernails, and toenails, or genitals were gilded, as there was much variation on this matter. After the complete covering of the body with a paste of resin and fat, the bandagers set to work. It is believed that there were individuals who specialized in wrapping certain parts of the body such as the fingers, arms, legs, and head. Each finger or toe was first separately swathed, then each limb. The body was first covered with a kind of tunic and the face covered with a large square bandage followed by the regular spiral bandages. Pads were placed between the bandages to aid in restoration and maintenance of the bodily contour. Lotus blossoms have been found between the layers of linen bandages. Some authorities claim that the living saved cloth all their lives to provide bandages for use as mummy wrappings. The bandages varied from 3 inches to 9 inches in width and up to 1,200 yards in length and were inscribed at intervals with hieroglyphics—indicating the identity of the enswathed person. Authorities believe that only one of ten mummies was prepared by the first method. The others were prepared by the cheaper methods, as described by the earlier writers. Another means of embalming used then was simple covering of the entire body with natron or molten resin. This latter process, while preserving the body, destroyed the hair and most of the facial features, fingers, and toes.

During the last 1000 years of Egyptian embalming practice, the emphasis gradually changed from producing a well-preserved body capable of withstanding decay for all eternity to creating an increasingly elaborate external appearance of the wrapped body. Wrapping patterns became quite elaborate and cartonnage and plaster were employed to present a sometimes fanciful external recreation of the deceased. During the terminal centuries of Egyptian embalming, portraits on a flat surface were painted and placed over the head area, which more faithfully resembled the dead.

Receptacles

The wrapped mummies were usually additionally encased and placed in boxes or coffins. An additional encasement, termed cartonnage, was made of 20 or 30 sheets of linen cloth or papyrus saturated in resin, plaster of Paris, or gum acacia and placed over the wrapped body while wet. To ensure a tight fit, the material was drawn together in the back of the body by a kind of lacing not unlike present-day shoe lacing. The cartonnage, when dry, was as hard as wood and was covered with a thin coating of plaster, then painted with a representation of a human head and other designs. Two or more wood cases of *Cedar* or sycamore might encase the cartonnage and each other. These coffins or mummy cases were of different shape, depending on the period when they were made. The outer wooden case was, at times, rectangular in shape with a cover resembling the roof of a house. Early coffined embalmed bodies were placed within the coffins lying on their side. The exterior of the coffin contained the representation of a pair of eyes on one side near the head of the coffin (Fig. 1.3). This indicated the position of the body facing outward at this point. Coffins shaped like the human form were termed anthropoid or mummiform (Fig. 1.4). If the deceased was a member of a great family, he might be enclosed within a stone sarcophagus that was a stone coffin or vault fashioned of marble, limestone, granite, or slate.

Even in Egyptian times, the tombs of the dead were plundered for their valuables. Many mummy cases were

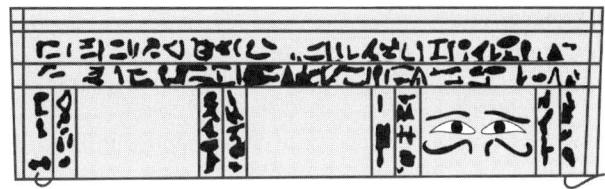

Fig. 1.3: Wooden coffin. The body placed inside and lies on its left side with the head at the end, where eyes are drawn facing eyes and thus looking outward.
Courtesy: Paul Johnson De Smet.

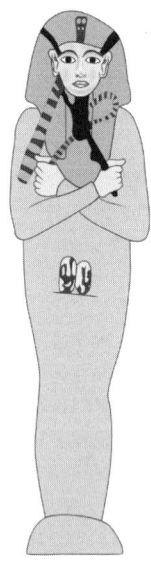

Fig. 1.4: Wooden anthropoid or mummiform coffin.
Courtesy: Paula Johnson De Smet.

broken open and the mummies themselves were damaged. The embalmers were called upon to repair the damaged mummies and to rewrap and recoffin them. This may explain, in part, the so-called faking of mummies. In the Field Museum of Natural History in Chicago, there are numerous X-ray pictures of unopened mummy cases and unwrapped mummies. Some of these pictures show damage that might have occurred prior to or during the course of embalming. One X-ray photo of a young child displays the complete absence of the anns and bilateral fractures of the femurs at about their midpoint, with the lower broken portion entirely missing. Museum authorities advance the theory that this was done to fit the child into a smaller mummy case. Another X-ray photo reveals a wrapped mummy lacking arms and the trunk of the body. The head was connected to the legs by a board and the body had been represented by padding of straw or lichen moss.

Additional faking may be the result of a curious custom of the early middle ages of using bits of mummies as good luck pieces and as a drug for internal consumption. This demand created a brisk business for the Arabs of North Africa, and as the supply of natural mummies was difficult to maintain, the Arabs began to produce their own from the bodies of the lepers and criminal dead.

Animals were also embalmed, wrapped, and coffined in a manner similar to humans. The variety of animals so treated was large and included baboons, monkeys, full-grown bulls, gazelles, goats, sheep, antelopes, crocodiles, cats, dogs, mice, rats, shrews, hawks, geese, ibis, snakes, and lizards. X-ray examination of these wrapped packages discloses an occasional falsity. Some of these false mummies are composed of straw or rags wrapped in the form of the animals they were to represent. G Elliot Smith, in his article on the Significance of Geographical Distribution of Practice of Mummification, states that knowledge of the Egyptian method of embalming was carried westward as far as the Canary Islands. He bases his decision on the similarity of the embalming procedures carried on in these areas of the world and the knowledge that the Egyptian method preceded those in all other known parts of the world.

PRACTICE OF BODY PRESERVATION OF VARIOUS ETHNIC GROUPS AND PLACES

Jewish

The Jews did not embalm but simply washed and shaved the body and swathed it in sheets between the folds of which were placed spices such as myrrh and aloes. The purpose of herbs and spices was to disguise the odor of decay of the body, not to preserve it.

Ancient Persians, Syrians, and Babylonians

Sometimes, the ancient Persians, Syrian, and Babylonians immersed their human dead in jars of honey or wax. Alexander the Great was said to have been so treated to preserve his body during the long journey from the place of death in Babylon in 323 BC (during a military campaign) to Egypt.

Ancient Ethiopians

The ancient Ethiopians eviscerated and desiccated their dead in a manner similar to the Egyptian method. The bodily contours were restored by applying plaster over the shrunken skin. The plaster-covered corpse was then painted with lifelike colors and given a coating of clear resin-like substance believed by some authorities to be a fossil salt and by others to be a type of amber, somehow rendered fluid at the time of application.

Canary Islands (from at least 900 BC)

In the Atlantic Ocean, about 4° South of the Madeira Islands, on the northwest coast of Africa, there is a cluster of

13 islands known as the Canary Island. These islands were not subdued by any European nation until the Spaniards overran them in the late 15th century. The original inhabitants, known as Guanches, are thought to have been descendants of the lost continent of Atlantis. It is believed that only prominent and influential families had the dead embalmed. The Guanches' method of embalming their dead is very similar to the Egyptian method.

The Guanche embalmers were both men and women who performed the services for their own sex. These embalmers were well paid, although their touch was considered contaminating and they lived in seclusion in remote parts of the islands. Upon the death of a person, the family bore the body to the embalmers and then retired. The embalmers placed the body upon a stone table and an opening was made in the lower abdomen with a flint knife called Tabona. The intestines were withdrawn, washed, cleaned, and later returned to the body. The entire body, inside and outside, was very thoroughly saturated with salt and the intestines were returned to th.e body along with numerous aromatic plants and herbs.

The body anointed with butter, powdered resin, brushwood, and pumice was exposed to the sun, or, if the sun was not hot enough, the body was placed in a stove to dry. During the drying period, the body was maintained in an extended position; the arms of men were placed along the sides of the body, while women's arms were placed across the abdomen.

The embalmers maintained a constant vigil over the body during the period to prevent it from being developed by vultures. On the 15th or 16th day, the drying process should be completed and the relatives would claim the body and sew it in goatskins. Kings and nobles were, in addition, placed in coffins of hollowed juniper logs. All bodies were deposited in caves in the hilly regions of the islands.

In another method of preparation described, a corrosive liquid believed to be juice of the spurge or euphorbia plant, was either introduced through the belly wall or poured down the throat; this was followed by the drying process described above. The mummies produced by these processes were called Xaxos and the method of embalming was believed to have been introduced from Egypt about 900 BC. In TJ Pettigrew's History of Egyptian Mummies, there is a description of a Xaxos as found by a sea captain in 1764. The author points out the "flesh of the body is perfectly preserved, but is dry, inflexible, and hard as wood not is any part decayed. The body is no more shrunk than if the person had been dead only 2 or 3 days. Only, the skin appears a little shriveled and of a deeply tanned; copper color". The Xaxos were extremely light in weight, averaging about 6-9 pounds for bodies up to 5½ feet in length.

Peru

Preservation of the body in Peru was practiced for at least a thousand years before the Spanish conquest in the early 16th century. It had for its motive a religious belief in the resurrection of the body. Most authorities agree that the Peruvians had no process of embalming, but—that their mummies were a product of the extremely dry climate of the region. There are reports that the Incas or ruling classes were embalmed, and because only mummies of the common people have been discovered, this report may be true. The manner in which the Inca rulers are believed to have been prepared was by evisceration. The intestines were placed in gold vases, the cavity filled with an unspecified resin, and the body coated with bitumen. The bodies were said to have been seated upon their thrones, clothed in their regal robes, hands clasped upon the breast, and head inclined downward. There is mention of the use of gold to plate or replace the eyes.

The usual Peruvian mummy, of which there are many specimens in the Field Museum at Chicago, was often found buried with the face toward the west, together with provisions of corn and coca contained in earthen jars. The mummies themselves were wrapped in cloth and tied with a coarse rope. The outer covering was of matting and followed a roll of cotton which, in turn, enveloped a red or varied-color wool cloth wrapped about the body. The innermost wrapping was white cotton sheet. The corpse was found in a squatting position, knees under chin, arm over breast, with the fists touching the jaws. The hands were usually fastened together, and on most mummies there was a rope passed three or four times around the neck. In the mouth, there was usually a small copper, silver, or gold disk. The greater part of the mummies was well preserved, but the flesh was shriveled and the features were disfigured. The hair was preserved with the women's hair braided. Nearly all types of animals and birds have been found mummified including parrots, dogs, cats, doves, hawks, heron, ducks, and llamas; vicunas and llamas wrapped in the manner of human mummies.

Ecuador

The Jivaro Indians of the Marano River region of South America had a method of preserving heads by shrinking them. Technically, this process does not come under the heading of embalming, but a brief general description of the process is of interest.

The bones of the skull were first removed through long slits in the scalp. The skin of the head, with the hair attached, was boiled in water containing astringent herbs. Upon completion of this process, hot stones of gradually diminishing size were inserted into the space formerly occupied by the skull bones. When the shrinking process was completed, the stones were removed and the incisions were sutured as were the mouth and the eyes. The finished shrunken head is about the size of a man's fist, with the features rather clear and retaining their proper proportions. It has been stated that this same process has been applied to an entire human body with equal success, although no such specimens have been found.

Mexico and Central America-Aztecs, To/tees, and Mayans

Upon Ute basis of information received from Dr Alfonso Caso, Mexico's outstanding anthropologist, there is no evidence of the employment of any artificial means of preservation of the body in the pre-Spanish era in these regions. There are accounts of finding mummies wrapped in matting and buried in the earth or in caves, but it is the opinion of Dr Caso and others that such mummification was the result of the natural climate of the region.

North American Indians

Although no proof exists to substantiate claims that some of the Indian tribes embalmed their dead, there are quotes from two accounts of embalming means recounted by Dr HC Yarrow in his *Study of Mortuary Customs of North American Indians* from 1880, collected from earlier publications. On page 185 of the History of Virginia (by Beverly, 1722), the below statement is found:

The Indians are religious in preserving the corpses of their kings and rulers after death. First they neatly flay off the skin as entire as they can, slitting only the back; then they pick all the flesh off the bones as clean as possible, leaving the sinews fastened to the bones, that they may preserve the joints together. Then they dry the bones in the sun and put them into the skin again, which in the meantime has been kept from shrinking. When the bones are placed right in the skin, the attendants nicely fill up the vacuities with very fine white sand. After this, they sew up the skin again, and the body looks as if the flesh had not been removed, they take care to keep the skin from shrinking by the help of a little oil or grease, which saves it from corruption. The skin being thus prepared, they lay it in an apartment for that purpose, upon a large shelf raised above the floor. This shelf is spread with mats for the corpse to rest easy on, and screened with the same to keep it from the dust. The flesh they lay upon hurdles in the sun to dry, and when it is thoroughly dried, it is sewed up in a basket and set at the feet of the corpse, to which it belongs.

Another account appeared on page 39, volume XIII of *Collection of Voyages* (Pinkerton, 1812), concerning the Werowance Indians.

Werowance Indian

Their bodies are first bowelled, then dried upon hurdles till they become very dry, an so about most of their joints and neck they hang bracelets or chains of copper, pearl, and such like, as they are used to wear. Their innards they stuff with copper beads, hatchets, and such trash. Then they lap them very carefully in white skins and so roll them in mats for their winding sheets.

The Indians are known to have wrapped their dead in cloth or leather and to have suspended the bodies in a horizontal manner in trees or buried them in the earth, in caves, or in the ground covered by rocks. This may have had a religious significance, but more likely it was done to prevent vultures or animals from devouring the dead.

Aleutian Islands and Kodiak Archipelago

It is believed that the inhabitants of Aleutian Islands and Kodiak Archipelago practiced preservation of their dead from at least AD 1000, although the custom did not prevail on the mainland. The internal organs were removed through an incision in the pelvic region and the cavity was refilled with dry grass. The body was placed in a stream of cold running water, which was said to have removed the fatty tissues in a short time. The corpse was removed from the water and wrapped in the fetal posture, knees under the chin, and arms compressed about the legs. This position was accomplished by use of force, breaking bones, if necessary. In this posture, the body was sun dried and, as a final gesture, was wrapped in animal skins and matting.

PERIOD OF THE ANATOMISTS (AD 650–1861)

With the Arabic conquest of Egypt and the fall of the Roman Empire, European and Mediterranean civilizations declined virtually to the vanishing point. The old world of law and order as the Romans and others knew it was replaced by anarchy. Geographical areas were ruled by bands of arm men with little stability of control. These Dark Ages were to continue until the year 1000 when a gradual elimination of unstable leaders left a few more wise and capable individuals in charge of substantial geographical divisions of Europe. With a return to a more normal civilized existence came the establishment of schools and colleges in what is today Sicily, Italy, France, and England and later in Germany, Holland, Belgium, and Switzerland. The schools were, in part, the product of the Catholic Church, which throughout the Dark Ages had maintained and served as a sanctuary for work in the fields of medicine, nursing, teaching, copying of manuscripts, and establishment of orphanages and poorhouses.

The medical schools that were established used some texts originally written during the glory era of Egypt. In Alexandria, on the Mediterranean at the mouth of Nile, there existed the greatest center for teaching that history had known. The library, before its destruction, was said to have contained more than half a million manuscripts on subjects varying from astronomy to mathematics to engineering to medicine. It was here that a famous teacher and practitioner of medicine, Claudius Galen (130–200 AD) born in Pergamum, Asia Minor, taught and wrote on the subject of anatomy. His textbook on anatomy described human anatomy principally from dissections of animals such as the pig or monkey. It must be obvious today that there are substantial differences or variations between the anatomical structure of the pig or monkey and that of the human being. Galen and others were not encouraged to dissect the human body as it was considered a mutilation and a crime under Egyptian law. Nevertheless, Galen's teachings and writings on human anatomy were to be considered as the unchallengeable authority for the next 1,000–1,200 years.

With the emergence of Europe from the Dark Ages came a craving for learning that had to that time been suppressed. The medical schools lacked the authority to legally acquire dead human bodies for dissection and anatomical study until 13th and early 14th centuries. Such authority was granted 1242 by Frederick II, King of the two Sicilies, and again in 1302 for the delivery of two executed criminals to the medical school at Bologna, Italy, each year for dissection. Such dissections were public affairs, often conducted in open areas or amphitheaters always during the cold months of the year as the dissection subjects were not preserved. The dissection itself was rapid, frequency confined to a 4-day period. In the actual procedure, the anatomy professor, who was seated, read from Galen's text on anatomy while pointing out (with a wand) the body structures mentioned by Galen. An assistant, a Barber-Surgeon, did the actual dissection as the lecture progressed. Obviously, there were frequent contradictions between Galen's description of a body part and its actual appearance as disclosed by the dissection. These most evident discrepancies encouraged the more intelligent student and medical practitioner to steal bodies from cemeteries and gallows for personal study and research. Every part of such a purloined cadaver was probed speedily for knowledge of its structure or function until it became too loathsome to conceal and had to be disposed of. In many cases, the soft tissues were thrown away and the bones boiled to secure the skeleton.

Military Religious Campaigns

During the period from 1095 to 1291, a series of military religious campaigns mounted by the Christian nations of Europe (termed Crusades) were conducted to recapture the Holy Land from the Muslims. The campaigns were successful early on, but with the passage of time, the Christian occupation forces in Holy Land became complacent and less martial and eventually—were expelled from the entire conquered territory. Many prominent members of the nobility, including King Louis XIX of France, died far from home during the crusades. To allow the return to their homeland of their remains, it was necessary to develop what became a gruesome procedure, as no certain means of embalming was available during the campaigns. The procedure consisted of disemboweling and disarticulating the body, cutting off all soft tissue and then boiling the bones until they were free of all soft tissues. The bones were then dried and wrapped within bull hides and returned to their homeland by the couriers who maintained the communication lines.

In 1300, Pops Boniface VIII issued a Papal Bull (a directive) that prohibited the cutting up of the dead for the purpose of transport and burial under penalty of excommunication. For a brief period, this Papal Bull was interpreted by some members of the medical profession to ban anatomical dissection. For example, in 1345, Vigevano stated that dissection was prohibited, and Mondino (1270-1326) said sin was involved in boiling bones. In any case, such interpretations were rare and were seldom given any regard by the majority of anatomists.

As the years passed, it became obvious that some system of preservation, even temporary, had to be contrived to permit a more careful and intensive study of body structure. Early efforts at preservation followed the ancient regimen of drying the parts, for moisture was and is the enemy of preservation. Preservation by drying of cadavers or their components was first sought by exposure to the natural heat of the sun. Later, use of controlled heat in ovens was employed to accomplish desiccation. Eventually, while probing the nature and extent of the hollow blood vessels, it was noted that warm air forced through the blood vessels removed blood and eventually dried out the tissue.

Reports of preservation attempts from the 15th century did not include injections of the blood vascular system. Such early injections into hollow structures of the body were made to trace the direction and continuity of blood vessels, or to inflate hollow organs so as to reveal their size and shape or to make internal castings of areas under study. As early as 1326, Alessandra Giliani of Italy injected blood vessels with colored solutions that hardened; Jacobus Berehgarius (1470-1550) employed as yr4lge and injected veins with warm water; Bartolomeo Eustaschio (1520-1574) used warm ink; Regnier De Graaf (1641-1673) invented a syringe and injected mercury; Jan Swammerdam (1637-1680) injected a wax-like material that later hardened—the great artist Leonardo Da Vinci (1452-1519), who is said to have dissected more than 30 corpses to produce hundreds of accurate anatomical illustrations, injected wax to secure castings of the ventricles of the brain and other internal areas.

Early Instruments for Injection

Early instruments for injection were crude and usually made in two parts—a container for the injection material and some form of cannula. The cannula was often contrived from a hollow straw, feather quill, hollow metal, or glass tube, which was attached by ligature to an animal bladder (stomach, or other intestine). The cannula was inserted into the hollow opening being studied and the bladder tied onto its free end. The bladder, in turn, was filled with a liquid and then tied to retain the bladder full. Entrance of the liquid material into the hollow area was secured by squeezing the bladder until it emptied.

As early as 1521, Berengarius wrote of using a forerunner of the modern syringe. Early syringes similar to the hypodermic syringes employed today were constructed. They were filled and then attached to a cannula in position within the opening to be injected. To refill the syringe, the operator had to detach the syringe from the cannula, refill it, and then reattach it. Bartholin (1585-1629) developed the first continuous flow syringe. It could be recharged during use without halting the injection process.

During the entire time from the end of the Egyptian embalming activity through the "Dark Ages" and into early medieval period, some members of the elite, clergy nobles, tradesmen, and landowners were embalmed, a procedure ordinarily neither contemplated by nor available to the average European. The embalming procedure, not surprisingly, was virtually identical to the Egyptian technique described by Herodotus and others, with the exception that far less time was consumed in its execution.

One of the best accounts of nonanatomical embalming for burial purposes is related by the Dutch physician Peter Forestus (1522-1597), who wrote about embalming. His account, in German, is contained as an appendix in the 1605 edition of Peter Offenbach's treatise on Wound Surgery. Forestus specifically described the embalming process and the materials used in five named cases between 1410 and 1548, two of which he personally performed:
- 1410—Pope Alexander V of Bologna, Italy
- 1511—Lady Johanna of Burgundy, Holland
- 1537—Bishop Magoluetus of Bologna, Italy
- 1582—Countess of Haute Kerken of the Hague, Holland
- 1584—Princess Auractus of Holland.

As these cases are essentially similar, only one embalming report is cited in its entirely.

Most of the above embalmings were performed in the room of the residence where the death occurred, a practice rather commonly followed later (well into the 20th century) in many countries including the United States.

The following is the full description of the Forestus embalming of the Countess of Haute Kerken. The others listed a quite similar with some individual variations such as opening the cranium and removing the brain and making long and deep incisions in the extremities to press out the blood, then filling the incisions with the powdered mixture.

I personally was bidden to embalm the Countess of Haute Kerken, who was a daughter of a nobleman of Egmont

(Holland) and who died of childbirth on January 9, 1582 in the Hague (Holland) before Johannes Heurnius (1543-1601), my good friend, and professor at Leyden in Holland was asked. Preceding all things, before the embalmment was begun, there was made the following preparation—1 took 2½ lbs aloes; myrrh, 1½ lbs; ordinary wermut, seven hands full; rosemary, four hands full; pumice, 1½ lbs; marjoram, 4 lbs; storacis calamata, 2 loht, the zeltlinalipta muscate, ½ loht. Mix all and reduce to a powder. Lay open the trunk of the body remove all the viscera, afterwards take such sponges, which were previously immersed in cold fresh water, afterwards dipped in aqua vita, and wash out the interior of the body by and with the sponge. This having been done, fill the cavities (of the body) with a layer of cotton moistened in aqua vita; sprinkle over it a layer of the previously mentioned powder place another layer of the moistened cotton and a layer of powder one over the other until the abdomen together with the chest is entirely full. Afterwards, see the above (abdominal walls) again together. Wrap around (the body) with waxed cloth and other things. Now having heard this you understand this embalmment was performed by me, the aforementioned Heurnius and Arnold the Surgeon on January 10, 1562, in the dwelling of the wellborn Count and Countess Von—Wassenaer in the Hague.

Ambroise Pare (1510–1590)

Born in France, Ambroise Pare was military Barber Surgeon an eventually surgeon to French Kings Henri II, Francois II, and Charles IX. He was famous for rediscovery and improvement of use of ligature of control bleeding after amputations, podalic version (changing the position of an unborn infant within the uterus) to facilitate delivery, and designing of artificial limbs. Pare, like many surgeons of the period embalmed the bodies of prominent military leaders and noblemen killed during military campaigns as well as similarly prominent civilians dying of natural causes.

In his book *The Works of Ambroise Pare*, translated into English and published in London in 1634, he devotes a portion of the 28th chapter on the manner how to embalm the dead.

But the body, which is to be embalmed with spices for very long continuance must first of all be embowelled, keeping the heart apart, that it may be embalmed and kept as the kinsfolkes shall think fit. Also the brain, the skull being divided with a saw, shall be taken out. Then you shall make deep incisions along the arms, thighs, legs, back, loins, and buttocks, especially where the greater veins and arteries run, first that by this means the blood may be pressed forth, which otherwise would putrefy and give occasion and beginning to putrefaction to the rest of the body; and then that there may be space to put in the aromatic powder; and then the whole body shall be washed over, with a sponge dipped in aqua vita and strong vinegar, wherein shall be boiled wormewood, aloes, coloquintida, common salt, and alum. Then these incisions, and all the passages and open places of the body and the three bellies shall be stuffed with the following spices grossly powdered. Radix pul rosar, Chamomile, Balsami, Methe, Anethi, Salvia, Lavendula, Rorismar, Marjoran, Thymi, Absinthi, Cyperi, Calami aromat, Gentiana, Irosflorent, Accavederata, Caryophyll, Nucis moschat, Cinamoni, Styracis calamita, Benjoini, Myrrha, Aloes, Santel, Omnium quod sut'ficit. Let the incisions be sowed up and the open spaces that nothing fall out; then forthwith, let the whole body be anointed with turpentine, dissolved oil of roses and chamomile, adding if you shall think it fit, some chemical oil of spices, and then let it be again strewed over with the forementioned powder; then wrap it in a linen cloth, and then in Cesare-clothes. Lastly, let be put in a coffin of lead, sure soudred, and filled up with dry sweet herbs. But, if there be no plenty of the forementioned spices, as it usual happens in besieged towns, the chirurgeon shall be contented with the powder of quenched lime, common ashes made of oak wood.

The procedure described by Pare was the most prevalent in use from the end of the Egyptian system to well past the discovery of arterial injection.

Discovery of a New Technique

Anatomical dissection, nonpreservative injections, and study continued until inevitably the technique of arterial injection of some preservative substance into the blood vascular system to secure an embalmed subject was stumbled upon. Contrary to popular belief, three men, all Dutch and all friends, were involved and must be recognized for their contributions to the technique—Jan Swammerdam (1637-1680), the original inventor or discoverer; Frederik Ruysch (1638-1731) the great practitioner who refined the technique; and Stephen Blanchard (1650-1720), the person who openly publish the method.

Swammerdam was educated in medicine but devoted the greatest part of his life to the study of insects and small animals. He perfect a system of injection to preserve even insects through tiny cannulae made of glass and manipulated by the aid of microscopes designed by Leeuwenhoek (the inventor of the microscope). His preservatives were said to have included various forms of alcohol, turpentine, wine, rum, spirits of wine (purer form of alcohol), and colored waxes. This injection technique was transmitted to Ruysch who applied it to human subjects, both entire bodies and portions thereof. His superb collections of anatomical specimens provided great teaching aids. His embalming of complete human remains included individuals such as British Admiral Sir William Berkley, who was killed during a sea battle of Holland in 1666, and whose body, was recovered from the sea in a decomposing condition. Ruysch was requested by the Dutch government to embalm the body "so that it might be returned to England for funeral and burial". It is said that the body was normal in appearance and color after his treatment.

In another episode, the Russian Czar Peter the Great, during one of his visits to Western Europe, visited the medical school of Leiden, Holland, and Ruysch's home, where his museum was situated. During the visit with Ruysch, it is elated that some domestic problem required Ruysch's attention and he left Czar Peter alone for a few minutes. Czar Peter began to explore the various rooms, and in opening, one door discovered an infant apparently asleep. Tiptoeing into the room, he contemplated the beautiful pink child, then bent down and kissed it, only to discover by its cold exterior lrtat, it was one of Ruysch's many preparations. Czar Peter purchased one entire museum collection from Ruysch, which some historian report was lost or destroyed. The truth is that it is still on exhibit in Leningrad today. Ruysch personally never did make a full disclosure of his technique or preservative. There are many who conjecture that his preservative was alcohol, turpentine, or even arsenic.

Blanchard, an anatomist of Leiden, published a book in 1688 entitled "*A New Anatomy with Concise Directions for Dissection of the Human Body with a New Method of Embalming*". Pages 281-287 and several diagrams of syringes and instruments constitute the appendix describing his method of embalming. He mentions the use of spirits of wine and turpentine. In one of his embalming treatments, he began by flushing out the intestinal tract by first forcing water from the mouth to the anus. Then he repeated the flushing with spirits of wine and retained it in place by corking the rectum. He opened large veins and arteries and flushed out the blood with water, then injected the preservative spirits of wine. *(This technique described in the book appears to be the earliest mention of injection of the blood vessels for the specific purpose of embalming.)*

Ludwig De Bils (1624–1671)

Ludwig De Bils was a Flemish anatomist and resident of Leiden who was also an embalmer. As with Ruysch, he never divulged his embalming methods and is said to have gone to great lengths to prevent accidental discovery of his method by visitors to his museum. Gabriel Clauderus, while viewing De Bils' specimens, shrewdly moistened his forefinger and applied it to the skin of an embalmed body and, tasting the moistened finger, disclosed a salty flavor, which led Clauderus to suspect that the principal ingredient in De Bils' fluid was salt. De Bils' wrote several books on the subject of embalming but failed to disclose his methods.

Gabriel Clauderus (Late 17th Century)

Gabriel Clauderus, a physician from Altenburg, Germany, was contemporary of De Bils. In 1695, he published a book, *Methodus Balsamundi Corpora Humani, Alique Majora Sine Evisceratione*, in which he described his method of embalming, which omitted evisceration. His fluid was made from 1 pound of ashes of tartar dissolve in 6 pounds of water, to which was added ½ pound of sal ammoniac. After filtration, it was ready for use and was denominated by Clauderus as his "balsamic spirit". He injected this fluid into the cavities of the body and then immersed the cadaver in the fluid for 6-8 weeks. The treatment was concluded by drying the corpse either in the sun or in a stove.

England's Customs and Achievements

While the British Isles are geographically grouped with Europe, they developed different customs and their scientific achievements advanced at a pace different from that in continental Europe.

Some individuals regard the Company of Barber-Surgeons of London to be the first group licensed to embalm. A brief examination of the background of this organization reveals that from about 1300 to 10, the Company of Barbers and the Guild of Surgeons were separate entities. In 1540, they received a charter form Henry VIII consolidating these two groups under the title of the Company of Barber-Surgeons and granting them the right to anatomize four executed criminals each year. In 1565, Queen Elizabeth I granted the same privilege to the College of Physicians. In 1745, the Surgeons and Barbers ended their joint relationship and again became two separate organizations. During the Barber-Surgeons period they were permitted to be the sole agency for embalming and for performing anatomical dissections in the city of London, although there is no record of any of the bodies for anatomy being embalmed.

This was never a well-respected or enforced monopoly. In their 200-year existence, there were fewer than ten complaints, and in several of the cases cited in the College of Barber-Surgeons records, no fine or other punishment is noted. In several cases, no conclusion of the case appears. Most complaints were lodged against members for performing private anatomical dissections not on the premises of the College. The more influential members such as William Cheselden and John Ranby simply ignored the rule and even withdrew from the organization as William Hunter did. *(The Barber-Surgeons made no progress in the development of licensing of embalmers as such and even today in the British Isles, no license or permit is needed from any governmental agency to pedon embalming and never has been so required.)*

William Hunter

William Hunter (1718–1783) was born in Scotland and studied medicine at the University of Glasgow and at Edinburgh. He finally settled in London where he specialized in the practice of obstetrics and taught anatomy. He became one of the great teacher of anatomy in English medical history and received many awards and appointments to honor societies, climaxed in 1764 by his appointment as Physician-Extraordinary to Queen Charlotte of England. He was the author of many brilliant treatises on medical subjects, perhaps the greatest being his *Anatomy of the Gravid Uterus*. His private collections of anatomical and pathological specimens, together with his lecture and dissecting rooms, occupied a portion of his home. All of this, plus a large sum of money, were donated to the University of Glasgow after his death.

Hunter was in the habit of delivering, at his private school at the close of the anatomical lectures, an account of the preparation of anatomical specimens and embalming of corpses. He injected the femoral artery with a solution composed of oil of turpentine, to which had been added Venice turpentine; oil of chamomile; and oil of lavender, to which had been added a portion of vermillion dye. This mixture was forced into the body until the s exhibited a red appearance. After a few hours during which the body lay undisturbed, the thoracic and abdominal cavities were opened, the viscera were removed, and the fluid was squeezed out of them. The viscera were separately arterially injected and bathed in camphorated spirits of wine. The body was again injected from the aorta and the cavities were washed with camphorated spirits of wine. The viscera were returned to the body intermixed with a powder composed of camphor, resin, and niter, and placed in the eyes, ears, nostrils, and other cavities. The entire skin surface of the body was then rubbed with the "essential" oils of rosemary and lavender. The body was placed in a box on a bed of plaster of Paris for about 4 years. When the box was reopened, and if desiccation appeared imperfect, a bed of gypsum was added to complete the process.

One of Hunter's admonitions to his students, which is still applicable to attainment of the finest results, was to begin the embalming process within 8 hours of death in the summer and within 24 hours in the winter.

Until the wartime aerial bombing of the Royal College of Surgeons Museum in 1941, the embalmed body of the wife of the eccentric dentist Dr Martin van Butchell, a pupil of William Hunter, was on exhibition. There was a letter in van Butchell's handwriting describing the embalming process. It is reproduced here verbatim:

- *12-January 1775*: At one-half past two this morning my wife died. At eight this morning, the statuary took off her face in plaster. At half past two this afternoon, Mr Cruikshank injected at the crural arteries five pints of oil of turpentine mixed with Venice turpentine and vermillion.
- *15-January*: At nine this morning, Dr Hunter and Mr Cruikshank began to open and embalm my wife. Her diseases were a large empyema in the left lung (which would not receive any air), accompanied with pleuropneumonia and much adhesion. The right lung was also beginning to decay and had some pus in it. The spleen was hard and much contracted; the liver diseased, called rata malpighi. The stomach was very sound. The kidneys, uterus, bladder, and intestines were in good order. Injected at the large arteries oil of turpentine mixed with camphored spirits, i.e. 10 ounces camphor to a quart of spirits, so as to make the whole vascular system turgid, put into the belly part 6 pounds of rosin powder, 3 pounds camphor, and 3 pounds niter powder mixed rec spirit.
- *17-January*: I opened the abdomen to put in the remainder of the powders and added 4 pounds rosin, 3 pounds niter, and 1 pound camphor. In all, there were 10 pounds rosin, 6 pounds niter, and 4 pounds camphor, 20 pounds of powder mixed with spirits of wine.

- *18-January*: Dr Hunter and Mr Cruikshank came at nine this morning and put my wife into the box on and in 130 pounds of Paris plaster at 18 d. a bag. I put between the thighs three arquebusade bottles, one full of camphor spirits very rich of the gum, containing 8 ounces oil of rosemary, and in the other 2 ounces of lavender.
- *19-January*: I dosed up the joints of the box lid and glasses with plaster of Paris mixed with gum water and spirits of wine.
- *25-January:* Dr Hunter came with Sir Thomas Wynn and his lady.
- *7-February*: Dr Hunter came with Sir John Pringle, Dr Heberden, Dr Watson, and about twelve more fellows of the Royal Society.
- *11-February*: Dr Hunter came with Dr Solander, Dr Mr Banks and another gentleman. I unlocked the glasses to dean the face and legs with spirits of wine and oil of lavender.
- *12-February*: Dr Hunter came to look at the neck and shoulders.
- *13-February*: I put 4 ounces of camphor spirits into the box and on both sides of neck and 6 pounds of plaster.
- *16-February*: I put 4 ounces oil of lavender, an ounce of rosemary and ½ ounce of oil of chamomile flowers (the last cost four Sh.) on sides of the face and 3 ounces of very dry chamomile flowers on the breast, beck, and shoulders.
- (The body was said to *resemble a Guanche* or Peruvian mummy and was very dry and shrunken.)

John Hunter

John Hunter (1728–1793) was born in Scotland, the younger brother of William Hunter, in whose anatomy classes he first proved so adept. After studying under the pat surgeons of his time, he was appointed to hospital staffs and lectured on anatomy. A region of the body, he described was named in his honor—"Hunter's canal". He served as a surgeon in the British army during the campaign in Portugal (1761–1763) and; upon his discharge from the service, settled in general practice in London. There he continued the collection and study of anatomical and natural subjects. He was the most brilliant and prolific writer on all phases of medicine and surgery and later founded his own private anatomy classes, which was unexcelled for the number of students who later distinguished themselves in medicine. Among these students were Jenner, Abernethy, Carlisle, Chevalier, Cline Coleman, Astley Cooper, Home, Lynn, and Macartney.

In 1776, Hunter was honored by appointment as surgeon-extraordinary to the King of England. In 1782, he constructed a museum between his homes in London to house his anatomical and natural history collections. These eventually contained nearly 14,000 items, and at his death were purchased by the British government for the Royal College of Surgeons. The main exhibit hall, measuring 52 by 28 feet, was lighted from above and had a gallery for visitors.

Many stories are told of body stealing for dissection and for securing specimens for collections. None would better illustrate this than John Hunter's acquisition in 1783 of the body of the Irish giant O'Brien, at a cost to him of about $2,500.00. O'Brien, about 7 feet 7 inches in height and dreading dissection by Hunter had, shortly before his death, arranged with several of his friends that his corpse be conveyed by them to the and sunk in deep water. The undertaker, who it was said had entered into a pecuniary agreement with Hunter, managed that while the escort was drinking at a certain stage of the journey to the sea the coffin should be locked in a barn. *Confederates*, which the undertaker had concealed in the barn, speedily substituted an equivalent weight of stones for the body. At night, O'Brien's body was forwarded to Hunter who took it immediately to his museum, where it was dissected and boiled to procure the bones. The skeleton was on exhibit until May 1941, when three-fourths of the museum of the Royal College of Surgeons, London, was destroyed by German bombers. Joshua Reynold's portrait of John Hunter displays the huge skeletal feet of O'Brien in the background.

Matthew Baillie

Dr Baillie (1761–1823) was a nephew of William and John Hunter. He was educated by his uncles and became famous as a physician and writer on medical subjects. He modified the Hunterian method of embalming, so as to provide as good preservation as ever in a shorter period. Using a solution of oil of turpentine, Venice turpentine, oil of chamomile, and oil of lavender (to which was added vermillion dye) he injected the femoral artery. He allowed several hours to elapse before he opened the body as in a postmortem examination and made a small incision in the bowel below the stomach, into which he inserted a small piece of pipe through which he introduced water to wash out the contents of the bowels. Then, ligating the rectum above the anus and the small bowels below the stomach, he filled the intestinal track with camphorated spirits of wine. The lungs were filled with camphorated spirits of wine via the trachea. The bladder was opened and emptied of its contents and a powder of camphor, resin, and niter was dusted over the viscera and the incision was dosed. The eyeballs were pierced and emptied of their contents and repacked to normal with the powder mixture, as were the mouth and ears. The body was rubbed with oil of rosemary or lavender and placed upon a bed of deep plaster.

Europe's Access to Cadavers

Continental European countries such as France, Germany, and Italy did not encounter the problems in supplying medical schools with cadavers as existed in Great Britain. Medical schools had access to bodies unclaimed for burial, a situation not present in the British Isles until after passage of the *Warburton Ad* in *1832*. The problem in continental Europe was different, consisting of securing a means to preserve Cadavers for dissection with nonpoisonous chemicals. In France, for example, medical schools in the North had scheduled anatomical dissection classes during the cold months of the year as the cadavers were unembalmed.

By the late 18th and early 19th centuries, France and Italy had a number of different techniques and chemicals for embalming proposed by members of the medical or scientific communities.

Baron Leopold Cuvier (1769-1832) of France was a comparative anatomist whose classification of mammals and ava forms the groundwork for present-day systems. Cuvier advocated the use of pure alcohol as a preservative agent.

Dr Francois Chaussier (1746-1828) of France recommended immersion of an eviscerated body in a solution of bichloride of mercury for preservation.

Dr Louis Jacques Thenard (1777-1857) of France was a brilliant teacher of and researcher in chemistry. He discovered the nature of hydrogen peroxide and made study of human bile and the preservative action of bichloride of mercury. In 1834, he advocated introduction of an alcoholic solution of bichloride of mercury into the blood vessels to preserve cadavers for anatomical dissection.

Dr G Tranchina (also spelled Tranchini or Franchini) of the early 19th century in Naples, Italy, openly advocated and successfully used arsenical solutions, arterially injected, to preserve bodies for both funeral and anatomical purposes. Tranchini's method of embalming varied, but the fluid was usually composed of 1 pound of arsenic dissolved in 5 pounds of alcoholic wine. He usually injected 2 gallons of this solution into the femoral artery without drainage of blood. At other times, he injected the same amount into the right common carotid artery, sending the fluid first toward the head and then downward toward the body, allowing some drainage through the jugular vein. This was followed by incision of the abdomen, opening, and emptying of the bowels, and moistening of the bowels with the injecting solution. The lungs were filled with the fluid via the trachea. A body prepared in this manner is said to have completely dried in 6 weeks.

Dr JP Sucquet of France (mid-19th century) was one of the earliest proponents of the use of zinc chloride as a preservative agent. He injected about 5 quarts of a 20% solution of zinc chloride in water through the popliteal artery and also introduced some of this solution into the abdomen. One body prepared in this way was buried for 2 years, then disinterred and found to be in an excellent state of preservation. About 1845, an agent representing Dr Sucquet sold the US rights to his method and chemical to Dr Charls D Brown and Dr Joseph Alexander of New York City.

Jean-Nicolas Gannal (1791-1852), a chemist in France (Fig. 1.5), began his life's work as an apothecary's assistant. From 1808 to 1812, he served in the medical department of the French Army, including the Russian campaign under Napoleon. After his discharge from the army, he re-entered the field of chemistry and was appointed assistant to the great French chemistry teacher Theaard. He later became interested in industrial chemistry and did research on methods of refining borax and improving the quality of glues and gelatins. In 1827, he was awarded the Montyon science prize for developing a method of treating catarrh and tuberculosis with chlorine gas. In 1831, he was asked to devote his time to devising an improved method of preserving cadavers for anatomical purposes. Close application to the problem resulted in success, which was recognized in 1836 by the JL Ward to Gannal of a second Montyon science prize.

His experiments included the use of solutions of acids (acetic-arsenous-nitric-hydrochloric), alkali salts

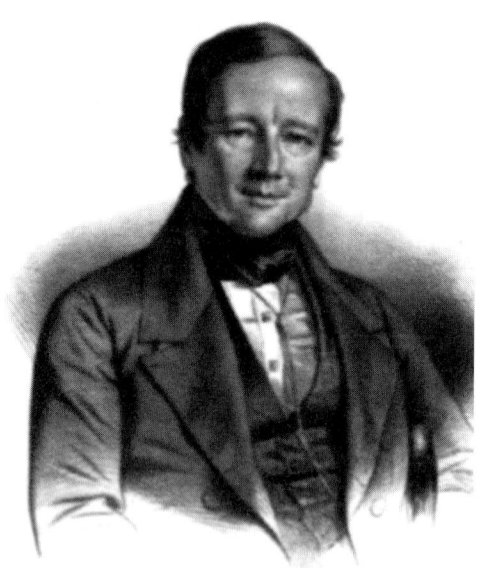

Fig. 1.5: Portrait of Jean-Nicolas Gannal of age 4U.
Courtesy: Ordre National des Pharmacien.

(copper–mercury alum), tannin–creosote–alcohol, and various combinations such as alum, sodium chloride, and nitrate of potash, and acetate of alumina and the chloride of alumina, the latter of which obliterated the lumen of blood vessels, is perfect method of embalming cadavers for anatomical purposes comprised the injection of about 6 quarts of a solution of acetate of alumina through the carotid artery without drainage of any blood. No evisceration or other treatment was used, although occasionally the bodies were immersed in the injecting solution until ready for dissection. Gannal used practically the same solution for embalming bodies for funeral purposes, although he did add a small quantity of arsenic and carmine to the solution. He injected about 2 gallons of this mixture, first upward and then downward in the carotid artery in less than one-half hour. No special treatment was given to the trunk viscera. In his book *History of Embalming*, he cited case histories of bodies he had embalmed and subsequently disinterred from 3 months to 13 months after burial. Gannal states that in every such case, the body was found in exactly the same state of preservation and appearance as when buried.

Gannal was involved in several precedent-making events. In mid-April 1840, a Paris newspaper published the following article:

- The young boy found murdered in a field near Villette not having been recognized and the process of decomposition having commenced, the Magistrates ordered it to be embalmed by JN Gannal's simple method of injection through the carotid arteries, so that this evidence of the crime may remain producible. This is the first operation of the kind performed by order of the Justices, and it was completed in a quarter of an hour.
- In his translation of Gannal's *History of Embalming* (1840) (Fig. 1.6), Harlan mentions that the Paris police have access to Gannal's embalming process to preserve bodies in the Paris morgue where murder has been suspected.
- Gannal was indirectly responsible for the passage of the first law prohibiting the use of arsenic in embalming solutions in 1846 (to which the use of bichloride of mercury was also prohibited in 1848).
- There are several versions of the story. In one, Gannal had omitted stating that a portion of arsenic was added to his alumina salts embalming chemical, and when this solution was analyzed and arsenic found, the medical community was enraged and compelled the law to be decreed. The other tale, never documented, relates that Gannal was retained to embalm the corpse of member of the nobility who died suddenly. The members of the nobleman's family accused the decedent's mistress of poisoning him with arsenic. Under French law, she was arrested and tried, the burden of her defense on her shoulders. Gannal followed the progress of the trial in the Paris newspapers and noted that the accused mistress was unable to prove her innocence. Finally at the last possible moment, Gannal appeared at the trial and requested permission to testify on her behalf. He states that in his opinion, the arsenic found in the body tissues of the deceased came there during the embalming with his embalming solution, as it contained arsenic. She was freed and the legal community petitioned for the abolition of arsenic in embalming solutions.
- Gannal had three sons—Adolphe, Antoine, and Felix who became physicians and continued the embalming practice after his death. They embalmed many famous people including De Lesseps who constructed the Suez Canal. The sons died in the early 1900s.
- *Richard Harlan (1796–1843)* of Philadelphia, Pennsylvania graduated from the Pennsylvania. Medical College in 1818 and was placed in charge of Dr Joseph Parrish's private anatomical dissection rooms in Philadelphia. After engaging in various projects in company with other Philadelphia physicians he became a member of the city health council. In 1838, he traveled to Europe and spent a portion of his time in

> HISTORY
> OF
> **EMBALMING**
> AND OF
> PREPARATIONS IN ANATOMY,
> PATHOLOGY
> AND NATURAL HISTORY;
> INCLUDING
> AN ACCOUNT OF A NEW PROCESS
> FOR EMBALMING
> By J.N. GANNAL
> Paris, 1838
>
> Translated From the French, With
> Notes And Additions
> By P. Harlan, MD
> PHILADELPHIA:
> PUBLISHED BY JUDAH DOBSON,
> NO. 106 CHESNUT STREET
> ....
> 1840

Fig. 1.6: Title page of Harlan's translation of the history of embalming.

P is visiting—various medical faculties and meeting local savants, among whom was JN Gannal. After being presented with a copy of Gannal's *History of Embalming*, he became so fascinated with it that he requested and received permission to publish an American edition translated to English. *The book, published in Philadelphia in 1840, became the first book devoted entirely to embalming procedures that was published in, the United States in English (Fig. 1.6)*.

OTHER PHYSICIANS AND ANATOMISTS

Girolamo Segato

A physician of Florence, Italy (17th century), Segato is known to have converted the human body to stone by infiltrating the bodily tissues with a solution of silicate of potash and succeeded in this treatment by immersion of the body in a weak acid solution. The exact modus operandi is unknown.

Thomas Joseph Pettigrew

A London physician and surgeon, graduate of Guys Hospital, and fellow of the Royal College of Surgeons, Pettigrew (1791-1865) was one of the great historians of the science of embalming. His treatise *History of Egyptian Mummies*, published in London in 1834, is a masterpiece revealing Pettigrew's ability to accurately observe and minutely describe objects and processes of interest to students and practitioners of the art of embalming. This volume is to this day considered one of the fine works on Egyptian embalming methods and customs. In 1854, he withdrew from the practice of medicine and devoted his entire energy to the study of archaeology.

Falconry

A French physician of the mid-19th century, Falconry employed a means of preservation of cadavers for anatomical purposes that are of interest because of its simplicity. The corpse was placed upon a bed of dry sawdust to which about a gallon of powdered zinc sulfate had been added. No injections, incisions, baths, or any additional treatment was used. The bodies so treated were said to have remained flexible for about 40 days, after which time they dried and assumed the appearance of mummies.

Thomas Marshall

Marshall was a London physician who published an account of a means of embalming in the *London Medical Gazette* in December 1839. His technique consisted of generously puncturing the body surface with needles or scissors and repeatedly brushing the body surface with strong acetic acid. A diluted acetic acid solution was introduced into the cavities of the body. The author claimed that the acetic acid would restore normal color even to gangrenous tissue.

John Morgan (Circa 1863)

A professor of anatomy at the University of Dublin, Dr Morgan made use of two principles, which are widely recognized as necessary to achieve the best embalming results—(1) the use of the largest possible artery for injection, and (2) the use of force or pressure to push the preserving fluid through the blood vessels. Also noted are his use of a preinjection solution (the earliest mention found) and his controlled technique of drainage. Dr Morgan cut the sternum down its center, opened the pericardium to expose the heat, made an incision into the left ventricle or into the aorta, and inserted a piece of pipe about 8-inches long. This injecting pipe was connected by 15 feet of tubing to a fluid container that was maintained 12 feet above the corpse, thereby producing about 5 pounds of pressure (Fig. 1.7).

The tip of right auricular appendage was clipped off to allow blood drainage. The first injection was composed of ½ gallon of a saturated salt solution to which was added 4 ounces of niter. After this solution was allowed to "rush" through the circulatory system, a clamp was fastened over the auricular appendage when the drainage stopped. Several more gallons of a solution of common salt, niter, alum, and arsenate of potash were injected until the body was thoroughly saturated with the fluid. No special treatment of the internal organs or viscera was mentioned.

At this time, there was virtually no embalming of the dead for funeral purposes available for the largest percentage of deaths.

Many books were written regarding the dangers of the living of exposure to the dead buried or entombed (unembalmed) in churches or in city cemeteries. There was also concern for those who handled the dead.

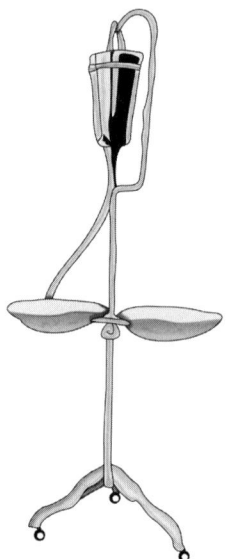

Fig. 1.7: Gravity fluid injection. The jar filled with arterial chemical could be elevated several feet above the corpse, thus creating pressure for injection.
Courtesy: Paula Johnson De Smet.

Bernardino Ramazzini

The founder of occupational medicine, Ramazzini (1633–1714) wrote the *Diseases of Workers* in 1700, and an enlarged edition of that text was published in 1713. The latter edition contained a chapter on the *Disease of Corpse Bearers*.

Numerous publications varying in size from leaflets to bound books were printed inveighing against existing burial practices. A few relevant titles are *considerations on the indecent and dangerous custom of burying in churches etc.* 1721, London, A Batesworth; *Blame of Kirk Burial, Tending to Persuade Cemeterial Civility,* 1606 NP; Rev William Birnie; *Gatherings from Graveyards, Particularly those of London etc.* 1830, GA Walker, surgeon, London; and *Sepulture, History, Methods, and Sanitary Requisites,* 1884, Stephen Wickes, Philadelphia. The astonishing accounts contained in these or similar works should convince even the most skeptical opponent of embalming of the sanitary value of the embalming process.

From Europe to the Colonies

The transfer of embalming knowledge from Europe to the colonies in what today is the United States was accomplished by several means.

Anatomical study in the colonies as early as 1676 in Boston and again in 1750 recorded that "Ors John Bard and Peter Middleton injected and dissected the body of an executed criminal for the instruction of young men engaged in the study of medicine". In 175, the NY Weekly Postboy carried an advertisement offering anatomy instruction by Dr Thomas Wood. From 1754 to 1756, William Hunter, physician and student of the famed anatomy teacher Alexander Monro I of Edinburgh, Scotland (and a relative of the Hunter Brothers), lectured on anatomy at Newport, Rhode Island. Doctors William Shippen and John Morgan of Philadelphia studied medicine in Europe and anatomy under British anatomists. Upon their return to the United States between 1762 and 1765, they became engaged in teaching medical subjects, especially anatomy, in Philadelphia.

In 1840 the translation of Gannal's book *The History of Embalming* into English was to provide the first text in English printed in the United States devoted to embalming. In the mid-1840s, the acquisition of Sucquet's embalming technique and chemicals as a franchise by Dr Charles D Brown and Dr Joseph Alexander of New York City added to the increasing amount of embalming knowledge transferred to the United States.

Modern Period

By the year 1861 and the onset of the Civil War, the transfer of embalming knowledge from Europe to the United States was virtually concluded. A small group of medically trained embalmers existed together with printed information such as Harlan's translation of Gannal's textbook and various European embalming formulas and techniques that had been acquired.

Until the Civil War, however, little or no embalming was performed for funeral purposes. Most preservation, such as it was, for brief periods was provided by ice refrigeration when available.

With the outbreak of the Civil War in April 1861, there began the raising of troops by the North and South to prosecute the war. Little if any embalming was available to the southerners during the war. Virtually all embalming was done by northerners. Since Washington, IX—was the capital city of the North, it became a center for troop concentration both to protect the city and to serve as a marshalling point for the armies moving against the south.

Northern troops composed of individual companies from small geographical areas and regiments from individual states as disparate as Vermont and Maine, Minnesota, and Wisconsin, and Ohio, Pennsylvania, and New York crowded into the Washington DC area. Civilian embalmers Dr Thomas Holmes, William J Bunnell, Dr Charles DeCosta Brown, Dr Joseph B Alexander, Dr Richard Burr, Dr Daniel H Prunk, Frank A Hu on, GW Scollay, CB Chamberlain, Henry P Cattell, Dr Benjamin Lyford, Samuel Rodgers, Dr EC Lewis, WP Cornelius, and Prince Greer are known to have embalmed during the Civil War. There are others who to this day remain anonymous.

None of the embalming surgeons, as they were called, were ever employed in the military as embalmers. Some had been or would become military surgeons but did not perform embalming while in the military service.

Civil War Times

At the beginning of the Civil War, as in all previous wars fought by the United States, there was no provision for return of the dead to their homes. In the Seminole Indian Wars (during the 1830s), the Mexican War (1846–1848), and the campaigns against the Indians up to the outbreak of the Civil War, the military dead were buried in the field near where they fell in battle. It was possible for the relatives to have the remains returned to their home for local burial under certain conditions.

- The next of kin was to request the disinterment and return of the body in a written request to the Quartermaster General.
- Upon military authority confirmation that the burial place was known and disinterment could be effected, the family was advised to send a coffin capable of being hermetically sealed to a designated Quartermaster Officer nearest the place of burial.
- Such Quartermaster Officer would provide a force of men to take the coffin to the grave, disinter the remains, and place them in the coffin and seal it. The coffined remains would then be returned to the place of ultimate reinterment.

During the early days of the Civil War and less frequently as the war dragged on, some family members of the deceased personally went to hospitals and battlefields to search for their dead and bring them home for burial. Civil War embalming was carried out with a variety of chemicals and techniques. Arterial embalming was applied when possible. An artery, usually the femoral or carotid, was raised and injected without any venous drainage in most cases. Usually no cavity treatment was administered. When arterial embalming was believed impossible because of the nature of wounds or decomposition, other means of preparation of the body for transport were resorted to. In some cases, the trunk was eviscerated and the cavity filled with sawdust or powdered charcoal or lime. The body was then placed in a coffin completely imbedded in sawdust or similar material. In other cases, the body was coffined as mentioned without evisceration.

Chemicals employed during the Civil War were totally self-manufactured by the embalmers and included, as basic preservatives, arsenicals, zinc chloride, bichloride of mercury, salts of alumina, sugar of lead, and a host of salts, alkalies, and acids. An example of fluid manufacture of one of the most popular embalming chemicals, zinc chloride, was the immersion of sheets of zinc in hydrochloric acid until a saturated solution was obtained. The resulting zinc chloride solution was injected without further dilution. Many of the injection pumps employed were quite similar to what would be described as greatly enlarged hypodermic syringes. Many require the filling of the syringe, the attachment of cannula, emptying of e syringe, unfastening of the syringe, and refilling. It was an extremely slow process! A few pumps were designed to provide continuous flow, aspirating the embalming chemical continuously from a large source into the pump during the injection process. Others, such as the Holmes invention, were designed to fit over a bucket that could hold a gallon or more of liquid.

On May 24, 1861, 24-year-old Colonel Elmer Ellsworth, commander of the 11th NY Volunteer Infantry, was shot to death in Alexandria, Virginia, as he seized a confederate flag displayed atop the Marshall House Hotel. He became the first prominent military figure killed in the war. His body was embalmed by Dr Thomas Holmes, who had set up an embalming establishment in Washington DC. Colonel Ellsworth had funeral services in the White House, in New York City, and in Albany, New York, with the burial in his home town of Mechanicsburg, New York. His funeral set a pattern to be followed by prominent members of the military, culminating in President Lincoln's historic funeral services. Colonel Ellsworth's embalming and viewable appearance were widely and favorably commented on in the press and did much to familiarize the previously uninformed public with embalming.

The Army issued only two sets of orders relative to fatal casualties in the early stages of the war, On September 11, 1861, War Department general order 75 directed the Quartermaster Department to supply all general and post-hospitals with blank books and forms for the preservation of accurate death records and to provide material for head-boards to be erected over soldiers' graves. On April 3, 1862, Section II of War Department general order 33 stated:

"In order to secure as far as possible the decent inter-ment of those who have fallen; or may fall in battle, it is made the duty of commanding generals to lay off lots of ground in some suitable spot near every battlefield, as soon as it may be in their power, and to cause the remains of those killed to be interred, with headboards to the graves bearing numbers, and when practicable, the names of the persons buried in them. A register for each burial ground will be preserved, in which will be noted the marks corresponding with the headboards.

This was the origin of what was to become the National Cemetery System.

Embalming Surgeons of the Civil War

Dr Thomas Holmes (1817-1900): Holmes was born in New York City in 1817 and educated in local public schools and New York University Medical College, though the records of the period are incomplete and document only his attendance, not his graduation. He did practice medicine and was a Coroner's physician in New York during the 1850s as numerous newspaper stories at. He apparently moved to Williamsburg (now Brooklyn) and experimented with a variety of chemicals for embalming and techniques.

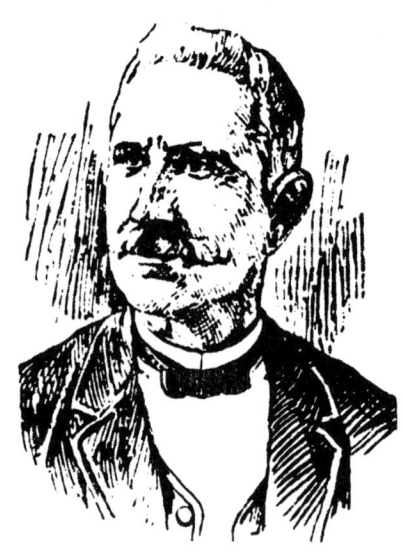

Fig. 1.8: Portrait of Dr Thomas Holmes.

When the Civil War broke out, he opened an embalming office in Washington, DC and Colonel Ellsworth became his first prominent client. Holmes subsequently embalmed Colonel ED Baker, a prominent politician and soldier killed in battle. This case brought more publicity both for Dr Holmes and for embalming (Fig. 1.8).

Holmes ultimately prepared about 4,000 bodies (including 8 generals), and patented many inventions relating to embalming during his lifetime. One in particular, a rubber-coated canvas removal bag, was far ahead of its time (Fig. 1.9).

When the war ended, Dr Holmes returned home to *Brooklyn* and only occasionally practiced embalming. He operated a drugstore and manufactured a variety of products as diverse as embalming fluid and root beer! He invested heavily in a health resort and lost the investment. He wrote little about embalming, did not teach, and had no children. After a serious fall in his home, he became periodically psychotic and occasionally required confinement. When he died in 1900, it was said that he wanted no embalming.

William J Bunnell (1823–1891): Bunnell was born in New Jersey, moved to New York City, and in the 1850s became acquainted with Dr Holmes and married his sister. Dr Holmes found him employment as an anatomy technician for some New York medical schools while teaching him embalming. When war broke out, Bunnell did not work directly with Dr Holmes but formed his own Embalming

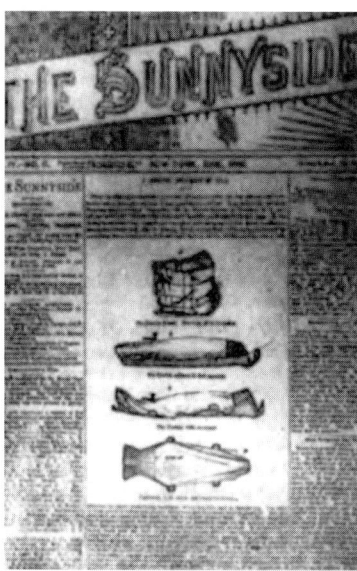

Fig. 1.9: Front page of The Sunnyside, June 1886, featuring an article on Dr Holmes removal bag, citing its all-around utility as a sleeping bag and stretcher, its ability to be inflated as a raft and of course its use as a corpse removal bag or coffin.

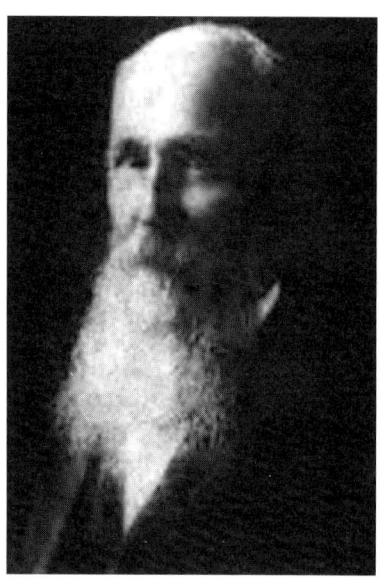

Fig. 1.10: Portrait of Henry P Cattell, an associate of Brown and Alexander, the embalming surgeons who embalmed Willie Lincoln in 1862 and President Lincoln in 1865.

Surgeon's Organization with Dr RB Heintzelman from Philadelphia as his active partner. Holmes and Bunnell did occasionally work together during the war at Gettysburg and at City Point, Virginia. After the war, it was reported that Bunnell was practicing medicine briefly in Omaha, Nebraska and eventually opened an undertaking establishment in Jersey City, New Jersey. He became a marshal at the funeral of General Grant and became prominent in Undertakers Associations. His son George Holmes Bunnell (1 1932) followed his father in the business and was given assistance by his uncle, Dr Holmes George H Bunnell had twin sons, Milton, who became a funeral director, and Chester, who became a physician.

Dr Charles DeCosta Brown, Dr Joseph B Alexander, and Henry P Cattell: Brown, Alexander, and Cattell were all active in the firm of Brown and Alexander, Embalming Surgeons. It is not known whether Brown and Alexander met in New York City in the late 1850s or in Washington, DC in early wartime. Cattell (Fig. 1.10) is believed to have been the stepson of Dr Charles Brown's brother, as his mother married a Dr Brown in 1860. In any event, he entered the employment of the firm that embalmed Willie Lincoln, son of the President Abraham Lincoln, and later embalmed the President himself in 1865. After the war Dr Brown abandoned embalming, returned to New York City practiced dentistry, and became very active in the Masonic Lodge. He died in 1896 and is buried in Greenwood Cemetery in Brooklyn.

Alexander died in 1871 in Washington, DC. HP Cattell halted his embalming practice after the war became a lithographer and then entered the Washington, DC police force. None of his family was ever aware that he had embalmed President Lincoln. He died in 1915 and is buried in Washington, DC.

Frank A Hutton Little is known of Hutton's personal biography. Born in or near Harrisburg, Pennsylvania, about 1835, he was a pharmacist by occupation. He had military service in the 110th Pennsylvania Volunteer Infantry ending in June 1862, was discharged in Washington, DC, and became a partner in the firm of Chamberlain and Hutton, Surgeons. This partnership did not last long and Hutton withdrew in February, 1863. He formed the firm of Hutton and Company with EA Williams, son of a Washington, DC undertaker as his partner. Hutton advertised in the Washington City Directory, taking a full page space to extol his embalming expertise. He was also issued Patent 38,747 for an embalming fluid on June 1, 1863. The formula included alcohol, arsenic, bichloride of mercury, and zinc chloride.

During mid-April 1863, Hutton became embroiled in an argument with a client over charges for shipping his son's body to him. The client complained to Colonel LC Baker, provost marshal of the Capitol, who, on April 20, 1863, arrested Hutton and seized the contents of his office as evidence. Hutton was confined in the Old Capitol Prison for about 10 days and then released. No details of his release or trial have been found. He subsequently relocated his quarters and continued in business with a much diminished clientele. Hutton is said to have returned to Harrisburg after the war ended and died there within a year.

Daniel H Prunk (1829-1923): Born in *Virginia* in 1829, Prunk and his family migrated to Illinois where he attended college. After attending medical school in Cincinnati, he began medical practice in Illinois and, in April 1861, moved to Indianapolis where he joined the 19th Indiana Volunteer Infantry as an assistant surgeon in September, 1861. He was transferred to the 20th Indiana Volunteer Infantry in June 1862, and was arrested in November of that year and incarcerated in the Old Capitol Prison in Washington, DC for about 3 months for conduct unbecoming of an officer. He was then dismissed from the service. From July to October, 1863 he was acting assistant surgeon at the 2nd Division Army Hospital at Nashville, Tennessee, and subsequently requested permission to provide embalming services in Nashville. The request was initially refused but finally granted late in 1863. He eventually had embalming establishment local not only in Nashville but also in Chattanooga and Knoxville in Tennessee, at East Point, Atlanta, Dalton, and Marietta in Georgia, and at Huntsville in Alabama (Fig. 1.11).

In 1865, Dr Prunk was licensed by the Army to practice embalming and undertaking. (He was also engaged in a wholesale grocery business, cotton trading, and money lending.) He made his own embalming fluid by dissolving sheets of zinc in muriatic acid (hydrochloric acid) until a saturated solution of zinc chloride was obtained to which a quantity of arsenious acid was added. The fluid obtained was injected quite warm without dilution or blood drainage.

Prunk sold all his embalming establishments in 1866 and returned to Indianapolis to practice medicine. It seems that he never engaged in embalming after his return to Indianapolis. He made one of the earliest written statements regarding the necessity of cavity treatment in a letter written in 1872 to Dr JP Buckesto of San Jose, California.

"If I were going to ship a corpse from San Jose to New York City, we have advised for sometime the puncturing of the stomach to give vent to gases, which accumulate at this time. In a subject with a large abdomen, where the bowels are discolored, the introduction of a couple of quarts into the peritoneal cavity by making a puncture near the umbilicus and throwing a thread of strong silk around it like a drawstring on a button cushion, which can be readily closed after you are thru injecting."

Dr Richard Burr: Although little biographical information other than his rumored origin in Philadelphia is available concerning Burr (who apparently practiced during the period 1862–1865), he has achieved immortality as the embalmer photographed by the Civil War photographer Brady in front of his embalming tent while injecting a subject (Fig. 1.12). WJ Bunnell complained about Burr's

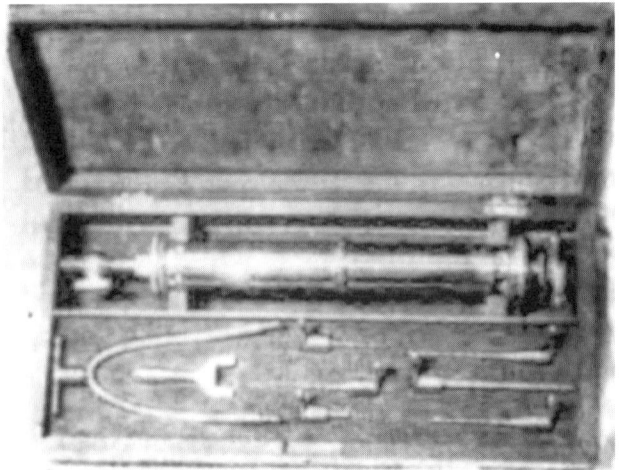

Fig. 1.11: Injection syringe and cannulas of Dr Daniel J Prunk, Civil War embalming surgeon.
Courtesy: The Illinois Funeral Director's Foundation.

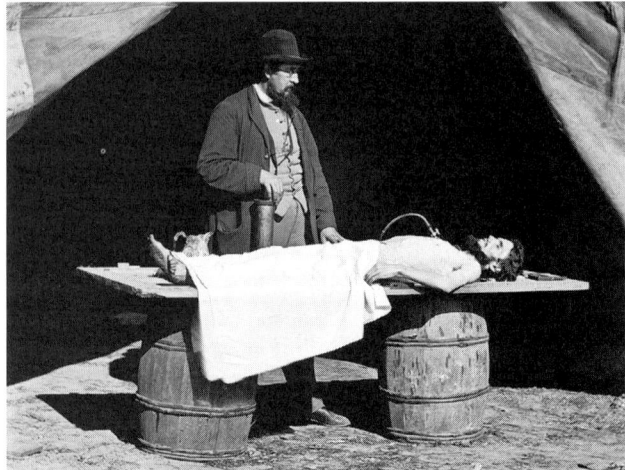

Fig. 1.12: Dr Richard Burr embalming near a battlefield during the Civil War.
Courtesy: Library of Congress.

unprofessional conduct, alleging that, among other things, he set Bunnell's embalming tent on fire! He was also one of the men against whom complaints had been issued regarding inflated prices and poor services, which resulted in all embalmers' being excluded from military areas by order of General US Grant in January 1865. This resulted in establishment of the first set of rules and regulations for the licensing of embalmers and undertakers in the United States.

The final Army order for embalmers contained some of the suggestions made by Dr Barnes, chief of the Anny Medical Service in December, 1863, to the effect that a performance bond should be posted by any embalmer desiring to practice. In addition, the requirement stipulated by the Provost Marshal General ordered the embalmer to furnish a list of his prices as charged for work or merchandise to the provost Marshal General, the medical director of the department, and the Post Provost Marshal.

US Army general order 39 concerning embalmers (March 15, 1865) read as follows:

- Here after no persons will be permitted to embalm or remove the bodies of deceased officers or soldiers unless acting under the special license of the Provost Marshal of the Army, department, or district in which the bodies may be.
- Provost marshals will restrict disinterments to seasons when they can be made without endangering the health of the troops. They will grant licenses only to such persons as furnish proof of skill and ability as embalmers, and will require bonds for the faithful performance of the orders given them. They will also establish a scale of prices by which embalmers are to be governed, with such other regulations as will protect the interest of the friends and relatives of deceased soldiers.
- Applicants for license will apply directly to the provost Marshal of the Army or department in which they may desire to pursue their business, submitting in distinct terms the process adopted by them, materials, length of time, its preservative effect can be relied on and such other information as may be necessary to establish their proficiency and success. Medical directors will give such assistance in the examination of these applications as may be required by the Provost Marshal.

In the Army of the Cumberland, the following additional requirements were stipulated:

- No disinterments will be permitted within the department between the 15th day of May and the 15th day of October.
- The following seal of prices will be observed from and after this date—at Nashville and Memphis—for embalming bodies each at $15.00 to disinter, furnish metallic burial cases, well-boxed marked and delivered to the express office each at $75.00, zinc coffins and the ABO listed services, each at $40.00. An additional charge of $5.00 may be made for embalming and also for either of the above styles of coffins at Murfreesboro, Chattanooga, Knoxville, and Huntsville, Alabama, or in the field.
- No person will be permitted to operate as an embalmer under any license issued to him until he shall have filed a bond in this office in the penal sum of $1,000 conditioned for the faithful observance of this order, and for the skillful performance of such work, as he shall undertake by virtue of his license. (Such licenses were not transferable from one individual to another).

By 1864, the Armory Square Military Hospital in Washington, DC had all its deceased patients routinely embalmed and the grave recorded, so that the body could be disinterred and sent to family or friends when requested.

CB Chamberlain: Chamberlain is said to have Philadelphia as his origin. Although very little is known of the man, he definitely was an early partner of FA Hutton. He and Hutton apparently were not compatible, and he formed a new partnership with Ben Lyford. They both can be documented as practicing embalming surgeons on the scene at Gettysburg after the battle. Chamberlain is listed in the Washington, DC City Directory as late as 1865 as a partner in Chamberlain and waters Embalmers at 431, Pennsylvania Avenue. He is mentioned by FC Beinhauer, Pittsburgh undertaker, as being in the Pittsburgh area prior to and during the Civil War. Joseph H Oarke also mentioned Chamberlain. As a teacher of embalming in the post-Civil War period.

GW Scollay: Judging from the various patents issued to him, Scollay was apparently from St Louis, Missouri. Very little personal information about him has been uncovered. He appeared to be an active embalming surgeon at the Gettysburg battlefield and in the area near Richmond. He has a listing in the 1865 Washington, DC City Directory as a member of the firm of Scollay and Sands-Embalmers of the Dead. Frank T Sands was a prominent undertaker in Washington, DC. Scollay patented two methods of embalming in the post-Civil War period, one in January

1867 and the other in October 1869. Both patents involved the use of gaseous compounds injected via the blood vascular system, one of the earliest recommendations for choice of gas rather than a liquid as a preservative introduced into the blood vascular system. In 1860, Scollay patented a two-piece cast glass coffin and, during the war, produced a number of different "sanitary" coffins.

Benjamin F Lyford: Born in Vermont in 1841 and receiving public school education there, Lyford attended and graduated from Philadelphia University's 6-month course of medical studies. He first appears on the Civil War scene as a partner of CB Chamberlain, who provided embalming after the Battle of Gettysburg. Later he had altercations with Provost Marshal General Rudolph Patrick of the Army of the Potomac. This series of disagreements stimulates him to accept appointment on July 1, 1864, as assistant surgeon of the 68th Regiment of Infantry US Colored Troops. He reported to the unit in Missouri and subsequently served Memphis. For a time, he served as commanding officer of a small cavalry and artillery contingent in southern Alabama.

He returned to his regiment stationed near New Orleans, Louisiana, and went on leave in New Orleans. He was arrested inside a bordello in full uniform and faced court martial charges. Apparently found innocent of the charges, he was discharged from the Army on February 5, 1866, traveled to San Francisco, and opened an office for medical practice. One of his early patients was a wealthy, widowed landowner who had an attractive daughter whom he fell in love with and married. The mother owned large tracts of land in Marin County across the bay north of San Francisco. Lyford built a health resort and dairy as well as his own home on this property and prospered.

In 1871, Lyford patented an improvement in embalming, which was a very complicated system consisting of the introduction through the blood vessels of specially distilled chemicals (including creosote, zinc chloride, potassium nitrate, and alcohol), while the body was enclosed in a sealed container. The container, to have the air within it, alternatively evacuated to create a vacuum and reversed to create pressure. Finally, the body was eviscerated and the trunk cavity filled with an arsenical powder. His final recommendation was the use of cosmetics to color the features; he was one of the first to make this recommendation. In 1870, a local newspaper carried a story describing a body he had successfully embalmed. Dr Lyford died in 1906 without issue and had a large well-attended funeral.

Dr EC Lewis, WP Cornelius, and Prince Greer: This most interesting account of the Civil War embalming surgeons relates the method of the transmission of embalming technique from a medically trained practitioner to an undertaker, who, in turn, trained a layman in the skill. Dr EC Lewis was a former US Army surgeon, WP Cornelius (1824–1910) was a successful undertaker in Nashville, Tennessee, and Prince Greer was a former orderly, body servant, and slave of a Colonel Greer of a Texas cavalry regiment who died in the fighting in Tennessee.

Dr Thomas Holmes wrote: In the forepart of the war, a young ex-Army doctor named EC Lewis called at my headquarters in Washington and wished me to instruct him in the embalming profession and sell him an outfit to go to the western Army and locate at Nashville. He offered as security a property holding m Georgetown, DC for any amount of fluid I would trust him for. I made a bargain with him and he used many barrels of fluid, I was often surprised at his large orders. (*Note*: Dr. Lewis headquarters were at Mr Cornelius undertaking establishment in Nashville.)

Cornelius stated: It was during the year 1862 that one Dr EC Lewis came to me from the employ of Dr Holmes and proposed to embalm bodies. It was new to me but I at once put him to work with the Holmes fluid and Holmes injector. He was quite an expert, but like many men could not stand prosperity and soon wanted to get into some other kind of business, which he did. When Lewis the embalmer quit, I then undertook the embalming myself with a colored assistant named Prince Greer.

Cornelius explained that Prince Greer had earlier brought the body of Colonel Greer of Texas cavalry regiment to Cornelius for shipment back to Texas. After shipping back, the body Prince Greer remained at Cornelius' premises and was asked what he wanted to do to earn his room and board. Prince Greer indicated he would do anything.

Cornelius continued: "Prince Greer appeared to enjoy embalming so much that he himself became an expert, kept on at work embalming during the balance of the war, and was very successful at it was but a short time before he could raise an artery as quickly as anyone and was always careful, always of course coming to me in a difficult case. He remained with me until I quit the business in 1871."

Prince Greer is the First Documented Black Embalmer in US History

Public and professional acceptance: With the ending of the war and the Assassination of President Lincoln, the Civil

War's last major casualty, the public had been familiarized with term embalming and obtained personal knowledge of the appearance of an embalmed body. This knowledge was acquired by the hundreds of thousands who viewed not only President Lincoln but other prominent military and civilian figures as well as the ordinary soldiers embalmed and shipped to their homes.

Despite, the end of the war and the establishment of peace there was no wide adoption of embalming by civilian undertakers of the United States. There were many reasons for this apparent reluctance to adopt a worthwhile new practice. Undertakers in the United States at the end of the Civil War were an unorganized, largely rural group of individuals lacking a professional body of knowledge and skills. Specifically, they lacked textbooks of instruction of embalming, instructors and schools of embalming, professional journals, and professional associations. Until these necessities became available embalming would not flourish.

The first step taken was to attempt to sale of embalming fluid to undertakers. Some Civil War embalming surgeons, such as Dr Thomas Holmes, engaged in this endeavor upon returning home. Holmes had a large local market (metropolitan New York City) for his preservative chemical, which he had named Innominata, and he promoted it well. Holmes, like other embalming chemical salesmen, realized quickly that the undertakers were interested in the preservative qualities of such chemicals but the clients were without knowledge of embalming techniques. Holmes therefore promoted the use of his Innominata as an external application to wash the body and to saturate cloths to place over the face. His fluid was also poured into the mouth and nose to reach the lungs and stomach. Holmes' early practices were duplicated by other purveyors of embalming chemicals.

In these early post-Civil War years, some instruction of undertakers in arterial embalming was imparted by the occasional knowledgeable traveling salesman who sold embalming chemicals. CB Chamberlain is reported to have done this in the late 1860s and early 1870s.

Examples of chemical embalming fluid patents include one issued to CH Crane of Burr Oak, Michigan, in September 1868. It was a powdered mixture of alum salt, ammonium chloride, arsenic, bichloride of mercury, camphor, and zinc chloride. It could be used as a dry powder or dissolved in water or alcohol to form an arterial solution and was named Crane's electrodynamic mummifier. In 1876, he sold the patent rights to this or a similar formulation to a Professor George M Rhodes of Michigan.

Another early embalming chemical manufacturer in 1877 was the Mills and Lacey Manufacturing Company of Grand Rapids, Michigan, whose embalming fluid featured arsenic as its preservative.

Instruments and chemicals available in the post-Civil War period included rubber gloves at $2 per pair (1 77); anatomical syringes and three cannulas m a case for $20–22; surgical instruments in cases for $4–5; Rulon's wax eyecaps and mouth closers at $1 each; and Segestor embalming fluid for $4.50 per dozen pint bottles (1873). Professor George M Rhodes was said to have sold 100,000 bottles of his dynamic Electro Balm in 1876 with more than 3,000 undertakers using the product. Egyptian Embalmer Fluid (1877) sold for $6.50 per dozen pint bottles and was also available in 5- and 10-gallon kegs as well as ½ and 1-gallon carboys at $3.00 per gallon.

Until the first quarter of the 20th century, embalming was most frequently carried out in the home of the deceased or, in some communities, in the hospital where death occurred. There were early attempts in some funeral homes in the 1870s to provide both a preparation room and chapel space for the wake and services. In issues as early as 1876 of both the Casket and the sunnyside, there were accounts reported of the installation of preparation rooms. For example:

- Maynard Funeral Home, Syracuse, NY, had a morgue fitted with marble slabs and running water for storing bodies.
- Hubbard and Searles Undertaking establishment at Auburn, NY, could provide seating for 100 persons at a service and had a cooling room with cement floor and marble slabs (2 × 8 feet) and running water connection.
- Knowles undertaking establishment at Providence, RI had a preserver room and a corpse room where surgical procedures and postmortems were made.
- The Douglas under asking Company of Utica, NY had a room for funeral services and a cooling vault in the cellar, which had walls 3-feet thick and also contained shelves for body storage.

Dr Auguste Renouard: In 1876, Dr Renouard (1839–1912) became a regular contributor to The Casket of articles on all phases of embalming knowledge, which greatly implemented interest in embalming. He was born on a plantation—in Pointe Coupee Parish, Louisiana, and received his early schooling locally. He is said to have attended to McDowell Medical school in St Louis, Missouri, and, at the outbreak of the Civil War, to have returned to Louisiana to enlist in the confederate Army. Despite his claim to military service in the confederate forces, no documented evidence has been found in some 50 years of searching. In the postwar period, he secured employment as a pharmacist in various cities such as New York, Memphis, and Chicago, where he was married. His son, Charles A, was born shortly before the Chicago fire of 1871. Losing everything in the fire, Renouard traveled to Denver, Colorado, and secured employment as a book-keeper for a combination furniture store and undertaking establishment. Because of its altitude, Denver at this time was regarded as a health resort for treatment of lung diseases. The undertaking section of the firm returned many bodies to the east and south for hometown burial, and Renouard became interested in the procedures employed at his firm for shipment of the bodies. After studying the existing rudimentary system, he suggested to his employer that he be permitted to prepare the bodies for postmortem by arterial embalming. This consent was given and it almost immediately produced a volume of letters from the receiving undertakers inquiring about the procedure used to create such beautiful corpses, which resembled a person asleep. Renouard graciously replied, explaining his chemicals and technique to the extent that it assumed the proportions of a correspondence course. Additionally, there were a number of individual undertakers who traveled to Denver to receive personal instruction in embalming from Renouard.

The publisher of The Casket urged Dr Renouard to write a textbook on embalming and undertaking for use by undertakers. In 1878, he published The Undertaker's Manual which contained 230 pages of detailed instruction anatomy, chemistry, embalming procedures, instruments, and details of undertaking practice (Fig. 1.13). This was the first book published specifically as an embalming textbook in the United States and would be followed by a hor4e of others. In 1879, notices appeared in The Casket that undertakers in states such as Connecticut and Pennsylvania were agents for the sail of Auguste Renouard's chemical formulas and techniques (Fig. 1.14).

In 1881, the doctor was requested to open a school of embalming in Rochester, New York, but for a variety of reasons, this did not become a reality until early 1883. In 1880, the state of Michigan was the first to form an Undertaker's Association, which, in 1881, changed the name to Funeral Directors.

Association: Other states quickly followed the Michigan lead and organized state associations. *The various state associations met in 1882 in Rochester and organized the*

THE

UNDERTAKERS' MANUAL:

A TREATISE OF

USEFUL AND RELIABLE INFORMATION

EMBRACING COMPLETE AND DETAILED

INSTRUCTIONS FOR THE PRESERVATION

OF BODIES

ALSO, THE

MOST APPROVED EMBALMING METHODS

WITH

HINTS ON THE PROFESSION OF UNDERTAKING

BY AUGUSTE RENOUARD

Rochester, N.Y.

A. H. Nirdlinger & Co. Publishers

1878

Fig. 1.13: Title page of Auguste Renouard's first edition of The Undertaker's Manual.

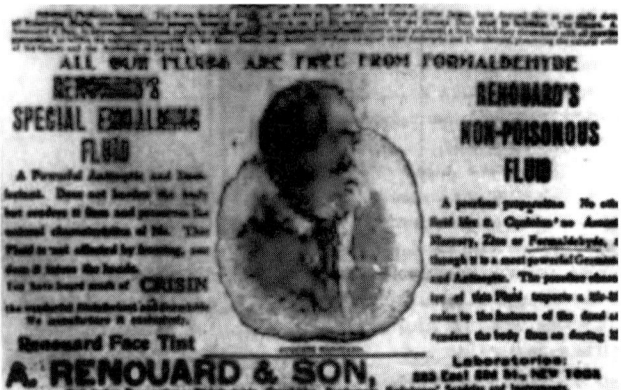

Fig. 1.14: Auguste Renouard's chemical formulas for embalming fluid.

National Funeral Directors Association, another important step toward professionalism. Renouard provided demonstrations of embalming in Rochester at the first national convention of the Association. This sets a pattern for many years of an obligatory embalming demonstration at state and national conventions. During the 1882 gathering, agents of an English firm (Dottridge Brothers, Funeral Supply Firm) offered Renouard a 5-year contract to teach embalming in London at $5000 per year, which he rejected.

The Rochester School of Embalming headed by Dr Renouard under the auspices of the Egyptian Chemical Company opened in 1883 and he continued his affiliation with this school until December 1884. He then entered into an agreement with Hallett and Company Undertakers in Kansas City, Missouri, to locate his school, the School of Embalming and Organic Chemistry, on the company's premises. By mid-1886, he terminated his school in Kansas City and returned to Denver. He then began to travel to distant points such as Fort Worth, Texas, and Toronto, and Montreal, Canada, providing embalming instruction for periods ranging from 3 days to 2 weeks.

In 1894, Dr Renouard made his final move to New York City and established the College of Embalming. The school had no fixed term classes and the student remained until he was able to embalm. In 1889, the doctor's son, Charles A was reported to be a shipping clerk with the firm of Dolge and Huneke-Embalming Chemical Manufacturers. Early in 1899, Charles opened the Renouard Training School for Embalmers in New York City and, in February 1900, Auguste Renouard closed the US College of Embalming and joined Charles at his school. Charles provided several months of embalming instruction in London, England, on behalf of the O.K. Buckhout Chemical Company of Grand Rapids, Michigan. In 1906, Auguste traveled to England and continental Europe where he was most graciously received and entertained.

Auguste Renouard died in his home in 1912. A monument paid for by voluntary subscription of his former students was an example of the esteem in which he was held by those he instructed. *He can, without question, be regarded as the first major figure to provide embalming instruction for undertakers in the United States.* His son Charles continued the Renouard Training School for Embalmers until his death in 1950.

Joseph Henry Clarke: Born in Connersville, Indiana, Joseph Henry Clarke (1840–1916) received his early education in Pharmacy and enrolled as a student in a medical college in Keokuk, Iowa. His studies, however, were interrupted by the Civil War. He volunteered for service with the Union Arm, 3, but was rejected because of physical defects. He was permitted to serve as a civilian and later held the position of assistant hospital steward in the 5th Iowa Infantry. After the death of his father, he returned home before the end of the war to support his family. He married and secured employment as a casket salesman. During the course of his travels, he became acquainted with a fluid manufacturer and became sufficiently interested in embalming to sell embalming fluids as a sideline. His interest in embalming grew as he realized the need to demonstrate the method of use of the fluid he hoped to sell to his patrons. This, in turn, led to his study of and experimentation with embalming chemicals to solve problems relating to preservation of the dead. He enrolled in an anatomy course conducted by Dr CM Lukens of the Pulte Medical College in Cincinnati, Ohio, which broadened into a lifetime friendship and professional partnership in the founding of the Clarke School of Embalming at Cincinnati in 1882 (Fig. 1.15).

The school lacked permanence because Mr Clarke traveled most of the year giving courses of instruction, each course varying in length from 2 days to 7 days. His second course of instruction away from Cincinnati was presented in New York City. One class member was Felix A Sullivan, who would later become a well-known teacher and writer in the embalming field. Sullivan and Clarke became rivals and bitter enemies. One major clash occurred when General and ex-President Ulysses S Grant died on July 23, 1885, at Mount McGregor, New York. Clarke had been advised by the Holmes Undertaking Company (no relation to Dr Holmes) of Saratoga, New York that the company would be retained to handle the funeral of General Grant and that they wanted Clarke to do the embalming.

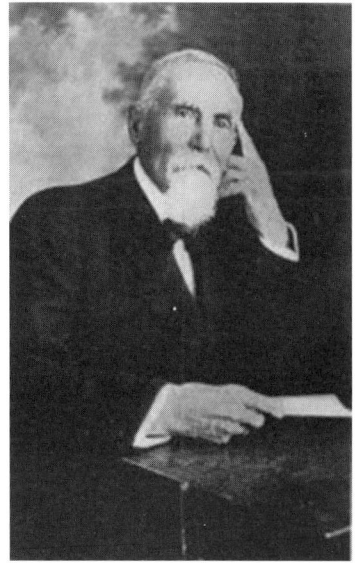

Fig. 1.15: Portrait of Joseph Henry Clarke—founder of the Cincinnati College of Embalming.

Clarke was in Baltimore on the day of Grant's death, but he became ill and went to his Springfield, Ohio, home where he was bedridden for 3–4 weeks. The embalming was accordingly performed by one member of the Holmes Undertaking Company family and a Dr McEwen using Clarke's proprietary embalming chemical.

After the body had been embalmed Rev Stephen Merritt, clergyman and undertaker of New York City and also General Grant's religious adviser, arrived together with Felix A Sullivan d an11ol!nced that they were to take charge. The Holmes personnel withdrew from the premises and Sullivan proceeded to re-embalm the body. He claimed he withdrew all previously injected arterial fluid and replaced it with the chemical made by the company he represented. Clarke rebuffed these claims in the professional journals. A reporter from the New York Times wrote that Mr Holmes (of Saratoga, New York) was too drunk to carry out the necessary preparation of the body. The New York Times was subsequently sued for libel and lost the case, and Mr Holmes was awarded several thousand dollars in damages.

The name of the embalming school was changed in 1899 to the Cincinnati College of Embalming and was established on a permanent basis. Mr Clarke conducted only occasional lecture tours at that time. He was ably assisted in the management of the school by his son—C Horace Clarke. In 1907, Charles O Dhonau became associated with him and later took over operation of the school. Mr Clarke was a capable teacher, lecturer, and author of several texts on embalming, and he held several patents in the embalming fields. He retired in 1909 to San Diego, California, where he died in 1916.

Felix Aloysius Sullivan (1843–1931): Sullivan was born in Toronto, Ontario, Canada, in 1843, the son of a Scotch immigrant undertaker and an Irish mother. He unquestionably had the most interesting, controversial, riotous, and successful career as a practitioner, writer, teacher, and lecturer of embalming and related subjects. His career was so full of incidents that it would be impossible to recount all but a few highlights. After the usual parochial school education and some experience working with his father, Sullivan, together with several other friends, crossed the border into the United States and enlisted in a New York cavalry regiment during the Civil War. Military records verify his service but reveal he deserted to service near the end of the war. He claims to have assisted in embalming while in the service, but the claim can neither be affirmed nor denied, as it lacks proof.

After the Civil War, he followed various occupations and traveled. He eventually drifted to New York City where he secured employment with various casket companies and finally became a funeral director for hire. He studied anatomy and other medical sciences and, by 1881, became an embalmer of some local repute. He was hired to go to Cleveland, Ohio, to re-embalm President Garfield, who died from an Assassin's bullet, and seems to have been successful in this venture. Sullivan attended Clarke's embalming class in New York City in 1882 to learn how such a class of instruction was conducted. Sullivan, together with Dr WG Robinson, opened the New York School of Embalming in 1884 and a year later was again involved in the embalming of a president, this time President Ulysses Grant (see previous information on Clarke's career). He then entered and left a long list of employers. In 1887, he was in Chicago when the anarchists who had bombed the police in 1886, killing and wounding police and civilians, were condemned to die. One exploded a dynamite cap in his mouth in jail and the others were hung. He prepared all bodies and was praised for his plastic surgery on the "mad bomber".

Sullivan continued his erratic employment or work habits, working for one firm, quitting, and then working for another. By 1891, he was again a lecturer/demonstrator, this time for the Egyptian Chemical Company. By 1892, he reached the height of his career as a lecturer, speaking, and teaching in more cities to larger classes than anyone previously had. He was expelled from the State Funeral Directors convention in 1893 in St Louis, Missouri, and a resolution was passed to forbid ever inviting his return. Sullivan settled in Chicago and opened a school of embalming. Local papers relate his arrest there together with a female companion (not his wife) on charges of adultery and wife and child desertion. When he finally settled the charges he underwent a cure for alcoholism and resumed teaching in a succession of short-lived appointments at various schools.

In 1900, the OK Buckhout Company of Michigan, a manufacturer of embalming chemicals, had Charles A Renouard under contract to lecture, and sent him to London, England, to present a 3-week course of instruction that was very well received. Renouard returned home to attend similar engagements in the United States. The Buckhout Company had to find someone to continue the successful course of instruction in England, and the position was offered to Sullivan, who immediately accepted. Sullivan began teaching in London on October 8, 1900, a career that would extend to 1903.

He lectured throughout the British Isles and helped to organize the British Embalmers Society as well as a journal entitled to British Embalmer.

He related that when Queen Victoria died in 1901, he was consulted about the possibility of embalming her. He recommended against it since it was impossible to guarantee perfect results. When he returned to the United States, he purchased an embalming school in St Louis, Missouri, but the venture proved unprofitable. He then moved to Denver and Salt Lake City and eventually back to St Louis, where he died. Sullivan wrote hundreds of articles plus eight books, taught thousands to embalm, and probably received more gifts from his classes than any other teacher before or since his time.

Increase in embalming schools: Some early "graduates" of embalming courses of instruction gave up regular employment at an undertaking establishment to provide embalming service to a number of undertaker who had no staff member trained to embalm. *This is how the terms embalmer to the trade or trade embalmer originated.*

Schools of instruction in embalming increased in number and activity by the beginning of the 20th century. Many manufacturers of embalming chemicals entered into the business of teaching embalming to maintain and increase the market for their products. Although the repair of injuries to the dead caused by disease or trauma had been dealt with since Egyptian times, it was not until 1912 that a systematic treatment for such cases was developed by a New York City embalmer, Joel E Crandall (1878-1942). From this time on the schools of embalming slowly began to adopt instruction in this special phase of embalming treatment. Today, the subject area is commonly referred to as *restorative art*. It would be impossible to list in this text every personality who became an embalming professor or every school that was established, but a few should be mentioned.

Carl Lewis Barnes: Born into a family that operated an undertaking establishment in Connellsville, Pennsylvania, Barnes (1872-1927) studied medicine in Indiana, opened an embalming school there, and moved it to Chicago. He manufactured embalming chemicals, wrote many books and articles on the subject, and had the largest chain of fixed location schools in history in New York, Chicago, Boston, Minneapolis, and Dallas. While serving overseas as a medical colonel in the US Army in World War I, his business failed. He never reopened the schools, continuing the practice of medicine until his death.

Albert H Worsham: Worsham (1868-1939) attended Barnes school and was on the faculty from 1903 to 1911 when he opened his own school in Chicago, with his wife Laura and brother Robert as faculty members. He lectured widely and was noted principally for contributing to the early foundation of postmortem plastic surgery.

Howard S Eckels: Eckels (1865-1937) was a manufacturer of embalming chemicals and the founder of Eckels College of Embalming in Philadelphia, Pennsylvania. (The school and chemical plant were in the same building, which was not on uncommon arrangement.) Eckels wrote many articles and books, was successfully sued for plagiarism, and was not adverse to engaging in prolonged debates in the press. After his death, his son John managed the school well into the post-World War II period when it closed after a period of affiliation with Temple University.

William Peter Hohenschuh: Born in Iowa City, Iowa, the son of an undertaker, Hohenschuh (1858-1920) took over the family business upon the death of his father and began to teach embalming, which he had learned by correspondence from Auguste Renouard in the mid-1870s. Hohenschuh was active in the Iowa State Association and was elected president of the National Funeral Directors Association. He operated an embalming school in Chicago and, in 1900, in partnership with Dr William S Carpenter (1871-1944), opened the Hohenschuh-Carpenter School of Embalming in Des Moines, Iowa. He also operated a funeral home. In 1930, Dr Carpenter moved the school to St Louis and merged it with the Moribund American college of Embalming owned by FA Sullivan. After Dr Carpenter's death his daughter Helen Craig and her son Golden Craig operated the school as well as the American Academy in New York City. This continued well into the post-World War II period.

Clarence G Strub: Born in Iowa March 1, 1906, Strub attended the University of Iowa in Iowa City, Washington University in St Louis, Missouri, and the Hohenschuh-Carpenter College of Embalming in Des Moines, Iowa. He became an instructor at Honenschuh in 1929. In 1930, the school was moved to St Louis where it merged with the American College of Embalming and operated under the name of the St Louis College of Mortuary Sciences. In 1934, he became a member of the staff of the Undertaker's Supply Company of Chicago and conducted clinics and demonstrations throughout the United States and Canada. He taught embalming and funeral management at the

University of Minnesota and the Wisconsin Institute of Mortuary Science and was the director of research for the Royal Bond Chemical Company for many years.

His greatest contributions to embalming lie in his ability to write clearly and simply, explaining embalming theory and practices. During his career, he published well over 1,000 articles, as well as many teaching outlines and quiz compendia. His little text, The Principles of Restorative Art, was the true prototype of all present-day texts on the subject. He also authored the monumental textbook, *Principles and Practice of Embalming*, published by LG "Darko" Fredericks, which became the standard embalming text used by most colleges of mortuary science. Strub also wrote several technical movies such as the *Conquest of Jaundice* and *The Eye Bank Story*, was well as many purely children's stories and movies. He was the architect of the Eye Bank System in Iowa, which set the national pattern, as well as the curator of the state of Iowa's anatomical donation program, he died in Iowa city, Iowa on August 6, 1974.

Women embalmers: Women as well as men were trained as embalmers and not only practiced embalming but founded tools of instruction. Among these women were *Mrs EG Bernard* of Newark, New Jersey, who founded the Bernhard School of Embalming; *Madame Lina Odou*, who founded the Odou Embalming Institute in New York City; (Fig. 1.16); and *Lena R Simmons*, who founded and operated the Simmons School of Embalming in Syracuse, New York, until her son Baxter took over the management.

Mortuary Colleges, as known today, are relatively recent in origin. The development of mortuary education has followed the general pattern common to all professional fields. It emerged slowly from a period in which knowledge was transmitted from preceptor to student by means of observation and informal discussion to its present academic status.

A system for national accreditation of mortuary schools was first introduced in 1927 by the Conference of Funeral service Examining Boards, a national association of state licensing boards. Higher standards governing qualifications of faculty, the curriculum, and teaching facilities were established and enforced.

The first teachers institute was held in Cincinnati in the spring of 1946. On November 8 and 9, 1947, the second teachers institute was held at the Pittsburgh Institute of Mortuary Science at which time the first curriculum in embalming was adopted (Fig. 1.17). The committee chairman was Professor Ronald F Hannum of the Cleveland College of Mortuary Science. A basic course content in anatomy was also adopted. This committee was chaired by Dr Emory S James of the Pittsburgh Institute of Mortuary Science. On November 10, in Pittsburgh, the National Association of Colleges of Mortuary Science met and adopted what became the Morticians' Oath, still administered today to graduates of mortuary science.

CONCERN FOR TREATMENT

Early embalming reports concerning arterial injection indicated some concern for special treatment of the trunk viscera. Most such treatments consisted of removal, treatment, and replacement of viscera in the trunk cavity

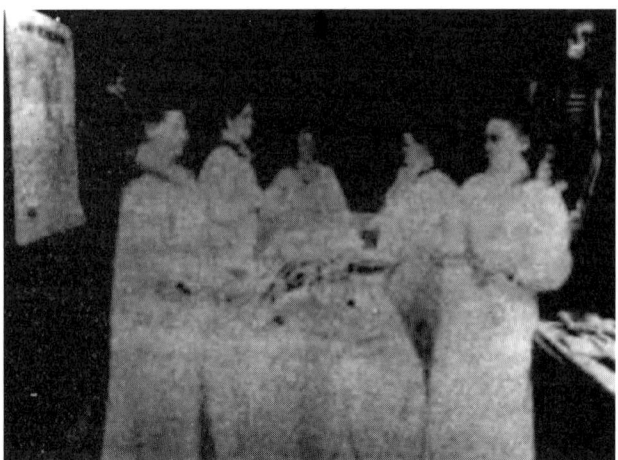

Fig. 1.16: Anatomy class at Odou Institute of Embalming, New York Circa 1900 (Professor C Odou at center of group).

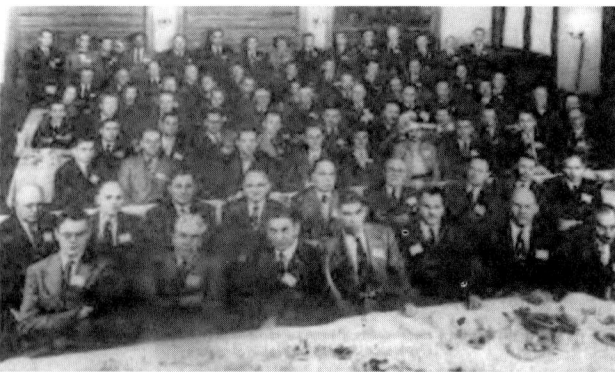

Fig. 1.17: Educators from across the United States gathered for the Second Teachers. Institute held in Pittsburgh, Pennsylvania, November 8 and 9, 1947 at this meeting the first curriculum in anatomy and embalming established and the Mortician's Oath was adopted. *Courtesy*: The Pittsburgh Institute of Mortuary Science, Pittsburgh Pennsylvania.

together with some preservative material, either powdered or liquid. Other reports, such as those of the Gannal–Sucquet era, indicate dependence for total preservation solely upon the arterial injection unaccompanied by any special treatment for the trunk cavities. Gabriel Clauderus had advocated preservation based upon introduction of his preservative chemical into the trunk cavity followed by immersion of the entire body in the preservative.

It was not until the mid-1870s that a "modern" system of treatment for the cavities was designed. The inventor of the trocar, Samuel Rodgers (listing Los Angeles, New York City, and San Francisco as his residence) secured two patents for the trocar, one in 1878 and the second in 1880. The 1878 patent described the trocar much as it exists today. The 1880 patent was issued for a system of embalming that consisted of introduction of his trocar, thrust through a single point in the navel into an the organs of the trunk to distribute a preservative fluid throughout the trunk viscera. The simplicity of this treatment and its modest success made it appealing to men who, for whatever reason, did not adopt arterial embalming, which required greater knowledge of anatomy and surgical skill. The inevitable result was a confrontation between "belly punchers" (cavity treatment advocates) and "throat cutters" r (arterial embalmers) concerning the merits of their respective means of preservation.

It slowly became evident that neither system was always completely successful and that combination of the two systems, arterial injection followed by cavity treatment, offered the greatest promise of embalming success. Although Rodgers did not mention aspiration prior to injection of preservative chemicals in his process, Auguste Renouard did specifically recommend this in his *Undertaker's Manual*. Rodgers' method of a single-entrance opening into the trunk cavity with a brilliant contept not followed by all his contemporary "authorities". Espy and Taylor's books of embalming instruction, for example, advocated multiple (three to four) points of insertion through the trunk wall for the trocar. Rodgers formulated an embalming preservative chemical named Alekton, which was believed to have phenol as its principal preservative. He also recommended cavity treatment followed by hypodermic injections utilizing his trocar, inserted into the limbs of the corpse.

Since, the introduction of arterial injection of the blood vessels in the late 17th century no other system of corpse preservation explored had ever been even seriously utilized. In 1884, a British physician, Dr BW Richardson, devised what he termed *needle embalming*. The process consisted of inserting a trocar (the needle), such as Rodger's invention, at the medial corner of the eye socket and forcing it into the brain area, where the injection process was repeated. After removal of the trocar from the brain area, cavity treatment, aspiration, and injection were carried out. This process was most often referred to as the eye process. Rodgers in his early patent had proposed insertion of his trocar through the nose to inject preservative chemicals into the brain area but did not suggest that this process would preserve the entire body as Richardson contented. It eventually was to be called the—nasal process. Professor Sullivan, ever alert for any new procedure to interest his students, adopted Richardson's eye process and exploited its simplicity to the maximum.

Carl Barnes offered a variation of the procedure by inserting the trocar through the neck and into the brain via the foramen magnum. TB Barnes, his brother and school instructor associate, inserted the trocar between dorsal vertebrae into the spinal canal. In this method, Dr Eliab Meyers drilled a hole through the center of the vertex of the skull, permitting direct access for a small trocar into the superior sagittal sinus. The process, regardless of point of access, is said to have delivered the preservative chemical eventually into blood vessels within the cranium and then to the rest of the body.

A dramatic test demonstration of the process is both described and illustrated in Barne's textbook, *The Art and Science of Embalming*. A severed head of a dissection room subject had trocars inserted into the brain area through the eye socket route. Rubber tubes connected the carotid arteries and jugular veins with collecting bottles. As fluid was injected through the trocars into the brain area, fluid flowed into the collecting bottles via the carotid arteries and jugular veins. The process achieved moderate popularity until about 1905 when it became extinct. Not all teachers of embalming were advocates of it, and JH Clarke was a vigorous critic.

A variation of the process was the short-lived attempt to insert the trocar into the left ventricle of the heart and inject the arterial system. The great difficulty encountered in positively locating the left ventricle quickly discouraged this procedure.

Professionalism in Embalming

Toward the end of the 19th century and on into the 20th century a number of events were to occur that would accelerate embalming toward the level of professionalism. A convergence of two movements became apparent about

1897, with the appearance of ads by embalming fluid companies stating that their fluid contained formalin. For some years, there had been arguments to eliminate arsenic and other poisons from inclusion in embalming fluid formulas for the same medicolegal reason that the French prohibited arsenic in 1846 and bichloride of mercury in 1848. Now that a powerful disinfectant, *formalin*, was available and reasonably priced, the opportunity to eliminate poisonous chemicals was at hand. The state of Michigan led the way in 1901 and was followed by other states.

The second movement was to require regulations for both licensing and governing those who practiced embalming, and in 1893–1894 the state of Virginia became the first state to do so. Formalin content fluids were not a total blessing and were not as favorably received as might have been expected. Embalmers of the period were unaccustomed to the very different characteristics of the new preservative. For example, bodies embalmed with arsenic were said to have been relatively supple, making dressing and positioning relatively easy. Many of the poisonous chemicals had bleaching qualities and left the body quite white. Only a few left any undesirable coloration, such as those reported to contain copper, which tended to produce a bluish color in the skin. Then too, little or no problem was reportedly encountered to the penetration of all the body tissues, with or without blood drainage. There was also the proven ability of such poisonous chemicals to preserve the body tissues. There were, of course, some negatives such as the possible absorption of poisonous chemicals through the embalmer's unprotected skin, various skin irritations, and thickened and cracked fingernails.

The embalmer, beginning to experiment with the formalin-based embalming fluids had to learn that he must remove the blood in all cases and began to use low-formalin-content or nonformalin fluids to wash the blood out before injection of the preservative formalin-based solutions. He also learned that he had to position the body properly before injection and the hardening effects of formalin or he would encounter serious problems later in trying to properly position hands together. To his astonishment, the embalmer also discovered that formalin reacted with the bile pigments present in the skin of jaundiced bodies to produce an unsightly green-colored skin.

The opponents of formalin fluids were highly critical of the formaldehyde fumes, which irritated mucous membranes, claiming these effects were more dangerous to health than the poisonous chemicals. Reason and science prevailed and the embalming fluid formulas were improved to overcome most of the early problems. With the eventual transfer of the site of embalming from the family home bedroom to the funeral home preparation room, proper ventilation tended to eliminate most of the irritation problem. Chemicals became more diverse. For example, different formulas were developed for specific uses, such as arterial and cavity, preinjection, coinjection, and for special purposes as in decomposing cases. The delivery of embalming fluids in concentrated form, to be added to water to create the desired dilution strength, was a distinct contrast to the former embalming chemical packaging, which was delivered in containers already combined with the water ready to inject. Thus, the embalmer had to become more experienced and intelligent in the mixing of the formalin embalming solution than he had formerly.

Utilization of New Devices

Over the years of embalming in bedrooms of the home of the deceased, little in the way t > f improvements was instituted in injection pumps or aspirating devices. With the transfer of the majority of embalming preparation to the funeral home, however, new devices could be used. In the last quarter of the 19th century, most embalming pumps or injectors were based on the gravity bowl, the handpump, or the rubber bulb syringe. The gravity bowl was simply a container suspended above the body and connected to the arterial tube by a length of rubber tubing. The height of the bowl above the body determined the pressure. Its main advantage was that it did not require the constant pumping by the embalmer and, therefore, left hands free to perform other tasks. The handpump could produce either pressure or vacuum for injection or aspiration into or from a glass container.

When the preparation of the body was moved to the funeral home, water pressure was used to create suction to aspirate. Special aspirators, such as the Penberthy, Worsham, and Slaughter, generated suction by water pressure and were made to attach to preparation room sink faucets, connected by rubber tubing to the trocar. Later in the 1950s, special electric motor-driven aspirators were devised and were found to overcome the aggravation encountered by low-water pressure during high-water-use periods. *Most communities today have requirements relating to the need for preventing suction of aspirated material into the water system.*

Falcon Electric Embalmer

At a New York state convention in 1914, a battery-powered electric pump, the Falcon Electric Embalmer for injecting embalming chemicals, was demonstrated but was not widely adopted. Some new instruments devised to simplify or improve certain embalming procedures were developed in the 1920s and 1930s. A new method of jaw closure was devised involving "barbed tracks" driven into the mandible and maxilla by a spring-propelled hammer. Wires attached to the "tacks" were then twisted together to sure the desired degree of jaw closure. A plastic, threaded, screw-like device called the trocar button became the most useful waterproof sea l for trocar punctures, bullet wounds, and even for intravenous needle punctures (when surgically enlarged). A metal dispensing device that was attached directly to any standard 16-ounce bottle of cavity fluid (by screwing it into the bottle opening in place of the cap) simplified cavity fluid injection.

The dispenser was connected to the trocar by a length of rubber hose and injection was accomplished by gravity after the cavity fluid bottle was elevated and inverted. It was not until the mid-1930s that electric-powered injection machines were available and in use. Some were simply electric motors with fittings to produce pressure or vacuum-connected to suitable containers by rubber tubing. In 1937, the Slaughter Company developed an all metal fluid injection tank equipped with a pressure gauge; in 1938, the Flowmaster electric-powered injection machine was announced; in 1939, the Frigid Fluid Company developed a pressure injector consisting of a metal container for holding embalming fluid complete with exit connection with shut off and carbon dioxide gas cylinder to create the necessary pressure to inject the fluid. *In mid-1939, the Turner Company announced the availability of the Porti Boy, which was to become the all-time most popular injection machine.* Several improvements over the years included a pulsator device, a larger fluid tank, and the ability to produce extreme high-pressure injections. By the 1960s, extreme high-pressure injection machines such as the Sawyer were available and in use.

Availability of More Materials

With the end of World War II, metal and other materials became available to produce various new embalming devices. The concept of utilizing externally generated agitation to assist in blood removal became popular. Some embalming table had such pulsating devices built in as an integral part of the structure. Other pulsating devices were devised to be attached to existing operating tables or were handheld devices to be applied to the body over the course of the major blood vessels. Disillusionment with this development came after a short period of the use. The vibrations produced by such devices made it impossible to keep instruments, and even the body itself, from sliding downward toward the foot of the table.

Another innovation was the development of a conventional embalming fluid by the Switzer Corporation of Cleveland that contained a large quantity of fluorescent dye. The dye was to act as a tracer or indicator of the degree of circulation or penetration of the embalming fluid when viewed under an ultraviolet light illuminator furnished with the embalming fluid. Although the system did indeed disclose the extent of the distribution of the embalming chemical and its fluorescent dye, it never was proof positive that area of the body beneath the skin was thoroughly embalmed.

In the wake of Hiroshima and Nagasaki and other major disasters such as airline crashes, earthquakes, mudslides, and building collapses, a search was instituted for some new means of quickly processing (preserving) huge number of dead. Over the years, different means of processing (preserving) the victims of such tragedies were devised, tested and found unsuitable for a variety of reasons. Experiments were conducted with processes utilizing ultrasound, radiation, atomic bombardment, and ultracold. No process tried seemed to be capable of preserving a tremendous number of bodies in a brief period. The search continues!

It is astonishing what has been achieved in the embalming field in nearly 5,000 years of growth of knowledge, skill, and experience. Naturally, what the future holds is unknown, but those working in the field feel it will be as exciting and rewarding as the past millennia.

BIBLIOGRAPHY

1. Beverly R. History of Virginia; 1922.
2. McClelland EH. Bibliography on Embalming (mimeo copy), National Association of Mortuary Science (limited to 100 copies). New York; 1949.
3. McCurdy CW. Embalming and embalming Fluids-with Bibliography of Embalming. Wooster, Ohio: Hearld Printing Co.; 1896.
4. Oatfield H. Literature of the Chemical Periphery-Embalming. Advances in Chemistry series, No. 16 (a key to pharmaceutical and medicinal chemistry literature). Washington, OC: American Chemical Society.

5. Pinkerton J. Collection of Voyages; 1812.
6. Townshend J. Surgeon General's Catalogue. Washington, OC: U.S. Army, 1883-1884. Grave Literature (a catalogue of some books relating to the disposal of bodies and perpetuating the memories of the dead), New York (private collection); 1887.

Egypt

1. Aliki. Mummies Made in Egypt. New York: Thomas J Crowell; 1979.
2. Arcieri GP. Note E Ricordi-Sulla Preservatione Del Corppo Umano. Rivista Di Storia Delle Scitnze Medicine E Naturoli No. 1, Florence, Italy; 1956.
3. Bardeen CR. Anatomy in America. Bulletin of University of Wisconsin, No. 115. Science Series. 1905;3(4):85-208.
4. Budge EAW. The Mummy. Cambridge: University Press; 1893.
5. Choulant L. History and Bibliography of Anatomical Illustration. New York; 1962 (reprint).
6. David AR. Manchester Museum Mummy Project. Manchester, England: Maney and Sons Ltd; 1979.
7. Harris JE, Weeks KR. X-raying the Pharaohs. New York: Charles Scribner's Sons; 1973.
8. Hemneter E. Embalming in Ancient Egypt. Ciba Symposia, 1(10): Summit, N.J. Ciba Pharm. Co.; 1940.
9. Herodotus. History (translated by George Rawl inson). New York: Dial and Tudor Presses; 1928.
10. Liebling R, et al. Time Line of Culture in the Nile Valley and Its Relationship to Other Countries. New York: Metropolitan Museum of Art; 1978.
11. Martin RA. Mummies. Anthropology Leaflet No. 36. Chicago, IL: Chicago Natural History Museum Press; 1945.
12. Mendelsohn S. Embalming. Ciba Symposia, 6(2): Summit, N.J: Ciba Pharm. Co.; 1944.
13. Moodie RL. Anthropology Memoirs, Vol. III: Roentgenologic Studies of Egyptian and Peruvian Mummies. Chicago, IL, Field Museum Press; 1931.
14. Pettigrew TJ. History of Egyptian Mummies. London: Longman; Rees; 1834.
15. Pons A. Les Origines de L'Embaumement et L'Egyte Predynastique. Montpellier, France: Imprimerie Grolier; 1910.
16. Smith GE, Dawson WR. Egyptian Mummies. New York: Dial Press; 1924.
17. Steuer RO, Saunders JB de CM. Ancient Egyptian and Cnidian Medicine. Berkley Los Angeles: University of California press; 1959.

Peru

1. Garcillaso de la Vega. Royal Commentaries of Peru (translated by Paul Rycant). London; 1688.
2. Prescott WH. History of the Conquest of Peru (2 vols). Philadelphia: JB Lippincott; 1882.
3. Rivero ME, Von Tschudi JI. Peruvian Antiquities (translated by Francis L Hawks). New York: George Putnam and Co.; 1853.
4. Von Hagen VW. Realm of the Incas. New York: New American Library of World Literature; 1957.

Alaska and Aleutian Islands

1. Quimby GI. Aleutian Islanders, Anthropology Leaflet, No. 35. Chicago: Natural History Museum; 1944.

North American Indians

1. Yarrow HC. Study of Mortuary Customs among the North American Indians. Washington, OC: U.S. Government Printing Office; 1880.

Ecuador-Jivaro Indians

1. Cottlow LN. Amazon Head Hunters. New York: Signet Book/Henry Holt and Co.; 1953.
2. Flotny B. Jivaro. New York: Library Publishers; 1954.

Canary Islands

1. De Espinosa A. The Guanches of Tenerife. London: The Hakluyt Society; 1907.
2. Hooton EA. The Ancient Inhabitants of the Canary Islands. Harvard African Studies, 2: Cambridge, MA: Harvard University Press; 1925.

Europe (Early Period)

1. Bradford CA. Heart Burial. London: Allen and Unwin Ltd; 1933.
2. Castiglioni A, Robinson V. The Anatomical Theater, Ciba Symposia, 3(4); 1941.
3. De Villihardouin G, DeJoinville I. Memoirs of the Crusades. New York: EP Dutton and Co.; 1938.
4. Dionis M. Cours D'Operations de Chirurqie. Paris: d'Houry Publishers; 1746.
5. Garrison FH. Introduction to the History of Medicine. Philadelphia; 1929.
6. Guichard C. Des Funerailles et diverses Manieres. Lyon, France: D'eosevelir; 1582.
7. Guichard C Funerailles. Lyon, France: Jean de Tovernes; 1581.
8. Greenhill T. Nekrokadeia-or The Art of Embalming. London: printed for author; 1705.
9. Guybert P. The charitable physician showing the manner to embalm a dead corpse, in The Charitable Physitian. London: Thomas Harper Printer; 1639.
10. Oauderus G. Methodus Balsamundi Corpora Humane Aliaque Majora sine Evisceratione et Sectione Hucusque Solita. Altenberg, Germany: G Richterum publishers; 1679.
11. Pare A. How to make reports and to Embalm the Dead (translated). London: Cotes and Young Publishers; 1634.
12. Pilcher LS. The Mondino myth (reprint.). Med Library Hist J. 1906;4:4.

13. The Art and Science of Embalming dead Bodies (taken from the 29th book of Peter Forestus and translated from the Latin into German) contained in A New Medical Treatise by Petrum Offenbach, M.D. Frankfort: Zacharian Palthenium Publisher; 1605.
14. Treece H. The Crusades. New York: Random House; 1962.
15. Walsh FF. The Popes and Science. New York: Fordham University Press; 1908.
16. Walsh II. The 13th-Greatest of Centuries. New York: Catholic Summer School Press; 1907.
17. Wellcome HS. The Evolution of Antiseptic Surgery. London: Burroughs Wellcome and Co.; 1910.
18. Young S. The Annals of tire Barber-Surgeons of London. London: Blades East and Blades; 1890.

Europe (Late Period)

1. Bailey JB. The Diary of a Resurrectionist 1811-1812. London: Swan-Sonnenschein and Co.; 1896.
2. Ball JM. The Sack-em-up Men. London: Oliver and Boyd; 1928.
3. Bayle DC. L'Embaumement. Paris: Adrien Delahaye Publishers; 1873.
4. Blanchard S. Anatomica Reformata-Balsamatione, Novus Methodus. Leiden: Boutesteyn and Lughtmans; 1687.
5. Cole FJ. A History of comparative Anatomy. London: MacMillan and Co.; 1944.
6. Coliez A. Conservation Artificielle des corps. Paris: Amedee Legarand; 1927.
7. Cope Z. The History of the Royal College of Surgeons. Springfield, IL: Charles C Thomas; 1959.
8. Dawson WR. Life and times of Thomas J. Pettigrew. Med Life. 1931;3:38.
9. DeLint JG. Atlas of tire History of Medicine, 1. London: HK Lewis and Co.; 1926.
10. Eriksson R (ed translator). Andreas Vesalius 1st public Anatomy at Bologna 1540. Uppsala: Almquist and Wikselle; 1959.
11. Gannal JN. Histoire des Embaumements. Paris: Ferra Librairie; 1838.
12. Gannal JN (as translated by R Harlan). History of Embalming. Philadelphia: Judah Dobson Publisher; 1840.
13. Gerlt-Wemich-Hirsch. Biographisches Lexikon Der Herrvorragenden Arzte Aller Zeiten und Volker. Berlin: Urban and Schwarzenberg; 1932.
14. Laskowski S. L'Embaumement, la conservatione des Sujets et les Preparations Anatomiques. Geneva: H Georg Publisher; 1886.
15. Mann G. The anatomical collections of Fredrik Ruysch at Leningrad. Bull Cleve Med Library, 11 (No. 1. January); 1964.
16. Nordenskiold E. The History of Biology. New York: Tudor publishing; 1928.
17. Paget S John Hunter. London: T Fisher University; 1898.
18. Peachy GC. The Homes of Hunter in London. London: Bailliere, Tindall and Cox; 1928.
19. Pettigrew JT. Frederik Ruysch, in Pettigrew's Medical Portrait Gallery. London: Whitaker and Co.; 1840.
20. Ramazzini B. de Morbis Artificum (ed 2, 1713). Diseases of Workers (translated by WC Wright). New York: Hafner Publishing Co.; 1964.
21. Richardson BW. The Art of Embalming in Wood's Medical and Surgical Monographs, 3. New York: 1889.
22. Sigerist HE. The Great Doctors. Garden City, NY: Doubleday and Co.; 1958.
23. Singer C. Studies in the History and Method of Science (2 vols), Oxford, England: Clarendon Press; vol I-1917, vol II-1921.
24. Sucquet JP. De L'embaumement et des Conservation pour L'etude de I' anatomie. Paris: Adrien· Delahaye Publishers; 1872.
25. Sucquet JP. Traits du visage L'embaumement. Paris: Adrien Delahaye Publishers; 1862.

United States

1. Barnes CL. The Art and Science of Embalming. Chicago, IL: Trade Periodical Co.; 1905.
2. Clarke CH. Practical Embalming: A recitation of actual experienced of the author and hundreds of the most expert embalmers of the world. Cincinnati, OH: CH Clarke, Year 1917.
3. Crane EH. Cranes' manual of instructions to undertakers embalming book. Crane Allen in Kalamazoo Michigan, Year 1888.
4. Dodge AJ. The Practical Embalmer. A Johnson Dodge Publishers; 1908.
5. Eckels HS. Practical Embalmer. Philadelphia: HS Eckels Co. Publishers; 1903.
6. Espy JB. Espy's Embalmer. Springfield, OH: Espy Fluid Co.; 1895.
7. Gallagher T. The Body Snatchers. Rockville, Maryland: Am Heritage; 1967.
8. Johnson EC. Civil War embalming. Funeral Directors Rev; 1965.
9. Johnson EC, Johnson GR. A Civil War Embalming Surgeon—The story of Dr Daniel H Prunk. The Director (NFDA publication); 1970.
10. Johnson EC, Johnson GR. Alone in His Glory. Unpublished manuscript, Civil War Mortuary Practices.
11. Johnson EC, Johnson GR. Prince Greer-America's First Negro Embalmer. Paris: Liason Bulletin, International Federation of Thanotopractic Association; 1973.
12. Johnson EC, Johnson GR. The Undtrtaurs Manual. Calgary: Canadian Funeral News; 1980.
13. Johnson EC, Johnson M, Rhodes DH. Conscientious Caretaker of Arlington National Cemetery. Am Funeral Director; 1984.
14. Johnson M. A Historic Precedent to the FTC Rules of 1977 (Civil War licensing for Embalmer Requirements). NFDA Bulletin; 1979.
15. Johnson M, Simmons LR. The Grande Dame of Early Embalmers. Am Funeral Director; 1977.
16. Johnson M. Lina Odou. Embalmer; 1977.
17. Johnson EC, Johnson GR, Johnson Williams M. Dr. Renouard's Role in Embalming History. Am Funeral Director; 1987.

18. Johnson EC, Johnson GR, Johnson M. Dr. Thomas Holmes-Pioneer Embalmer. Am Funeral Director; 1984.
19. Johnson EC, Johnson GR, Johnson Williams M. History of Modern Restorative Art. Am Funeral Director; 1988.
20. Johnson EC, Johnson GR. Johnson Williams M. The Trial, Execution and Embalming of Two Civil War Soldiers. Am Funeral Director; 1986.
21. Keen WW. Addresses and Other Papers. Philadelphia: WB Saunders; 1905.
22. Lukens CM and Clarke JH. The Faculty of the Cincinnati School for Embalming. Textbook on Embalming. Springfield, OH: Limboc'ker Printer; 1883.
23. Mendelsohn S. Embalming Auids. New York: Chemical Publishing Co.; 1940.
24. Mills and Lacey Mfg. Co. (no author stated). Practical Directions for Embalming the Dead. Grand Rapids, MI: Stevens, Cornell and Dean· Printers; 1881.
25. Myers E. Champion Textbook on Embalming. Springfield, OH: Chemical Co.; 1908.
26. Oarke JH. Reminiscences of Early Embalming. New York: The Sunnyside; 1917.
27. Renouard A. Undertakers Manual. Rochester, NY: A Nirdlinger and Co.; 1878.
28. Renouard CA. Taylor's Art of Embalming. New York: HE Taylor and Co.; 1903.
29. Samson H, Crane ON, Perrigo AB, et al. Pharmaceutical, Anatomical and Chemical Lexicon (the NFDA official textbook). Chicago, IL: Donohue and Henneberry Publishers; 1886.
30. Strub CA, Frederick LG. The Principles and Practice of Embalming, 4th edition. Dallas, TX: LG Frederick Publisher; 1986.
31. Sullivan FA. Practical Embalming. Boston: Egyptian Chemical Co. Publisher; 1887.
32. War Department. General Order 33; 1862.
33. War Department. General Order 39; 1865.
34. War Department. General Order 75; 1861.
35. Wightman SK. In search of my son (Civil War). Rockville, Maryland: Am Heritage; 1963.

Chapter 2

Environment and Personal Health Considerations*

Robert G Mayer

INTRODUCTION

The art and the multidisciplinary science of embalming have historically encompassed the principles and practices of public health concern of preserving and disinfecting human remains. The epidemiological basis for this concern has been established and documented by several related studies.

The practitioner of embalming is professionally responsible for a three-tiered spectrum: (1) Public health safety (2) Personal involvement dealing with the embalmer's immediate family, and (3) the community served by the embalmer.

The first level of responsible practice involves the maintenance of a work environment that is hygienically dean and safe. The embalmer must constantly be aware of the necessity for the use of (1) protective barrier attire, (2) disinfection and decontamination chemistry, and (3) practices and the identification of primary work environment reservoirs of actual and potential infectious disease hazards.

The "at risk" nature of preparing human remains for disposition demands the implementation of effective personal health and safety measures if funeral service is to offer acceptable standards of quality assurance and quality control.

FAULTY THEORIES

In recent years, critics of the practices of conventional and traditional funeralization involving embalming and in-state viewing have alleged that embalming is of little value in terms of accomplishing public health protection. Surprisingly, even individuals with educational and practical backgrounds in the physical and biological sciences argue that unembalmed remains are harmless and do not constitute reservoirs of classical or opportunistic pathogens. Several of the critics of embalming erroneously maintain that "germs die with the host", a most dangerous assumption on the part of anyone responsible for the handling and preparation of human remains.

An extensive review of literature pertinent to the public health hazards associated with human remains was conducted in 1968 by Maude R Hinson, a medical research librarian, and sponsored by the Embalming and Chemical Manufacturers Association. The review included abstracts of 88 bound references and 265 journal publications which repeatedly referred to the persistence and survival of pathogenic microbial agents in unembalmed remains. The review also indicated that the absence of antemortem cellular and chemical body defense mechanisms contributes to increased virulence factors associated with postmortem microflora.

CONFIRMED STUDIES

Laboratory studies involving the postmortem microbiological evaluations of specimens procured from remains certified to have died from causes other than an infectious disease have confirmed except that *unembalmed remains constitute an ideal environment for microbial growth and proliferation.*

---

*From Robert G Mayer. Embalming: History, Theory, and Practice. Connecticut: Appleton and Lange; 1990, with permission.

The normally operative antemortem epithelial, fascial, and other tissue barriers which tend to maintain systemic and/or anatomic localization of host microflora during life may undergo:

- Loss of structural integrity soon after somatic death. [This loss of structural, systemic compartmentalization of endogenous microflora characteristic of a given functional system (upper respiratory tract, genitourinary tract, gastrointestinal tract) contributes to the postmortem translocation and redistribution of host microflora on a hostwide basis.]
- The reticuloendothelial system (RES), another nonselective barrier to antemortem translocation, contributes to the same phenomenon of microbial relocation after death.
- The blood-brain barrier, an example of one of the antemortem anatomic defenses against microbial invasion of the central nervous system, becomes inoperative soon after death.

ENDOGENOUS INVASION

Endogenous invasion of cerebrospinal fluid by bacterial agents associated with the colon occurs within 4–6 hours of death. The colon, designated as the postmortem origin of "indicator" organisms recovered from extraintestinal sampling sites, seems to be the primary source of many of the translocated microbial agents. The isolation of "indicator" organisms as well as nonindicator organisms from such sampling sites as the left ventricle of the heart, the lungs, the urinary bladder, and the cisterna cerebellomedullaris indicates the extent to which microbial agents of low, moderate, and high virulence can translocate within a relatively brief postmortem interval of 4–8 hours.

The postmortem multiplication of systemic and translocated recoverable microbial agents may begin within 4 hours of somatic death and reach peak densities of 3.0–3.5×10^6 organisms per milliliter of body fluid or per gram of body tissues within a 24- to 30-hour postmortem interval.

Postmortem factors contributing to the translocation of endogenous microflora include chemical and physical changes, movement and positional changes of the remains, passive recirculation of blood from contaminated body sites, thrombus fragmentation and relocation, and the inherent true motility of many of the intestinal bacilli.

The relocated organisms may exit from body openings, natural and other, and become associated with adjacent animate and inanimate surfaces. They may also become airborne particulates in the form of aerosols (droplet infection particle) or dried particles (droplet nuclei) and constitute sources of body surface, either upper respiratory or other body site, contamination of living tissues.

LACK OF INFORMATION

A factor not to be ignored by the embalmer is the all too frequent lack of information related to deaths caused by reportable contagious or communicable infectious diseases. Throughout the United States there seems to be considerable inconsistency on the part of healthcare facilities (acute, general, and extended) to alert to receiving funeral director or funeral home that an infectious disease was the primary or a contributing cause of death.

Preparation of the remains may often precede access to the death certificate and the notification of the embalmer of the increased risk, either by "Red Tagging" of the remains and/or direct communication with the funeral service firm. This would enable the embalmer to exercise all appropriate personal health protection measures. Such a reporting system is to be encouraged within our healthcare delivery systems and agencies at the national, state, and local levels. The current deficiencies in the notification scheme make it incumbent on the embalmer to consider each embalming as a potential public health risk and to employ maximal personal protection measures as recommended for a margin of safety against any density or level of recognized or opportunistic infectious agents. In his 1895 manuscript entitled "The Embalmer as Sanitarian: Embalming and Embalming Fluids", Dr Charles W McCurdy wrote: "In the disposal of the dead, that process is most natural, most scientific which protects the living from disease, death and anguish of soul". The history of funeral service parallels the history of preventive medicine in the United States. More than a century of preventive medicine has been recorded since its recognition in 1859. It has always reflected a progressive evolution in regard to the causes, the prevention, and the control of infectious disease.

ESTABLISHMENT OF BOARDS OF HEALTH

The first boards of health, established in Massachusetts and California in 1869 and 1870, respectively, were followed by 32 other state boards of public health by the turn of the century. This added much impetus to the branch of science related to the regulation of public health and the prevention of infectious diseases. The "undertakers" of this earlier era were considered to be sanitarians and practitioners of public health and, at the time, these responsibilities were classified as the primary professional obligations of funeral service. Funeral service practitioners protected "the living from disease" during the pandemic occurrences of influenza in 1918, 1938, 1958, and beyond, during the epidemic of poliomyelitis in the 1950s, the epidemic of tuberculosis, herpetic infections, serum hepatitis, and several other infectious diseases of past and current concern.

Infectious disease risks have always been present in the professional practices of funeral service. Hepatitis (types A and B), systemic mycoses, upper respiratory infections of viral and bacterial etiology, bacterial and viral encephalitides, human immunodeficiency virus (HIV), and acquired immunodeficiency syndrome (AIDS) are examples of a few of the infectious diseases that place the embalmer in an "at risk" but very important public health protection role.

EFFECTS OF PATHOGENS

Many deaths are caused by the direct effects of recognized or opportunistic pathogens and by the indirect effects of infectious agents. Embalmers must learn to effectively employ acceptable standards of public health protection techniques on all remains, no matter what the indicated cause of death may be. Under these conditions of practice, the risk of transmitting an infectious "dose" of a pathogenic agent from a victim of infectious disease is minimized.

Example: Studies have indicated that the number of small diameter microbial aerosols necessary to cause upper respiratory infections via the respiratory alveoli is small, often less than 10 viable organisms. The do age with larger-diameter biological particles may be as high as 1,000–10,000 or more. The causes of diphtheria, streptococcal pharyngitis, measles, or influenza, for example, involve inhalation of the larger particles. Several observers have discussed the risk of aerosol dissemination of tubercle bacilli in the postmortem environment. If a victim of tuberculosis could originate an infected particle for every 200 ft^3 of air prior to *and* during the embalming process, an embalmer breathing about one-third of a cubic foot of air per minute might inhale an infectious dose during a relatively short exposure period. This example of airborne biological contaminants emphasizes the importance of an efficient air handling system in the preparation room *a minimum of 6 and preferably as many as 20 complete air exchanges per hour.*

PUBLIC HEALTH GUIDELINES

Public health guidelines were prepared on behalf of and published by the Memorial Affairs Division, Air Force Logistics Command United States Air Force, for implementing by assigned personnel, military and civilian, at all installations involved in the preparation of remains of deceased military personnel or their dependents. These guidelines were reviewed and approved by the National Institutes of Health (Environmental Services, NIH), the Occupational Safety and Health Administration (OSHA)-Air Force, and the Surgeon General's Office-Air Force. These guidelines, with updating revisions, are recommended as the basis for developing personnel health policies and public health practices in all funeral service firms. They have been recommended by several State Boards of Examiners in Mortuary Science to all licensed funeral service practitioners in their respective states of jurisdiction.

The guidelines were reviewed by the staff of the Environment Safety Branch (ESB), the National Institutes of Health in 1978, and an opinion was expressed by the chief of the ESB: It is our opinion that such guidelines and regulations are most important from a public health standpoint. There must be proper protection for the mortician, pathologist, and others, as well as the community. We believe this because of the problems of emerging pathogens (Oviatt, 1978).

The public health guidelines are as follows:

Purpose

To provide procedural guidelines in the areas of public health, personal hygiene and safety as they pertain to the practices of personal and environmental disinfection and decontamination by practitioners of mortuary services. Prevention of the following is a reasonable expectation of the proper practice of the guidelines.

- The transmission of actual (recognized) and/or opportunist pathogens from human remains to the embalmer
- The transmission of pathogens from the embalmer to susceptible hosts within the mortuary facility environment or to members of the embalmer's family
- The transmission of pathogens from the preparation room environment to family and friends of the deceased, and/or other visitors to the mortuary.

Premise

Many of the infectious agents associated with the medical and the paramedical environments are categorized as "opportunistic" pathogens or microbial agents normally considered to be of low virulence. The increasing association of "opportunistic" pathogens with infectious disease has all but eliminated the reference, "nonpathogenic". There seems to be general agreement that a "nonpathogen" is simply a microbial agent that has not yet overcome the defense mechanisms of a suitable host. Such opportunistic organisms are always a part of the postmortem microflora to which the embalmer is exposed and against which appropriate environmental control measures should be taken.

CONCURRENT DISINFECTION AND DECONTAMINATION

Human Remains

- Thoroughly cleanse and sanitize the body surface and body openings with a suitable generic category of chemical disinfectant, e.g. 150–200 ppm of an iodophor, 0.5% use-dilution of a phenylphenol, one of the latest generations of a quaternary ammonium compound complex, 1,000–5,000 ppm of sodium hypochlorite, etc. The case analysis evaluation of the remains conducted during the sanitizing procedures may indicate a need for chemical disinfectant concentrations higher than routinely recommended. For example, evidence of gas gangrene should alert the embalmer to increase the recommended use-dilution level.
- Thoroughly rinse the sanitized body surfaces and body openings, especially if there has been body surface contamination with radioisotopes, natural or artificial.
- The injection and drainage protocol should include the following recommended guidelines, as discussed previously:
  a. Multipoint or multi-site injection and drainage
  b. Intermittent (restricted) drainage
  c. The use of a minimum of a 2.0% v/v concentration of nonformaldehyde preservative/disinfectant
  d. The chemical treatment of the primary body cavities (thoracic, abdominal, and pelvic) with one pint (16 fluid ounces) of concentrated cavity chemical per cavity or a minimum of three pints per adult case.

Embalmer

- Always wear an outer, protective garment, preferably one which is impervious to the penetration of liquids and aerosols, such as a rubber or plastic wrap-around apron or gown.
- Always wear rubber or plastic gloves during the handling of human remains. The gloves should be discarded after each use.
- Wear protective head and shoe coverings, especially in the handling of autopsied and/or septic disease cases.
- Wear a protective oral-nasal mask designed to prevent the inhalation of infectious or hazardous chemical particulates.
- Rinse gloved hands in appropriate dilution of chemical disinfectant periodically during the preparation of the remains to minimize transfer of contaminants to skin surfaces of the embalmer.
- Concurrently immerse instruments in separate pan or container of chemical disinfectant between actual uses during the preparation of the remains.

Air Handling in the Preparation Room

- The use of an efficient air exhaust system or air purification system is highly recommended during the preparation of the human remains to maintain a non-hazardous level of airborne contamination. Respirable contaminants usually include those microbial agents measuring 5.0–100 μm in diameter.
- The air handling system should also prevent the accumulation of formaldehyde vapor and/or paraformaldehyde aerosol concentrations in the preparation room environment by creating a minimum of six air exchanges per hour. Formaldehyde concentrations exceeding 2.0 ppm constitute a potential health hazard to the embalmer (Fig. 2.1).

TERMINAL DISINFECTION AND DECONTAMINATION

Preparation Room

- Cleanse and disinfect all instruments, the operating table surfaces, aspirating equipment and appurtenances, preparation room floor and wall surfaces, water faucet handles on sinks, door knobs, waste receptacles, etc. In cases of known or confirmed reportable infectious disease, contagious or communicable, and/or instances of gas gangrene, instrument, including trocars

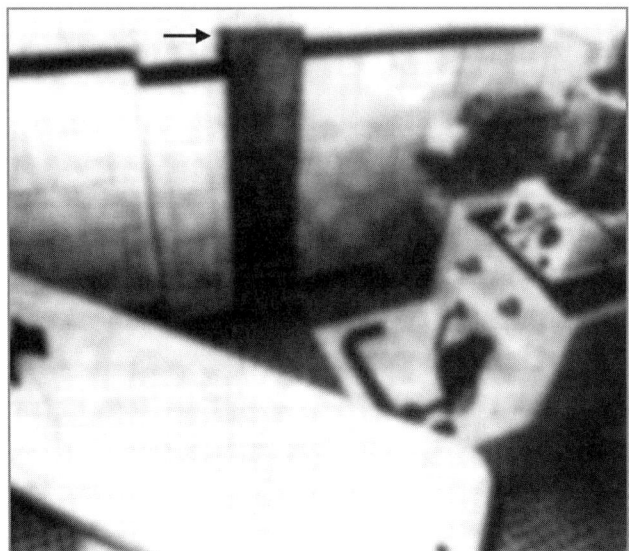

Fig. 2.1: The exhaust duct against the back wall. It exhausts fumes from the floor level.

and drainage tubes, should either be steam sterilized (autoclaved) or immersed in a suitable cold chemical sterilant, e.g. 2.0% acid glutaraldehyde (Sonacide) or alkalinized (Cidex) glutaraldehyde, Bard-Parker solution (8.0% v/v formaldehyde in 70% ethanol or isopropanol), 400–500 ppm of an iodophor, 5,000 ppm of hypochlorite solution, or other suitable disinfectant.
- Incinerate all incinerable fabric or plastic body coverings, e.g. bandages, dressing, sheets, towels, or other patient-associated items placed in direct contact with the remains.

Funeral Coach/Service Vehicle(s)

- Cleanse and sanitize the mortuary cot or tray. Use freshly cleansed and sanitized cot or tray covers on each transfer of remains.
- Cleanse and sanitize the internal surfaces of the funeral coach/sanitize vehicle following each transfer of remains.

Embalmer(s)

- Remove and dispose of gloves. Gloves are a single-use accessory and should not be considered reusable items. Scrub hands and forearms with a suitable medicated liquid soap or 200 ppm of an iodophor or other suitable germicide.
2. Shower-cleanse entire body surface, including the germicidal shampooing of the hair.

GENERAL GUIDELINES

Vacuum Breakers

The potential hazards associated with biologic and chemical contaminants encountered within the preparation room environment must not be allowed to enter any network of plumbing cross-connections within the preparation room. Vacuum breakers must be installed in all involved water lines to prevent the back-siphoning of contaminated liquids into potable water supply lines.

Physical Examination

Funeral service personnel should receive a thorough medical/physical examination at least annually, and preferably biannually.

Immunization

Funeral service personnel should adhere to an effective program of preventive prophylactic immunization schedules. All embalmers should follow the recommended booster periodicity for typhoid fever, influenza, tetanus, etc.

Mantoux Skin Test for Tuberculosis

All embalmers should be skin tested for tuberculosis on an annual basis until they convert from skin test negative to skin test positive. At the time of conversion, a chest X-ray should be performed every 2–3 years.

Rubella Vaccination

All embalmers, male or female, should be vaccinated against German measles (rubella) if it is known that they do not possess protective antibody level against the virus. Women of pregnancy age may sustain a teratogenic effect from exposure to the virus during the first trimester of pregnancy; males may transmit the virus to susceptible females.

Hepatitis B (Serum Hepatitis) Vaccination (Heptavax B)

All embalmers not immune to hepatitis B should be vaccinated against it. Hepatitis B may be transmitted to the embalmer via any body fluid originating from the deceased victim of the viral disease. Embalmers sustaining accidental skin penetration during the preparation of an hepatitis A (infectious hepatitis) or hepatitis B (serum hepatitis) victim and are known to be susceptible, should promptly seek the administration of immunoglobulin (specific antibody preparations against the viral diseases).

Administration of Prophylactic Antibodies

Embalmers involved in the preparation of known deaths related to bacterial meningitis (meningococcic meningitis) should contact a physician, clinic, or emergency center for the administration of preventive/prophylactic antibiotic(s).

Oral-Nasal Masks

All embalmers involved in the preparations of known victims of systemic fungal infections, e.g. histoplasmosis, coccidioidomycosis, blastomycosis, or known victims of hepatitis B, AIDS (HIV), viral encephalitis, bacterial meningitis, etc., should always take the precaution of wearing an oral-nasal mask designed to entrap biologic particulates of minute diameters, 0.1 μm or greater.

At the present time, nearly 90% of clinical infections occur in four body sites: (1) urinary tract, (2) skin and subcutaneous (wound), (3) upper respiratory tract, and (4) vascular system (bacteremia/septicemia). There is an increasing number of immunocompromised hosts whose susceptibility to infection may be two to three times greater than that of the average member of the community. The majority of infections originate from endogenous sources: hands, nasopharyngeal secretions, fomites, and the contaminated surfaces of preparation room equipment.

Airborne transmission may involve the etiologic agents of such infectious diseases as tuberculosis, whooping cough, measles, Legionnaires' disease, chickenpox, and fungal infections. Newly identified and recognized infectious agents and the mode(s) of transmission of the same can be anticipated. As the number of immunocompromised hosts, the "walking wounded", increase the clinical presentations of infections and the causative agents involved will change. There will always be a constantly changing cast of microbial "actors" with new and different epidemiologic costumery.

The best defense against the emergence of new pathogens and the environmental selection of increased microbial resistance to inactivation is to effectively interrupt the direct and indirect modes of transmission within the "at risk" environment.

The public health guidelines that should be a part of every funeral home's personal health policies should be accompanied by a set of minimum standards for the preparation of human remains for in-state viewing. The implementation of the following standards together with the previously listed public health guidelines will more consistently ensure the public health quality of our professional practices.

RECOMMENDED MINIMUM STANDARDS FOR THE EMBALMING OF HUMAN REMAINS

The voluntary adoption and implementation of minimum professional practice standards in embalming is a necessary first step in the provision of quality control and quality assurance in the preservation and disinfection of human remains. This is especially important in terms of providing more precise definitions of the public health values of embalming. It is to be highly recommended that when embalming is performed, a measure of uniformity of minimum professional skills be employed by all practitioners. The experimental studies completed to date confirm that *embalming is effective when the commercially available embalming chemicals are used in proper concentrations and in adequate total volumes, and are administered under conditions of proper techniques.*

The following professional profile of minimum standards of embalming practices is based on laboratory evaluations and post-embalming observations.

Multi-site Injection and Drainage

Multi-site (two or more) injection and drainage methodology ensures a more consistent distribution of the disinfection and preservation chemical solutions to all receptive tissue areas, both deep and superficial; maximal chemical perfusion of receptive tissues is necessary to ensure the effectiveness of embalming. This more consistently provides the public health protection expected and eliminates any environmental impact hazards in earth interment.

Rate of Flow of Arterial Injection Chemicals

A moderate rate of flow (10–15 minutes/gallon) and sufficient injection pressure to maintain the moderate rate of flow (2–10 psi) are companion recommendations for the assurance of distribution and diffusion of the injection chemicals. Occasionally, it may be necessary to initiate and to maintain drainage. These conditions may be applicable to the first gallon of injection solution only, after which the moderate conditions should be employed. The injection pressure(s) should exceed vascular resistance and create moderate movement of the injection solution. Injection pressure(s) and rate(s) of flow should not, however, cause excessive short circuiting and loss of the injection solution or undesirable tissue distortion.

Use of Intermittent (Restricted) Drainage

One of the most effective methods of ensuring adequate distribution of the arterial injection solution is the use of intermittent drainage. It is especially recommended after surface discoloration has been removed, for example, after the first gallon of arterial injection solution has been injected. If proper drainage has been accomplished, this technique will not impede further drainage. Solutions under pressure tend to follow routes of least resistance. This method should produce maximum preservation and disinfection effects from the injected chemicals.

Total Volume of Arterial/Injection Solution Employed

Consideration should be given to employing a minimum of 3–4 gallons of arterial injections solution for the average adult weighing from 125 pounds (lb) to 175 lb. Injection and drainage techniques may involve the removal of 4–6 quarts of blood and body fluids. To properly restore the loss of body fluids and overcome the loss of preservative and disinfecting arterial injecting chemicals, especially in the use of continuous drainage, it is necessary to employ the total injection solution volume of 3–4 gallons, for example, 1 gallon/50 lb of body weight, exclusive of primary injection solution(s) (By today's standards this rule would be better to read: inject 1 gallon of properly prepared arterial solution for every 40 lb of body weight).

Use of Supplemental Chemicals

The enhancement of the distribution of the injected disinfectant/preservative solution may often require the use of supplemental chemicals, for example, modifying and surface active additives, primary injection chemicals, and water conditioners. The use of such additives may increase the efficacy of injection solution distribution and drainage.

Concentration (%) of Preservative/Disinfectant in the Injection Solution

Data from extensive laboratory evaluations indicate that the concentration of formaldehyde preservative/disinfectant in the arterial injection solution should never be less than 2.0% v/v. Formaldehyde in concentrations ranging from 2.3% to 3.0% v/v inactivates existing bacterial populations in excess of 95%. It is known that formaldehyde concentrations less than 2.0–3.0% may produce tissue fixation, but may not reduce microbial densities (microbicidal effect) by more than 50%. Significant reductions should be a minimum of 70% or greater. Formaldehyde is classified as a "high-level" disinfectant when used in concentrations of 3.0–8.0% v/v. The recommended use of a 2.0% v/v concentration of formaldehyde in arterial injection solutions, and preferably a 3.0% v/v concentration, is based on investigative documentation.** It may be necessary to begin arterial fluid injections using a 1.25 to 1.50% v/v concentration for the first gallon—or often until all intravascular discolorations are cleared and fluid is distributed through most body areas. The solution strengths can then be increased to 2.0–3.0% strength. Use of restricted cervical injection may also be necessary. This would allow for injection of the stronger arterial solutions into the trunk areas and the use of a milder arterial solution for the head and facial tissues. This may be necessary because many arterial fluids would produce too much facial dehydration when used at a 2.0 to 3.0% v/v concentration, and it may be difficult with some fluids to establish good distribution.

**Preinjection fluids* are those fluid formulations whose primary purpose of injection into the vascular system is vascular preparation. *Arterial fluids* are those compositions and fluid formulations whose primary purpose after injection into the vascular system is the preservation and disinfection of tissue. Herein, those concentrations are expressed in formaldehyde concentrations by volume as follows: low concentration—up to 1% formaldehyde; moderate concentration—1–2% formaldehyde; high concentration—2% formaldehyde or above. Co-injection fluids are those compositions and fluid formulations whose primary purpose is to accompany, supplement, and enhance the action of the other two fluids.

Use of Cavity Treatment Chemicals

Thorough and adequate treatment of the thoracic, abdominal, and pelvic cavities should include the aspiration of liquids and semisolids that can be aspirated from the nonautopsied remains and the injection of 1 pint (16 ounces) of concentrated cavity chemical into each of the major cavities. When body weight exceeds 200 lb, it is recommended that the embalmer used 1 pint of concentrated cavity chemical per 50 lb of the body weight. The cavity treatment techniques employed should ensure maximal tissue contact as a result of pretreatment trocar separation and perforation of all organs in each of the three primary body cavities.

Performance Procedures

The preceding minimum standards of performance include disinfection and decontamination procedures that are important to the public health protection of the embalming practitioner, that is, concurrent disinfection of the remains gloved hands of the embalmer, and all adjacent contact surfaces and the terminal disinfection of these and other direct and indirect contact sites in the preparation room.

All items of attire, soiled clothing, healthcare gowns or pajamas, and postsurgical or skin and subcutaneous wound dressings should be immersed in a disinfectant solution or steam sterilized (autoclaved). Incineration of these items is no longer permitted.

The body surfaces of the remains should always be cleansed and sanitized and the body orifices treated with an appropriate disinfectant and packed with cotton previously saturated with disinfectant. Contaminated disposable items may be placed in a waste receptacle lined with an impervious, autoclavable plastic bag. The plastic bag with contaminated contents should not be transferred from the preparation room to a site of disposition until steam sterilization has been completed.

A professional framework of practical and reasonable minimum standards for the practice of embalming will contribute significantly to the accomplishment of our public health goals and obligations.

The recommended set of minimum standards for the preservation and disinfection of human remains should, when implemented: enhance the distribution of the arterial injection chemicals throughout the entire cardiovascular system. Protocols include (1) multi-site injection and drainage, (2) restricted drainage, (3) adequate total volume of injection solution, and (4) the use of supplemental chemicals. The structural mediator of the delivery of the injection chemicals to receptive tissue sites is the fundamental and simplest division of the blood vascular system, the capillary. In this sense, arterial embalming might be referred to as capillary embalming. These simple endothelial tubes with an average diameter of 7–9 μm connect the terminal arterioles and the venules.

The surface area of the capillary network in the human body approaches 6,000 m^2 or 64,585 ft^2. This vast membrane of over 1.5 acres is the permeable barrier that controls the delivery of preserving and disinfecting chemicals to deep and superficial body tissues. The closed circulatory system of humans normally contains 5–6 quarts of blood, 8.0% of the body weight, 85% of which is contained within the capillaries. Obviously, thorough perfusion of the soft tissue sites with appropriate concentrations of injection chemicals involves far more than filling the aorta and its primary branches. The long-term preservation and disinfection of human remains require the embalmer to utilize such standards of technique as to effectively transform routine "injection" into "capillary embalming".

RISKS OF INFECTION

Most embalmers, pathologist, and epidemiologists readily agree that human remains constitute an "at risk" reservoir of infectious agents and pose a continuing occupational health hazard. Although the public health significance of embalming has been adequately documented, recorded public health statistics confirming the high incidence of infections, among embalmers are minimal. The lack of such confirmatory vital statistics has, unfortunately, discouraged appropriate recognition of embalming as a public health function and the "at risk" role of the embalmer by public health agencies—local, state, and national.

**It would take 12.8 ounces (or 13 ounces) of a 20 index fluid to make 1 gallon of a 2% solution or 18.7 ounces of a 20 index fluid to make a 3% solution. With a 30 index fluid, 8.5 ounces would be needed for a 2% solution or 12.5 ounces of concentrated fluid to make 1 gallon of 3% solution.

The increasing incidence of herpes simplex virus, hepatitis B virus, and the HIV or AIDS virus infections has caused many public agencies to re-evaluate the potential infectious disease risks assumed by morticians, e.g. the Office of Biosafety, Centers for Disease Control, Atlanta, Georgia. Morticians, pathologists and anatomists are often unknowingly exposed to hepatitis B because the virus may remain dormant in carriers. Further, the hepatitis B virus in serum or plasma may be transmitted indirectly via inanimate environmental surfaces.

The author is aware of service embalmer who was hospitalized for hepatitis B and died. The postmortem diagnosis was infectious jaundice or leptospirosis, a spirochetal infection against which there are effective therapeutic antibiotics. In this instance, misdiagnosis needlessly took the life of an embalmer who sustained a needle penetration of the skin during embalming. Although the incidence of tuberculosis has declined in the United States, a study of 129 cases in which tuberculosis was considered to be the primary cause of death indicated that diagnosis did not occur until autopsy in 33% of the cases. Such retrospective diagnoses tend to underline the potential for transmission of infectious disease to the embalmer.

SANITATION SURVEY

A sanitation survey involving more than 2,000 responding mortuary science licensees was conducted by the Champion Chemical Company in 1975. More than 18% of the respondents indicated that they had sustained one or more serious infections during their careers in the funeral service profession.

Tuberculosis (14%), viral upper respiratory infections (44%), infectious hepatitis (13%), fungal infections (19%), bacterial septicemias (17%), and bacterial wound infections (14%) were the most frequently reported funeral service-associated infections. The incidence of infectious disease among funeral service licensees was two to three times higher than the incidence in the general population. The incidence of tuberculosis, infectious hepatitis, and fungal infections among pathologists is approximately 16%, slightly above the incidence associated with funeral service practitioners. The higher incidence in the funeral service profession may be well indicative of careless and/or negligent practices employed in the preparation of human remains.

Table 2.1 summarizes the basis for the protective measures recommended in the section entitled Public Health Guidelines. Methods of chemical and physical decontamination must be employed to eliminate "reservoirs" or infectious agents and to prepare preparation room surfaces, instruments, and equipment hygienically safe for reuse and the re-exposure of the embalmer-host.

Chemical and physical decontamination is a very important weapon in the fight against infectious diseases,

Table 2.1: Breaking the cycle of transmission of infectious agents in the preparation room: Public health guidelines for the at risk embalmer "host".

Portal of "host" entry	*Infectious agent*
Skin or mucous membrane, *respiratory tract, alimentary tract*, body openings—natural and/or artificial (abrasions cuts, laceration wounds), proper "barrier" attire, aseptic technique(s), handwashing, gloves, disinfection and decontamination	Bacteria, fungal (molds and yeasts), viruses, rickettsia, protozoa Personal health practices Personnel health policies Environmental sanitation Disinfection and decontamination
Modes of transmitting the infectious agent	Reservoirs of infectious agents in the preparation room
Direct contact (aerosol or droplet infection) and indirect contact (air, contaminated surfaces) and objects or fomites body fluids and exudates, insects	Remains, equipment (e.g. hydro-aspirators, trocars, razors), instruments, adjacent hard surfaces, air, contaminated linens, bandages solid and liquid wastes
Proper "barrier" attire Handwashing, gloves Proper disposition of wastes Effective air handling system Concurrent and terminal disinfection	
Asepsis bactericidal bacteriostatic	A condition free of germs, destructive to bacteria, inhibiting the growth or multiplication of bacteria (no destruction of viability implied)

Contd...

Contd...

Portal of "host" entry	Infectious agent
Cleaning	Removal of infectious agents by scrubbing and washing, as with hot water, soap, or suitable detergent
Disinfectant	An agent, usually chemical, applied either to inanimate objects/surfaces or living purpose of destroying disease causing microbial agents, but usually not bacterial spores
Germicide	An agent, usually chemical, applied either to inanimate objects/surfaces or living tissues for the purpose of destroying disease-causing microbial agents, but usually not bacterial spores
Sanitizer	An agent, usually chemical, that possesses disinfecting properties when applied to a precleaned object/surface
Sterilization	Total destruction of all living microbial agents and their products

Note: Prope "barrier" attire may include whole body covering, head cover, shoe covers, oral-nasal mask and eye protection (safety glasses)

Table 2.2: Chemical and physical methods for controlling microbial contamination.

Method of decontamination	Temperature requirement	Minimum interval of exposure (min) 0, 2, 10, 12, 15, 20, 90, 120, 150, 180
Sterilization: complete destruction of all forms of microbial life	285°F (140°C)	--: (Instant)
Saturated steam under pressure (autoclaving)	270°F (132°C) 250°F (121°C)	----------------: ----------------: 30 min for hepatitis viruses 2–12 h
Ethylene oxide gas	130°F (54°C)	--------------------------------------: 2 h or more
Hot air, e.g. oven	320°F (160°C)	--------------------------------------: or more
Chemical sporicide solution, e.g. 8.0% formaldehyde plus 70% isopropanol, glutaraldehyde*		3–12 h or more
Disinfection: Killing of disease-producing microbial agents, but not resistant spores		
Boiling water or free-flowing steam, chemical germicide solutions, e.g. iodophors, phenylphenols, quaternary ammonium compounds	212°F (100°C) Room temperature	------: or more, 30 min for hepatitis viruses -------: or more
Sanitization: Chemicals aided by physical methods of soil removal	Maximum of 200°F (93°C)	------------------------:

*Recommended for high-level disinfection.
Source: Modified from a chart copyrighted in 1967, Research and Development Section, American Sterilizer Company. Erie, Pennsylvania.

especially in environments exposed to a multitude of actual and potential pathogens. It should be emphasized that chemical and physical disinfection is no substitute for good housekeeping and practical cleaning procedures. The following terms are applicable to the function of environmental control, utilizing methods of disinfection and sterilization.

Primary disinfection is the application of disinfection and decontamination measures prior to embalming. *Concurrent disinfection* is the application of disinfection and decontamination measures during embalming of the body. *Terminal disinfection* is the application of disinfection and decontamination measures after completion of the preparation of the remains. Primary, concurrent, and terminal disinfection require the application of physical and chemical methods for the control of microbial contamination (Table 2.2).

"High", "intermediate", and "low" levels of antimicrobial activity are recognized for the proper disinfection of critical, semicritical, and noncritical environments and objects. As shown in Table 2.3, an essential property of a *high-level disinfectant* is effectiveness bacterial spores: suitable reagents include aqueous 2.0% glutaraldehyde,

Table 2.3: Levels of disinfection activity.

	Bacteria		Fungi		Viruses	
Level of activity	Vegetative	Tubercle bacillus	Spores	Lipid and medium-size	Nonlipid and small	
High	+	+	+	+	+	+
Intermediate	+	+	−	+	+	+
Low	+	−	−	+	+	−

+: positive mircobicidal effect; −: negative microbicidal effect.
Source: Adapted with permission from Block SS. Disinfection, Sterilization, and Preservation, 3rd edition. Philadelphia, PA: Lea and Febiger; 1983.

Table 2.4: Activity levels of selected microbicides*.

Liquid microbicide	Use-concentration	Activity level
Glutaraldehyde, aqueous, e.g. Cidex, Sonacide, Sporicidin	20%	High
Formaldehyde + alcohol	8.0% + 70.0%	High
Stabilized hydrogen peroxide	6.0–10.0%	High
Formaldehyde, aqueous	3.0–8.0%	High to intermediate
Iodophors, e.g. Betadine, Wescodyne, HiSine, Iosan	75–200 ppm	Intermediate
Iodine + alcohol	0.5% + 70.0%	Intermediate
Chlorine compounds, e.g. sodium hypochlorite as in chlorine bleach	1,000–5,000 ppm	Intermediate
Phenolic compounds, aqueous, e.g. Amphyl, Staphene, O-Syl	0.5–3.0%	Intermediate to low
Quaternary ammonium compounds, e.g. Phemoral, Zephiran chloride, Diaparine chloride	0.1–0.2% aqueous	Low
Mercurial compounds organic and inorganic, e.g. merthiolate, mercurochrome, metaphen	0.1–0.2%	Low

*Trade names of certain microbicides are given.
Source: Adapted with permission from Block SS. Disinfection, Sterilization, and Preservation, 3rd edition. Philadelphia, PA: Lea and Febiger; 1983.

8.0% formaldehyde solution in 70.0% alcohol, 6.0–10.0% stabilized hydrogen peroxide, and ethylene oxide gas.

Intermediate-level disinfectants do not necessarily kill large numbers of bacterial spores in a relatively short time, but they do inactivate the tubercle bacillus. These disinfectants are also effective against fungi as well as lipid and nonlipid medium-size and small viruses; examples include 0.5% iodine, 70–90% ethanol and isopropanol, chlorine compounds (free chlorine as derived from sodium or calcium hypochlorite), and some phenolic ("tamed" phenols) and iodophor-based disinfectants.

Low-level disinfectants cannot be relied upon to destroy bacterial spores, the tubercle bacillus, or small nonlipid viruses. These disinfectants, such as quaternary ammonium compounds and mercurials, may be useful in actual practice because they can rapidly kill vegetative forms of bacteria and fungi as well as medium-size lipid-containing viruses. The disinfecting levels of iodophors ("tamed" iodines) and phenolic compounds may be classified as intermediate or low depending on the concentration employed (Table 2.4).

Noncritical items within the preparation room environment may include walls, floors, and furnishings. Many embalmers rely on low-level disinfectants for application to such surfaces, used either alone or in addition to cleansing with detergent system. Blood, mucus, or feces, when present on items to be disinfected, may contribute to the failure of a given disinfectant or sterilization procedure. The organic contamination may occlude microbial agents and prevent penetration of the disinfection chemical(s). Or, the organic material may directly and rapidly inactivate certain disinfection chemicals such as chlorine- and iodine-based disinfectants and quaternary ammonium compounds. This effect is correspondingly greater with weak concentrations and with low-level disinfectants than with strong concentrations and high-level disinfectants.

This emphasizes the necessity of thoroughly cleansing contaminated instruments such as trocars, hydroaspirators, and forceps prior to chemical disinfection. In fact, physical cleaning may be the most important step in a disinfection process, which by definition, does not include the possible "overkill" factor of a sterilization procedure.

The chemical agents listed in Table 2.4 are categorized by type rather than by specific formulation. Whenever there is a choice between "cold" chemical sterilization (high-level activity) and sterilization by heat (autoclaving), the latter is preferable.

Specific recommendations, grouped by types of objects to be disinfected or sterilized, are presented in Table 2.5. The numbers designate the specific procedures that are acceptable in each situation; the key to the numbers is given at the bottom of the Table 2.5; exposure times for each situation are included. If should be noted that certain

Table 2.5: Acceptable antimicrobial procedures/exposure intervals.

Object	*Vegetative bacteria and fungi, influenza viruses*	*Tubercle bacilli, enteroviruses except hepatitis viruses, vegetative bacteria and fungi, influenza viruses*	*Bacterial and fungal spores, hepatitis viruses, tubercle bacilli enteroviruses, vegetative bacteria and fungi, influenza viruses*
	Disinfection	Disinfection	Sterilization
Smooth hard surface objects	A-10 min D-5 min E-10 min F-10 min H-10 min L-5 min M-5 min	B-10 min D-10 min G-10 min H-10 min L-10 min M-10 min	D-18 h J K L-9 h M-10 h
Rubber tubing rubber catheters	E-10 min F-10 min H-10 min	G-10 min H-10 min	J K
Polyethylene tubing Polyethylene catheters	A-10 min E-10 min F-10 min H-10 min	B-10 min G-10 min H-10 min	D-18 h J K L-9 h M-10 h
Lensed instruments	E-10 min F-10 min H-10 min K M-10 min	K M-10 min	K
Hypodermic needles	Sterilization only	Sterilization only	J
Thermometers*	C-10 min K	C-10 min K	D-18 h L-9 h M-10 h
Hinged instruments	A-20 min D-10 min E-20 min F-20 min H-20 min L-10 min M-10 min	B-30 min D-20 min G-30 min H-30 L-20 min M-20 min	J K L-9 h M-10 h
Floors, furniture, other appropriate room surfaces	E-5 min F-5 min H-5 min I-5 min	G-5 min H-5 min	Not necessary or practical

*Investigate thermostability when indicated.

chemical agents tend to cause some materials to corrode or rust; recommendations for prevention of corrosion are footnoted below the Table 2.5.

CONCLUSION

The dictates of logic, reason, and research all demand that the dead human body be considered a source of pathogenic microorganisms. Embalmers are charged by the same dictates and by law with the responsibility to implement protective and thorough procedures to ensure that the potential for contagion thorough exposure to the body is minimized. This chapter has presented a set of public health guidelines and minimum standards that if followed by the embalmer, will accomplish this objective.

Key Terms and Concepts for Study and Discussion

- Define the following terms:
  - Opportunistic pathogens iodophor
  - Concurrent disinfection
  - Terminal disinfection
  - Capillary embalming
  - Translocation
  - Droplet nucleus
  - Cisterna cerebellomedullaris
  - Disinfectant
  - Germicide protective barrier attire
  - Primary disinfection
- At what concentration do airborne formaldehyde monomers constitute a potential health hazard to the embalmer?
- Bacterial spores require high-level disinfectants for effective treatment. Name two other microbial agent and of current public health importance that also required this level of activity for proper treatment.
- What is the incidence of infectious disease among funeral service personnel compared with the (1) general population and (2) pathologists?
- Tuberculosis is an airborne respiratory infection. How is it possible for an embalmer to contact tuberculosis from human remains via the respiratory route of transmission?
- Several critics of embalming maintain that germs die with the host. Why is this an erroneous assumption?
- Why is multi-site injection and drainage preferable to single-site injection and drainage in the recommended minimum standard for embalming?
- Specify three conditions that commercially available embalming chemicals must fulfill for embalming process to be effective.
- List the three areas of public health safety for which funeral service practitioners are professionally responsible.
- Describe five methods for breaking the cycle of tranmission of infectious agents in the preparation room.

Key

- Isopropyl alcohol (70–90%) plus 0.2% sodium nitrite to prevent corrosion
- Ethyl alcohol (70–90%)
- Isopropyl or ethyl alcohol plus 0.2% iodine
- Formaldehyde (8%)-alcohol solution plus 0.2% sodium nitrite to prevent corrosion
- Quaternary ammonium solutions (1:500 aq) plus 0.2% sodium nitrite to prevent corrosion
- Iodophor—75 ppm available iodine plus 0.2 sodium nitrite to prevent corrosion
- Iodophor—450 ppm available iodine plus 0.2% sodium nitrite to prevent corrosion
- Phenolic solutions (2% aq) plus 0.5% sodium bicarbonate to prevent corrosion
- Sodium hypochlorite (1:500 aq—approximately 100 ppm)
- Heat sterilization—see manufacturers' recommendations
- Ethylene oxide gas—or technical literature
- Aqueous formalin (40%)
- Activated glutaraldehyde (2% aq).

Note: 1,000 ppm of available chlorine is recommended for inactivation of hepatitis B virus and 5,000 ppm for inactivation of HIV (AIDS) virus. Thoroughly rinse all inanimate surfaces of any excess formalin prior to application of the hypochlorite disinfectant. Keene cautions that when formaldehyde reacts with hydrochloric acid, the compound bis (chloromethyl) ether (BCME) may be formed. BCME is a highly toxic, carcinogenic compound.

BIBLIOGRAPHY

1. Benenson AS. Control of Communicable Diseases in Man, 12th edition. Washington DC: American Public Health Association; 1975.
2. Block SS. Disinfection, Sterilization, and Preservation, 3rd edition. Philadelphia: Lea and Febiger; 1983.

3. Burke PA, Sheffner AL. The antimicrobial activity of embalming chemicals and topical disinfectants on the microbial flora of human remains. Health Lab Sci. 1976; 13(4): 267-70.
4. Du Moulin GC, Paterson DG. Clinical relevance of postmortem microbiologic examination: a review. Hum Pathol. 1985;16(6):539-48.
5. Finegold SM, Kirby WM. Changing patterns of hospital infections: implications for therapy. Am J Med. 1984; 77(1B):1-2.
6. Fuerst R. Frobisher and Fuerst's Microbiology in Health and Disease, 15th edition. Philadelphia, PA: Saunders; 1983.
7. Hinson MR. Final report on literature search on the infectious nature of dead bodies for the Embalming Chemical Manufacturers Association. Cambridge, Massachusetts; 1968.
8. Hockett RN, Rendon L, Rose GW. In-use evaluation of glutaraldehyde as a preservative-disinfectant in embalming. Abstracts of the Annual Meeting of the American Public Health Association, Session 449, Contributed Papers: Microbiology-Immunology. Washington, DC: American Public Health Association; 1973.
9. Isolation techniques for use in hospitals. US Department of Health, Education and Welfare, Public Health Service, Washington, DC: DHEW Publication No. (HSM) 71-8043; 1973.
10. Junqueira LC, Carneiro J. Basic Histology, 3rd edition. Los Altos, CA: Lange Medical Publications; 1980.
11. Keene BR. Chemistry in Britain. 1973.
12. McCurdy CW. The Embalmer as Sanitarian: Embalming and Embalming Fluids. Wooster, OH: University of Wooster; 1895.
13. Oviatt VR. Chief, Environmental Safety Branch, National Institute of Health, Public Health Service, Bethesda, MD; Letter dated January 25, 1978.
14. Rose GW, Rendon L. Coping with the present and the future: minimum standards for performance of embalming. The National Reporter. Evanston, IL: National Research and Information Center; Vol. 2, No. 9, 1979.
15. Rose GW, Wetzler TF. A public health view of embalming. The Director, Milwaukee, WI: National Funeral Directors Association; 1969.
16. Sanitation survey results. Champion Expanding Encyclopedia of Mortuary Practice, No. 459. Springfield, Ohio: The Champion Company; July-August 1975.
17. Teaching Outline for Occupational Safety and Health in the Funeral Service Profession. New York: Ad Hoc Committee, The American Board of Funeral Service Education, Inc.; April, 1977.

---

*Must be thoroughly wiped preferably with tincture or soap, before disinfection or sterilization. Alcohol-iodine solution will remove markings on poor-grade thermometers.

Chapter 3

Death and Postmortem Changes

TD Dogra, A Sinha, ML Ajmani

INTRODUCTION

Conventionally, death means complete cessation of the activities of the three vital and interdependent systems of the body:
1. Circulatory
2. Nervous
3. Respiratory.

Death occurs when one or more of these systems completely fail. Many medicolegal experts classify the mode of death on the basis of these three systemic failures:
1. Syncope—failure of function of the circulatory system.
2. Asphyxia—failure of function of the respiratory system.
3. Coma—failure of function of the nervous system.

According to Spitz and Fisher, after a person is legally dead, the individual muscle fibers and other cells may continue to live for varying amount of time. Because of this phenomenon, the death of the person as a whole has come to be referred to as somatic death and the ultimate death of all of the cells of the body is described as cellular death.

There are two types of death: (1) somatic and (2) molecular death. Somatic death means the death of the whole organism. It progresses in orderly form from clinical death to brain death, then to biological death, and finally, to molecular death.

Somatic death means permanent and irreversible cessation of the following three organs that constitute "Tripod of Life":
1. Brain
2. Lung
3. Heart.

Failure of any one of these organs will result in loss of integration of the body systems.

However with the invent of cardiorespiratory resuscitative measures and in view of organ transplantation, it has become difficult to establish progression of the stages of death. Moreover with recent medical advances, it is now possible to keep the body alive by artificial supportive measures.

In clinical death, there is spontaneous cessation of respiration and heartbeat. If resuscitative measures are taken at this stage, life may be fully restored otherwise death will be established within a maximum of 5–6 minutes after the failure of respiration or circulation. This is a reversible stage of somatic death.

Brain death occurs in steps, so as the body. The cells die because of oxygen starvation (anoxia). The first part of the brain to die is the cerebral cortex (after 5 or 6 minutes), followed by midbrain and brainstem. Therefore, brain death can be:
- Cortical or cerebral death with an intact brainstem
- Brainstem death with the cerebrum intact and functionally cut-off
- Whole brain death.

Therefore, it is possible to have death of higher center, i.e. cerebrum without damaging the brainstem. In this condition, the patient remains unconscious but the respiratory system and heart may function for years. After brain death, biological death occurs. Now, the death of individual cells begins and results in cessation of the life processes of the various organs and tissues of the body. It is an irreversible phase of the somatic death.

Molecular death varies depending upon metabolic activity of the cells. It continues till there is a complete biodegradation of total tissue mass. The process of molecular death occurs in "bits and fragments" because more highly specialized and more active cells of the body react faster to a decrease in oxygen and nutrient contents, whereas less-specialized cells continue to live in the body for hours after somatic death are given in Table 3.1.

Table 3.1: Lifespan of less-specialized cells after somatic death.

Cells	Lifespan
Cells in brain and nervous system	5 minutes
Muscle cells	3 hours
Blood cells	6 hours

AGONAL PERIOD

This is the period just prior to commencement of somatic death. This period has been greatly prolonged by medical science. Long-agonal period provides more time to disease process and secondary infections to act upon the body organs. Two types of thermal changes occur during the agonal period:
1. *Agonal fever*: It is an increase of body temperature just prior to death. It hastens the onset of rigor mortis and decomposition process after death. It is more often seen in infectious bodies.
2. *Agonal algor*: It is a cooling or lowering of the body temperature just prior to death. This is because metabolism and circulatory system have slowed down. It slows the onset of rigor mortis and decomposition and is good for the embalming procedures.

POSTMORTEM CHANGES

The postmortem changes occur in a sequential manner, which depends upon many factors like environmental conditions (temperature, humidity, weather, land, and water), manner of death, and time passed since death. After death, the body undergoes a number of physical and chemical changes. The longer the time between death and embalming, the more changes will occur and embalming process may not be successful. On the other hand, embalming conceals the postmortem changes. The postmortem changes can be divided into three groups:
1. *Immediate (somatic death)*:
   - Insensibility and loss of voluntary power
   - Cessation of respiration
   - Cessation of circulation.
2. *Early changes (cellular death)*:
   - Pallor and loss of elasticity of skin
   - Changes in the eye
   - Cooling of the body (Algor mortis)
   - Postmortem lividity
   - Primary flaccidity of muscles
   - Rigor mortis
3. *Late changes (decomposition, autolysis, and decay)*:
   - Putrefaction and autolysis
   - *Modified putrefaction*:
     - Adipocere formation
     - Mummification.

Immediate Changes

Insensibility and Loss of Voluntary Power

Early signs of death can be found in cases of prolonged vagal inhibition, epilepsy, catalepsy, narcosis, electrocution, etc.

Cessation of Respiration

Complete stoppage of respiration for more than 5 minutes usually causes death. It may stop for short period as in Yoga, Cheyne–Stokes breathing, drowning, and newborn infants.

Cessation of Circulation

Stoppage of heart for more than 3–5 minutes is irrecoverable and is considered as evidence of death.

Early Changes

Changes in Skin

It becomes pale and there is loss of elasticity.

Changes in Eye

Loss of corneal reflex, opacity of the cornea, flaccidity of eyeball, pupillary changes (pupil dilation and no response to light), changes in blood vessels, and chemical changes.

Algor Mortis

It is a postmortem cooling of the body. Normal pathways of heat loss are circulation, respiration, and excretion. After death, these are no longer functioning and there may be slight rise in body temperature. It takes time for the body to cool to the temperature of the surrounding environment. In the first few hours after death, the body usually cools faster and thereafter, cooling slows as the body assumes the temperature of the surrounding environment. Normally, the dead body cools to temperature of the surrounding environment within 12–14 hours. The internal organs cool much slower than the surface tissues of the body and contribute to the putrefaction and autolytic changes at a rapid rate. The fall of temperature is further influenced by the following factors:
- Temperature difference between body and environment
- Individual physique—larger persons cool slowly; thin persons cool faster.

- Age of the individual—younger body cools much faster than an adult.
- Body coverings—the amount of clothing on the body also affects algor mortis.

Postmortem Caloricity

In this condition, there is a rise of body temperature after death in first few hours. Cellular metabolism continues in the body after somatic death and releases heat and energy. This reaction continues until the entire oxygen present in the tissues is used; the heat released is trapped in the tissues because the normal pathways of heat loss circulation, respiration, and excretion are no longer functioning. This results in a slight rise in temperature. The heat loss is slowed, if the body is clothed or environment is warm.

Cadaveric Lividity, Hypostasis, and Suggillation for Postmortem Staining

It is a discoloration of skin due to the accumulation of the fluid blood into the capillaries and small veins of the rete mucosum in the most dependent parts of the body. Postmortem staining begins to form within an hour after death and is well marked in 4–12 hours. It starts as patchy mottling of the skin, which fuses to produce the discoloration of dependent parts. In the first few hours after death, these patches will disappear and new ones will form on the dependent parts on changing the position of body. Later on, fading is slow and incomplete due to its inability to flow in well-marked lividity. The coagulation of blood commences in 6–12 hours after death when the postmortem staining is fixed and pressure does not blanch the area. The color of hypostasis may depict the cause of death.

- Cherry red in carbon monoxide and sometimes in burns cases.
- In hydrocyanic acid poisoning and sometimes in burns, the color is bright red.
- Poisoning by nitrates, potassium chlorate, or potassium bicarbonate, color is reddish brown or deep blue.
- In phosphorus poisoning, color is dark brown.
- In asphyxia, the color may be bluish violet or purple.
- Dead body exposed to cold in refrigeration may become pink in color.
- In septic abortion due to *Clostridium welchii* the color may be grayish brown. Internal hypostasis may occur on the dependent part of the internal organs. It is likely to be confused with antemortem congestion and is required to be differentiated from contusion/bruise.

Primary Flaccidity of Muscles

This stage occurs in somatic death period immediately after death, all muscles are relaxed. This is called primary flaccidity. This is the best period for embalming the body because the body proteins will react best with formalin and produce firm tissues.

Rigor Mortis

Rigor mortis is a postmortem stiffening of all body muscles (voluntary and involuntary) with slight shortening. Individual cell death (muscle cell) takes place at this stage. Rigidity is well established in smooth muscles before it is apparent in the skeletal muscles.

After death, during primary flaccidity phase, the body tissue pH is slightly alkaline or neutral. In rigor mortis, tissues gradually become acidic with pH 5.5. As rigor passes the tissues again become alkaline because of decomposition of muscle proteins and formation of alkaline product (Table 3.2).

Table 3.2: Postmortem staining and contusion of body.

Postmortem staining	Bruise/contusion
Occurs on extensive area of most dependent part	Can occur anywhere on body
Involves superficial layers	Involves deeper tissues
Sharply defined edges of skins	Edges not sharply defined
Does not appear elevated above surface	Appear raised above surface
Cuticle intact	Cuticle may be abraded
Uniform color, may become green on putrefaction	Exhibits changes of color
Pressure prevents postmortem staining color	Pressure gives it a lighter color
On cut section, no effusion of coagulated or liquid blood in subcutaneous tissues	On cut section, infiltration of the tissues with coagulated or liquid blood

During life, the pliability of the muscles depends on the union between the muscle protein, actin and myosin, and adenotriphosphate (ATP). ATP stores and releases energy for use in cellular processes. Dephosphorylation of ATP by the action of ATPase produces adenodiphosphate (ADP) and phosphate, and the ATP is replaced by resynthesis. After death, oxygen is no longer available to the cells, as a result ATP is depleted and there is no resynthesis of ATP. When the ATP is reduced to critical position, actin and myosin filaments combine as rigid link of actomyosin, which is viscous and inextensible producing rigidity of muscles. During life, glycogen stored in the muscles and liver is broken down to produce ATP, energy, and pyruvic acid. In the absence of oxygen, the pyruvic acid is reduced to lactic acid.

Therefore, there is rise in lactic acid and fall in hydrogen ion concentration due to glycolysis. After cellular death, the lactic acid content of muscle becomes very high. Thus rigor mortis marks the end of muscle cell life.

The time of onset of rigor mortis is variable depending on the local temperature and humidity. The rigor mortis is also affected by age, nature of death, muscular state, etc. It is likely to be apparent within 1–2 hours after death and takes 1–2 hours to develop. In temperate countries, the onset is within 3–6 hours and takes further 2–3 hours to develop. In India, usually it lasts 24–48 hours in winter and 18–36 hours in summer. It lasts for 2–3 days in temperate region. When rigor sets in early, it passes off quickly. In rigor, stiffness of the muscle mass is stronger than in normal muscle contraction. This is because in rigor all the muscle fibers contract and contraction is stronger than the normal muscle. The acid present in rigor inhibits bacterial activity thus preventing decomposition.

Rigor mortis appears first in eye then progresses to the face, lower jaw, upper limbs, trunk, and lower limbs affecting lastly the legs and feet. It passes off from the body in the same order as it appears, i.e. firstly from the face and lastly from the legs and feet. Refrigeration or cold may delay the onset. Heat will hasten the onset.

Rigor mortis is required to be differentiated from heat stiffening (muscles are shortened causing flexion of the joints), cold stiffening (in cold body fats solidify, giving the tissues rigor like firmness), cadaveric spasm (as in violent death—the position of the body remains as it is at the time of death and the rigor may not affect all the muscles of the body), gas stiffening, etc.

Secondary Flaccidity

When the rigor passes off in the unembalmed body, the muscles become soft and flaccid. Autolysis occurs and muscle protein starts breaking down and shows evidence of decomposition. The reaction of the muscle becomes alkaline.

Late Changes

Putrefaction

The putrefaction commences immediately after death at the cellular level, which is not evident to the naked eye. It is defined as decomposition of proteins. It is an anaerobic process brought about by the action of enzymes and results in the formation of foul smelling products. The proteolytic enzymes produced by bacteria break down complex proteins. The changes are brought by microorganisms and fungi such as *Penicillium, Aspergillus, Streptococci, Staphylococci, Balantidium proteus, Balantidium coli, Balantidium aerogenes capsulatus*, etc. These bacteria produce enzymes causing break down of body tissues. Lecithinase produced by *C. welchii* most important as it hydrolyses the lecithin, which is present in all cells including blood cells and is responsible for the postmortem hemolysis of blood. Putrefaction may appear after disappearance of rigor mortis but during summer, it may commence prior to the disappearance of rigor.

Autolysis

The process of self-digestion or self-destruction of the body cells and tissues by enzymes produced within the cells when living is called autolysis. In dead human body, the enzymes of decomposition have two sources—(1) saprophytic bacteria and (2) lysosomes. The saprophytic bacteria are normal inhabitants of the gastrointestinal tract. After death, they translocate and increase in number. They thrive on dead organic material. During life, lysosome, a cell organelle contains the digestive enzymes of a cell. As the pH changes from alkaline to acidic, the membrane surrounding the lysosome ruptures or is destroyed and their enzymes are released, which digest the surrounding cellular material, thus autolysis occurs. In this process, the proteins break down into peptones and amino acids, which reverse the pH to alkaline and stop the enzyme activity. Alkaline nature of the embalming fluid further weakens the action of the enzymes. The proteolytic, glycolytic, and lipolytic action of enzymes causing autodigestion and disintegration of various organs without bacterial effect is seen in parenchymatous and glandular tissues and brain. Autolytic fermentation results in maceration of dead fetus in uterus. Autodigestion of gastric mucosa by gastric juice may be seen resulting in softening and rupture of the stomach.

Putrefactive Changes

Putrefaction occurs at different rates in various body tissues and depends upon their moisture content. Three main changes are noticed during putrefaction:
1. Changes in color
2. Liberation of gases
3. Liquefaction of tissues.

Color changes: The color change is due to hemolysis of red blood cells. The liberated hemoglobin of blood is converted into sulfmethemoglobin by the combination of hydrogen sulfide formed in large intestine. The color change appears in 6–12 hours in summer and in a period of 1–2 days in winter. The pigment stains the tissue greenish. In unembalmed body, the first greenish discoloration appears over the right lower quadrant of the abdomen, i.e. the area of the cecum. Slowly the discoloration spreads to the entire trunk, genitalia, chest, neck, face, arms and legs, and then these patches become green, later coalesce and the whole skin of the body is discolored. The blood present in the superficial veins gradually breaks down and stains the surrounding tissues. The outline of the veins on the surface of the skin can be easily marked. The superficial veins especially over the shoulder, upper chest, neck, groin, and lower abdomen are stained greenish brown or purplish red due to hemolysis of red blood cells, which stain the wall of vessels and infiltrate into the tissues giving a "marbled" appearance. This occurs early but is more prominent in 36–48 hours. The early discoloration that occurs due to hemolysis of red blood cells is the "postmortem stain". This staining of the tissues is extravascular and cannot be removed by arterial injection and blood drainage.

Liberation of foul-smelling gases: As decomposition progresses, gases are formed in the viscera, firstly in the stomach and intestine and later in the body tissues. This is due to reduction of the complicated proteins and carbohydrates, which split into simple compounds like amino acid, ammonia, carbon dioxide, hydrogen sulfide, methane, and mercaptans. The gases have characteristic smell of their own; hydrogen sulfide smells like a rotten egg; hydrogen phosphate like garlic and ammonia smells urinous. Gases collected in the gastrointestinal tract in 6–12 hours in summer and the abdomen becomes tense and distended. On opening the abdomen, at times gases may escape with explosive noise. As a result of the pressure from the gas, the contents of the stomach and the lungs are compressed and forced through the oral and nasal cavities. Such an evacuation is called "purge". The purge material from stomach is a foul-smelling liquid and contains acid and is described as coffee ground in color. Purge from the lungs is generally frothy. The gases are noninflammable in the early stages, but later on, there is enough collection of hydrogen sulfide, which can be ignited to burn with a blue flame.

The eyeballs become soft and yielding. Cornea becomes white, flattened, and later it collapses, 18–36 hours after death, the gases collect in body tissues and cavities causing considerable pressure and the features become bloated. The subcutaneous tissues become emphysematous giving an appearance of corpulence to a thin body. Certain areas such as breast, scrotum, and eyelids easily distend with gases. Eyeballs bulge out of sockets, tongue is forced out between the swollen lips, the sphincters relax and urine and feces may escape. Gases may accumulate in tissues, giving crepitant sponge like feeling on touch and spread to inflate the body. The gas formation in the blood vessels may force fluid, air, and liquid fat between epidermis and dermis developing small blisters. Blisters contain blood-stained fluid. These gradually enlarge, coalesce, and rupture causing large area to be denuded of the cuticle. The break down of vessel wall and cell membranes lead to water logging of tissues, which further facilitates to the spread of bacteria. The anus and uterus may prolapse in 48–72 hours. Postmortem delivery of a fetus has been known to take place.

Hypostasis stain may get displaced in any direction after 3 days. The face is so discolored and bloated that identification becomes very difficult.

Hair become loose and are easily pulled out in 48–72 hours, the nails are also loose. In 3–5 days or more, the sutures of skull especially in children are separated and brain gets liquefied. The skin of the hand and feet shows slippage and may come out in the glove in stocking fashion.

Luminescence of dead body may occur due to contamination of bacteria like photobacterium fischeri, luminescent fungi, armillaria mellea, etc.

Small military plaque consisting of calcium fat endothelial cells and bacteria, which may be mistaken for inflammatory lesion 1–3-mm size are seen on endothelial surface of pleura, peritoneum, pericardium, and endocardium in advanced stage of decomposition. Colliquative putrefaction begins after 5–10 days of death and skeletonization may occur depending upon circumstances of the dead body.

Internal Phenomenon

The order of decomposition of the various organs and tissues of the body varies depending upon their moisture

content. The organs containing muscular and fiber tissue resist putrefaction longer than the parenchymatous organs with the exception of intestine and stomach, which may get decomposed rapidly. The order of tissue decomposition is given below:
- Soft tissue
- Firm tissue
- Hard tissue.

The blood-rich organs and organs close to source of bacterial infection putrefy rapidly. Vascular system is one of the last systems to decompose. The common sequence of decomposition changes is as follows:
- Larynx and trachea—infant brain—stomach—small intestine
- Large intestine—spleen—mesentery and omentum—liver
- Adult brain—heart—lungs—kidneys—urinary bladder—esophagus
- Pancreas—diaphragm—veins—arteries—prostate nonpregnant uterus.

Factors Affecting the Rate of Putrefaction

External factors: Temperature—putrefaction commences at 10°C and is optimum between 21°C and 38°C. It is arrested below 0°C and above 48°C. Other factors are moisture, air, clothing, etc.

Internal factors: Age, sex, condition of the body, cause of death, and mutilation.

Putrefaction in Water

It is rapid in warm water and slow in cold and salted water. In buried bodies, it is slower than in bodies exposed to air and water due to the anaerobic conditions. If buried immediately after death, the rate of putrefaction is slow; if buried after putrefaction has set in, it is rapid. As a general rule, body decomposes in air twice as rapidly as in water and eight times as rapidly as in earth. Putrefaction is slow in old and aged bodies due to more fibrosis and less of moisture content. It is rapid in women and obese persons because of more fat and moisture.

Modified Putrefaction

Adipocere (saponification/grave wax): It is soft, whitish, greasy material consisting mainly of fatty acids formed by the hydrolysis and hydrogenation of body fats. Ultimately, fat is converted into palmitic, stearic, and hydroxystearic acid and mixture of these substances forms adipocere. It first begins in the subcutaneous fat in the buttock, breast, cheek, lower abdomen, and thigh. The presence of moisture is necessary for the formation of adipocere. Warmth enhances the formation of adipocere. Once the adipocere starts to form putrefaction is retarded because of the acid formed, which inhibits the bacterial activity. Its medicolegal importance is that the surface features are preserved and body can be identified years after burial. Adipocere formation starts within days of death and take 3-6 months to become visible. Time required for adipocere formation in India observed is within 3 days. In temperate climate, it is about 3 weeks.

Mummification: It is the complete dehydration, desiccation, and shriveling of the dead body due to evaporation of moisture. Mummification begins in the exposed parts such as hands, feet, and the face and then extends toward the trunk. It resists decomposition due to lack of moisture. This occurs in hot and dry atmosphere. Embalmed body can become mummified by the simple process of dehydration, if left uncared.

DISPOSAL OF THE DEAD

The methods of the disposal of the dead vary with the religion and social and economic status of the deceased. Most of the bodies are disposed off unpreserved. The most commonly practiced method of disposal in India is either burial or cremation. The body is wrapped in cloth and buried in the soil in a particular community. In the large cities, incineration is done in the welt designed electricity operated crematorium. The cremator maintains a high degree of temperature around 600–700°C for total combustion of the body. It takes about 1–2 hours to fully consume an average adult body. In towns and villages, the incineration is done in an open place by burning the body. The energy for heating is obtained from burning the dry wood.

In India embalming is not necessary for burial or cremation. People prefer the traditional way of quick method of disposal of the dead within the shortest possible time after doing the last rites. Preservation is required only when the body has to be transported or when the preservation is desired pending the arrival of the next of kin. Embalming is done solely by anatomy departments of the medical schools in India. Medical schools are located only in big cities.

With the improvement in educational standard and change in the social pattern, people are becoming more and more aware about the science of embalming and possibility of preserving the cadaver for variable length of times after death.

Chapter 4

Mummification

ML Ajmani

HISTORICAL BACKGROUND

It is a riddle as old as the pyramids—how, exactly, did the ancient Egyptians mummify the bodies of their rulers to preserve them for thousands of years? Perhaps it is the mystery, if the remains of a person who lived perhaps 3,000 years ago and is still recognizable as a person. In some sense, he did achieve his goal of immortality. Mummification developed slowly over several thousand years, from naturally preserved bodies in Egypt and deserts to—advanced mummification that reached a peak in Egypt's New Kingdom period (1559-1070 BC). The ancient Egyptians did this entire procedure because they believed in resurrection that the body would reanimate in the next world, so it had to be preserved. Mummification, which is so closely identified with ancient Egypt, is often taken as evidence that the Egyptians were preoccupied with death. The truth is quite the opposite. The Egyptians loved life so much that they developed to elaborate embalming rituals and techniques in order to prolong it. The goal of mummification was not to preserve a dead body, but to prepare it for an eternal life.

My fellows asked, why do you want to do the same, which has already been done 3,000 years ago? Something is happening to man that has not happened in the past 3,000 years, I replied. Egyptians were one of the first to study anatomy, medicine, mummification, and embalming. Replicating mummification will increase understanding of anatomical preservation and provide remarkable record of that civilization in advancing man's knowledge of anatomy and surgery. It is believed that a learning by doing process will increase knowledge about an ancient past. It is worth doing because its history, "said Amy Wray, producer of the mummy show". Like any historical research, the more we understand the better. Moreover, ancient Egyptians did not leave detailed description on how to perform mummification. Most information came from the recorded observations of Herodotus, the Greek historian who travelled to Egypt, and from scattered hieroglyphics and artifacts found in ancient tombs. Much has also been learned in recent years by using modem advances, such as X-rays and computerized tomography (CAT) scan, to study ancient mummies.

Still some practical matters remain a mystery. For example, no one has known precisely that how the Egyptians remove brain? It was also not certain whether they used natron in a liquid or powdered form. In the absence of historical records and artifacts, the best way to answer some of these questions may be through hands-on approach. As a major research, institution dedicated to developing new knowledge, we also have a commitment to verifying the old. This represents a unique opportunity to provide information about an ancient process lost to mankind.

For perhaps, the first time in modern times, a faithful recreation of the mummification techniques, the Egyptians used centuries ago, is being attempted.

WHAT IS MUMMIFICATION?

Mummification is the complete dehydration of a body so as to form a dry, brown, and hard structure, which is light in weight and resistant to decomposition.

Mummification occurs naturally when the air and/or soil are extremely dry and the temperature consistently above (120° or more) or below (32°F or less) the point where bacterial activity cannot take place. In other words, atmospheric conditions must be consistently hot and dry or cold and dry.

Mummification begins in the exposed portions such as the hands, the feet, and the face, which become sunken, shriveled, dry brown, and hard. The entire body loses weight and becomes stiff and brittle. If adequately protected, it will be preserved for years or even for centuries.

Mummification results in permanent preservation because me of the basic necessities for bacterial growth, water has been eliminated from the body. The change occurs naturally in hot desert areas and in some cold mountainous regions. It is difficult in high-humidity regions. In cases of newly born children, mummification may occur if the body is wrapped in absorbent clothes or paper and placed in a trunk or cupboard where the air is hot and dry.

Procedure

Question comes how to obtain a body and what type of body is preferred for this process? Best results can be obtained from a young man whose body had not been damaged by long-term disease, who did not die by accident and who had not undergone surgery. As soon as body is received, put him into a freezer. If the body is donated one, it is not mandatory to tell the family of donors exactly how the body will be used. Family members may object, if they know the peculiar way their loved one will be used.

As far as possible, use fresh body for the procedure. Cadaver is weighed, washed, and photographed (face and body) before starting the procedure. Later, drape the body with linen cloth.

Removal of Brain

During the old kingdom period (2613–2181 BC), embalmers left the brain inside the skull. Later, they developed the technique described by Herodotus and remove the brain in small pieces through the nostrils. The brain was one of the few parts of the body, the embalmers threw away. Apparently, they thought, it had no important function and thus did not have to be preserved. The ancient Egyptians believed that a person thought with his heart, not with his brain. In excitement, it is the heart that beats quickly, not the brain.

The most difficult part of the procedure is removal of the brain through the nose. An entry was made through the cribriform plate of the ethmoid via the right or both nostril into the cavity of skull. No great force was needed to breakthrough the bone. An artificial foramen of 1.5 cm in diameter was created. The brain tissue was macerated by slow rotation of rod and the tentorium cerebelli and falx cerebri were torn away to produce a contiguous cavity between both sides and the posterior cranial fossa. The brain was then evacuated through the nostrils in head turned face downwards position of the body. This method was slow. The brain was more easily and quickly aspirated through a wide-bore catheter/cannula and piston type syringe. After complete evacuation, the interior of the skull was irrigated with water, which flushed the macerated tissue rapidly through the nostrils. The cranial vault was swabbed with the palm wine and stuffed in frankincense. The cranium was then repacked with linen strips soaked with resin bitumen. If possible, take X-ray of skull with tool inside the cranium.

Removal of Other Organs

A line was drawn on the left side of the lower abdomen. Later, an incision was given on the line with obsidian or flint knife or scalpel. All the organs were removed except the heart, which the Egyptians believed was the most important. The rest of the organs were cured with salt and put on plates to be stored around the body for use in after life.

- Removal of liver—wash and place in dish with natron
- Removal of intestines (at rectum)—flush intestines to evacuate; place in dish with natron
- Removal of stomach—wash and place in dish with natron
- Removal of spleen, pancreas, etc.—wash and place in dish with natron
- Removal of kidneys—wash, dry, and place in dish with natron
- Cut diaphragm and remove lungs—wash and place in dish with natron.

Body was surrounded by pottery of different shapes and sizes, each piece containing one of the man's organs. The viscera wrapped in linen and soaked in a weak solution of natron (or preserved in 10% formalin solution) were preserved in canopic jars. These jars were made especially for this purpose. These jars were highly ornamental and made of various material, most commonly limestone. The jars were capped with lids in the shape of heads appropriate to the four sons of Horus, the son of Osiris. The four sons were the guardians of entrails. Imset with a human head looked after the liver and gallbladder; happy with a baboon head cased the lungs and heart. Qebehsenuef with falcon head (Hawk head) guarded the large intestines and other viscera; Duamutef with a jackal head—the stomach and small intestines. Embalmers left the heart and kidneys inside the body and preserved the remaining viscera.

After removing the organs, the body cavities were washed and swabbed with palm wine and myrrh. Insert two sticks retractor to keep incision open. Packed the body cavities with packets of natron (natron salt wrapped in linen) and frankincense and myrrh to dehydrate the body from inside.

Also cavities were packed with linen soaked in resin, so that the body would retain its original shape.

The incision through which the viscera were removed drawn dose and stitched with thread or plate or struck together with resin or wax (we can use metal wire for stitching or a metal dips). The incision was engraved "Eye of Osiris", this being so named after the Egyptian god of death, Osiris. The face was padded with linen in the cheeks and under the eyelids.

Now body is placed on a wooden board or mummifier table. The whole body except the feet was covered by a mound of mixture of salt and baking soda compound, i.e. artificially prepared natron salt. Following composition has been mentioned in Table 4.1 and used for preparing the artificial natron salt.

Natron (Table 4.1)

Dimensions

- 26 cm long × 148 cm width, boards 3 cm thick
- Four battens 6½ × 4 cm in section.

It was tried to make the same composition as was in ancient Egyptian riverbed, Wadi el Natron. The man's feet were covered with surgical shoe cover filled with mixture of natron. The whole body was covered with natron in such a way that his ankles emerge out of the mound. The caustic action of natron would cause the nails of the fingers and toes to loosen and come off. Each nail was tied on by a thread or wire, so that it would remain intact during the preliminary cleaning and dehydration of the body. For the 45 days, the body was covered and surrounded by 600 pounds of powdered natron, an artificially prepared salt for drying the body to turn the man into a mummy. Any change in skin color of the ankle indicates that the drying process is working. At the end of 45 days prescribed by the ancient Egyptian, body is inspected for the process of mummification. Once the drying process is completed, the natron was swept and shoveled away revealing a cadaver that was leathery brown and almost skeletally thin—both the results of the moisture having been drawn from the body. He also emitted an unpleasant acrid smell that forced us to wear surgical masks. Body contains approximately 75% water and is a fairly large object. Therefore, the process of dehydration took a long time. Herodotus and other Greek workers have mentioned 70 days time for dehydration. The Bible mentions 40 days, when Joseph and the physicians embalmed his father, Israel, it took 40 days to complete and there was a 70 days mourning period (genesis 50:2-3).

After 45 days, the body is cleaned and wrapped head to foot in 500 linen strips that have been smeared with resin that the ancient Egyptians used in place of glue. The layers of lenin were fastened together with gum or glue and fitted to the body, still damp and pliable. First each finger and toe was individually wrapped. Each nail was tied on by a tiny thread or wire, if it has become loosen during the preliminary cleaning and dehydration process.

The head was done next, bound very tightly to show the contours of the face.

The number of linen strips was prescribed; four on the forehead, two on top of the head, two around the mouth, four on the neck, until there were 22 pieces on each side of the face.

Arms and legs were bandaged next. Hand was wrapped in linen folded six times. Similarly, trunk was bandaged with number of linen bandages.

After the mummy is wrapped, it is unknown exactly what will become of the mummy. After completing the process, there should be checks on the mummy every 6 months to a year to see how the preservation has worked. I plan to keep it for at least 2 years to see—if the preservation technique worked. Later I will store it in a sarcophages for public viewing. Although I am confident that experiment will succeed, yet I am worried that if we wrap this up and 1 or 2 years from now there is decay, we will know that we missed something and there was something else key to the process. Presumably, Egyptians may have taken some of their secrets with them. The Egyptians were involved in magic. There were secret things that were never written

Table 4.1: Mummifier's table.		
Sodium carbonate	36.9%	84.7%
Sodium bicarbonate	8.3%	
Sodium chloride	9.9%	1.5%
Sodium sulfate	33.9%	13.8%
Matter insoluble in water (largely quartz sand)	5.4%	100%
Water, free and combined (by difference)	5.6% 100.0	—

down if this does not work, we may never know how they really did it.

BIBLIOGRAPHY

1. Breasted James Henry. The Edwin Smith Surgical Papyrus. Chicago: University of Chicago Press; 1930. p. 12.
2. Bob B. Ancient Egyptian Magic. Mummification. New York City: William Morrow Paperbacks; 1972. pp. 67-95.
3. Budge EA. Wallis. The Mummy. New York: Cause way Books; 1974. p. 195.
4. Dawson WR. "Making a Mummy". J Egypt Arch. 1927;13:40-7.
5. Derry DE. "Mummification" II-Methods Practiced at Different Periods". Ann Du Sent. Antiq Eg. 1942;41:244-5.
6. Gray PK. "Embalmers' Restorations". J Egypt Arch. 1969;58:138-40.
7. Herodotus of Halicamassus. The Histories. New York: Penguin; 1972.
8. Leek FF. The Problem of Brain Removal During Embalming by the Ancient Egyptians. J Egypt Arch. 1966;52:112-6.
9. Lucas A. Ancient Egyptian Materials and Industries. London: Edward Arnold; 1945. p. 320.
10. Lucas A. "The use of Natron in Mummification". J Egypt Arch. 1932;18:125-40.
11. Moodie RL. "Roentgenologic studies of Egyptian and Peruvian Mummies". Chicago: Field Museum of Natural History; 1931. p. 23 and Plate XIV.
12. Paabo S. "Molecular Cloning of Ancient Egyptian Mummy DNA". Nature. 1985;314:644-6.
13. Peet TE. The great Tomb Robberies of the Twentieth Egyptian Dynasty. Hildesheim: George Olms; 1977. pp. 48-9.
14. Ruffer A. "Notes on Two Egyptian Mummies dating from the Persian occupation of Egypt" in studies in the Paleopathology of Egypt. Chicago: University Chicago Press; 1921. pp. 127-38.
15. Smith GE, Warren RD. Egyptian Mummies. London: George Allen and Unwin; 1924. p. 61.
16. Smith GE, Warren RD. Egyptian Mummies. London: Kegan Paul; 1991. p. 145.
17. Strub CG, Frederick LG. The Principles and practice of Embalming, 4th edition. 27- Australia: National Library of Australia; 1967. p. 29.
18. Thompson DL. The Artists of the Mummy Portraits. Malibu: J Paul Getty Museum; 1976. p. 12.
19. Winlock HE. "The Materials used at the Embalming of King Tut-Ankh-Amun". New York: The Metropolitan Museum of Art; 1941. pp. 5-18 Plate 1-X.
20. Zaki A, Zaky I. "Materials and Method used for Mummifying the body of Amentefneksht, Saqqara, 1941". Annal du service Antiq Egypt. 1941;42:223-55.

Chapter 5

Anatomical Considerations

ML Ajmani

HEART

Heart is a muscular pump. It is somewhat larger than the closed fist of the individual. It has four chambers—the right and left atria and the right and left ventricles. The atria are separated from the ventricles by a groove that completely encircles the heart and is called the coronary or atrioventricular sulcus. The ventricles are separated from each other by the anterior and posterior interventricular sulci. The notched anterosuperior part of each atrium resembles a dog's ear and is called the auricle. Atrial chambers are separated from each other by interatrial septum. Similarly, the ventricular chambers are separated by the interventricular septum (Fig. 5.1).

The heart has three surfaces—(1) sternocostal (anterior), (2) diaphragmatic (inferior), and (3) left surface; it also has an apex and a base. The sternocostal surface is formed mainly by the right atrium and right ventricle, and partly by the left ventricle and left auricle. The diaphragmatic surface is formed in the left two-thirds by the left ventricle, and right one-third by the right ventricle. The left surface is formed mostly by the left ventricle and at the upper end by the left auricle. Apex is the lowest and left most point formed by the left ventricle. It is situated in the left fifth intercostal space 9 cm lateral to the midsternal line, just inner to the midclavicular line.

Heart is the most important organ of the blood vascular system. The left side of the heart controls the systemic circulation that one is to say arterial blood, while the right controls the venous blood. The systemic circulation starts from the left ventricle of the heart. Oxygenated blood is pumped from the ventricle into the aorta, which is an arched structure, arising from the left ventricle. It gives out several branches, which feed every part of the body. Deoxygenated blood is conveyed back to the right atrium of the heart via the superior vena cava, inferior vena cava, and coronary sinus.

The pulmonary circulation commences at the right ventricle. Deoxygenated blood is propelled into the pulmonary trunk, pulmonary arteries, and finally to the lung tissue where an interchange of gases takes place in the lung alveoli. The blood at this stage is oxygenated. It is then conveyed to the left atrium by the four pulmonary veins.

The portal circulation is a filtration process for the blood coming from the stomach, small and large intestines, spleen, etc. Venous blood is collected from these organs by the tributaries of the portal vein, which convey it to the liver. In the liver, the nutrients contained in the portal blood are deposited in the substance of the liver. Blood is retrieved from the liver by small veins terminating in the hepatic veins, which convey it to the inferior vena cava.

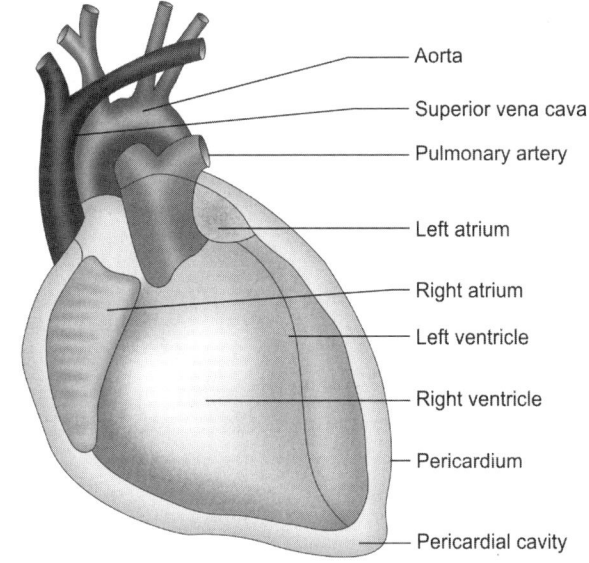

Fig. 5.1: Heart.

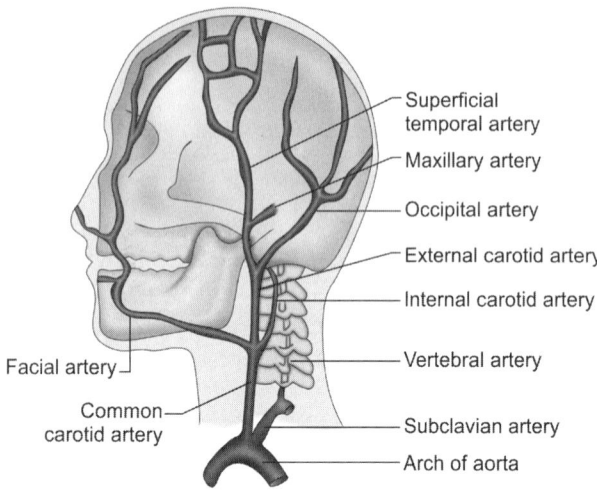

Fig. 5.2: Arteries of the head and neck.

parotid glands behind the neck of the mandible by dividing into superficial temporal and maxillary artery.

The artery is overlapped at its commencement by the medial border of the sternocleidomastoid muscle. The internal jugular vein first lies lateral to the artery and then posterior to it.

Branches

- Superior thyroid artery
- Ascending pharyngeal artery
- Lingual artery
- Facial artery
- Occipital artery
- Posterior auricular artery
- Superficial temporal artery
- Maxillary artery.

ARTERIES OF THE HEAD AND NECK (FIG. 5.2)

Arteries of Neck

Common Carotid Artery

The right and left common carotid arteries are the principal arteries of this region. They differ in origin, the right arising from the brachiocephalic artery, while the left arises directly from the arch of the aorta. The right common carotid begins at the level of the right sternoclavicular joint and extends to the superior border of the thyroid cartilage. The left common carotid begins at the level of the second costal cartilage and extends to the superior border of the thyroid cartilage. There are no branches of the common carotid, except the terminal bifurcation into the external and internal carotid arteries at the upper border of the thyroid cartilage.

The common carotid artery is embedded in the carotid sheath throughout its course and is closely related to the internal jugular vein and vagus nerve. The common carotid arteries are located posterior to the medial border of the sternocleidomastoid muscle. The internal jugular vein is lateral to the artery within the carotid sheath.

External Carotid Artery

It is one of the terminal branches of the common carotid artery. It begins at the level of the superior border of the thyroid cartilage and terminates in the substance of the

Internal Carotid Artery

It begins at the level of the upper border of the thyroid cartilage and ascends in the neck to the base of the skull. It enters the cranial cavity through the carotid canal. The internal jugular vein lies lateral to the artery within the carotid sheath. The artery does not give off any branch in the neck.

Branches of the intracranial portion of the internal carotid artery:

- Ophthalmic artery
- Anterior cerebral artery
- Middle cerebral artery
- Choroidal artery
- Posterior communicating artery.

The ophthalmic artery supplies the eye. Remaining branches of the internal carotid artery join with the posterior cerebral artery, a branch of the vertebral artery, and form the arterial anastomosis known as the circle of Willis, which gives off branches to the brain tissues (Fig. 5.3).

Subclavian Artery

The right subclavian artery arises from the brachiocephalic artery, behind the right sternoclavicular joint. The left subclavian artery arises from the arch of the aorta, behind the left common carotid artery. These arteries pass upwards and laterally at the root of the neck and become continuous with the axillary artery at the outer border of the first rib. The subclavian artery is divided into three parts by the presence of the scalenus anterior muscle.

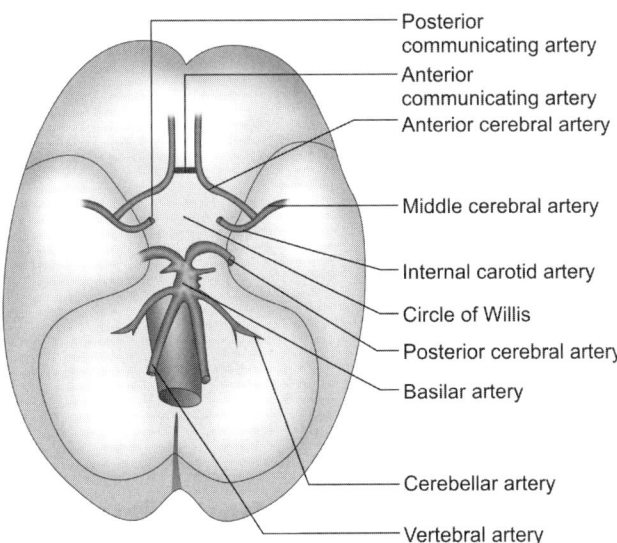

Fig. 5.3: Circle of Willis.

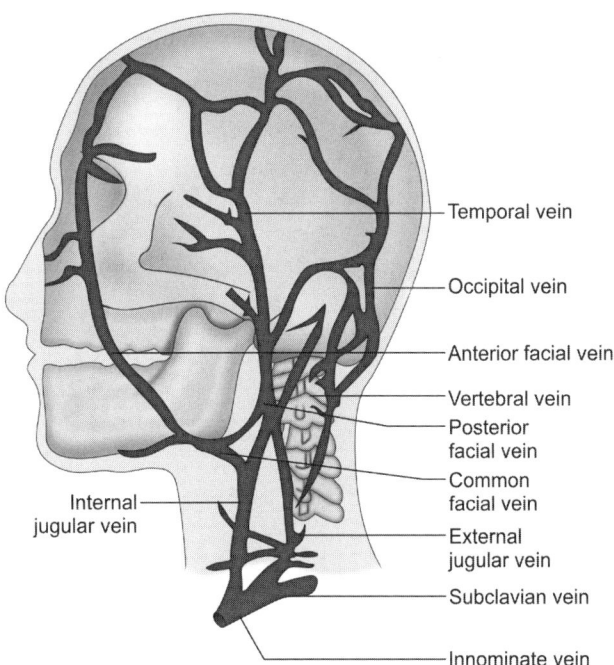

Fig. 5.4: Veins of the head and neck.

The branches of the first part of the subclavian artery are as follows:

Vertebral artery: It ascends in the neck and passes through the foramina of the transverse processes of the upper six cervical vertebra. It ascends into the skull through the foramen magnum and joins the opposite artery at the lower border of the pons to form the basilar artery. This artery ascends to the upper border of the pons and then subdivides to form the two posterior cerebral arteries.

Thyrocervical trunk: It gives off three branches:
1. Inferior thyroid artery
2. Superficial cervical artery
3. Suprascapular artery.

Internal mammary artery: The branches of the second part of the subclavian artery are as follows:
- *Costocervical trunk*: It gives off two branches:
  1. Superior intercostal artery
  2. Deep cervical artery.

VEINS OF THE NECK (FIG. 5.4)

Superficial Veins

These veins lie superficial to the deep fascia of the neck.

External Jugular Vein

It begins just behind the angle of mandible by the union of the posterior auricular vein with the posterior division of the retromandibular vein. It descends obliquely across the sternocleidomastoid muscle and enters the posterior triangle and drains into the subclavian vein.

Anterior Jugular Vein

It begins just below the chin, by the union of several small veins. It descends close to the midline of the neck and just above the suprasternal notch, the veins of the two sides are united by a transverse trunk, called the jugular arch. The vein then runs laterally and passes deep to the sternocleidomastoid muscle to drain into the external jugular vein.

Deep Veins

These veins lie deep to the deep fascia of the neck. They are as follows.

Internal Jugular Vein

The internal jugular vein receives the blood from the brain, the face, and the neck. It begins at the jugular foramen in the skull as a continuation of the sigmoid sinus. It descends through the neck in the carotid sheath and joins the subclavian vein behind the medial end of the clavicle to form the brachiocephalic vein. The internal jugular vein has two dilatations, one at its upper end called the superior bulb, and another near its termination, called the inferior bulb (Fig. 5.4).

The internal jugular vein follows a parallel course to the internal and common carotid arteries in the neck and is embedded in the carotid sheath. The arteries lie medial to the vein.

Tributaries
- Inferior petrosal sinus
- Facial vein
- Pharyngeal vein
- Lingual vein
- Superior thyroid vein
- Middle thyroid vein.

Subclavian Vein

It begins at the outer border of the first rib as continuation of the axillary vein. At the medial border of the scalenus anterior, it joins the internal jugular vein to form the brachiocephalic vein. At its angle of junction with the internal jugular vein, the left subclavian vein receives the thoracic duct and the right subclavian vein receives the right lymphatic duct.

It is related anteriorly to the clavicle, behind and above with the subclavian artery, separated from it by scalenus anterior muscle. Below, it rests on the upper surface of the first rib.

ARTERIES OF THE UPPER LIMBS (FIGS. 5.5A AND B)

Axillary Artery

It begins at the outer border of the first rib as a continuation of the subclavian artery and ends at the lower border of the teres major muscle where it continues as the brachial artery. Throughout its course, the artery is closely related to the cords of the brachial plexus and is enclosed with them in a common fascial sheath, called the axillary sheath. The pectoralis minor muscle crosses in front of axillary artery and divides it into three parts:
1. First part extends from the outer border of the first rib to the upper border of the pectoralis minor. Axillary vein lies medial to it. It gives off a branch, known as superior thoracic artery.

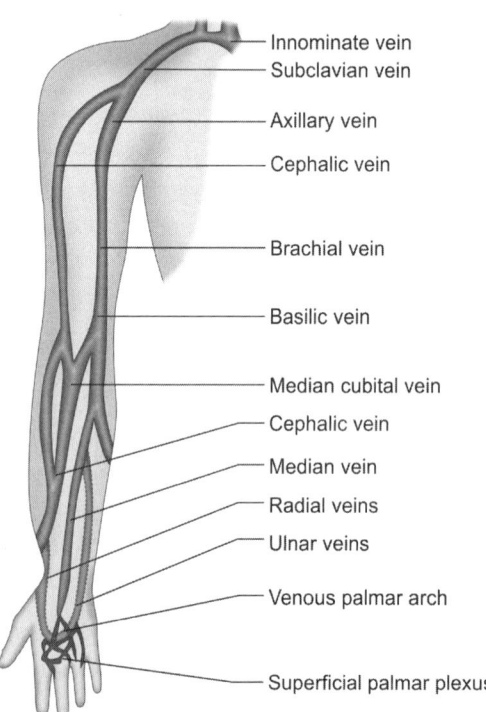
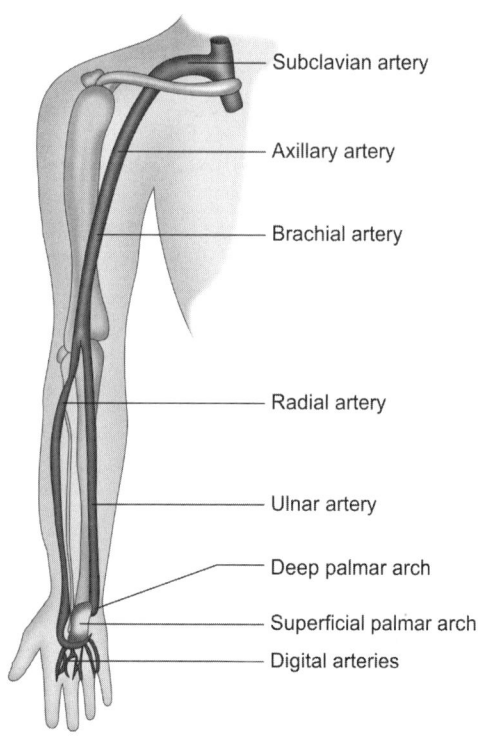

Figs. 5.5A and B: Arteries and veins of the upper limb.

2. Second part lies behind the pectoralis minor. Axillary vein lies medial to it. This part of artery gives off two branches—(1) lateral thoracic and (2) thoracoacromial.
3. Third part extends from the lower border of the pectoralis minor to the lower border of the teres major muscle. Axillary vein lies medial to it. It gives off three branches—(1) subscapular artery, (2) anterior circumflex humeral artery, and (3) posterior circumflex humeral artery.

The axillary artery supplies tissues of the anterior thoracic wall, lateral thoracic wall, back, shoulder region, axilla, and upper arm.

Brachial Artery

It begins at the lower border of the teres major muscle as a continuation of the axillary artery. It terminates opposite the neck of the radius by dividing into the radial and ulnar arteries. The vessel is superficial and overlapped by coracobrachialis and biceps muscles in its upper part and bicipital aponeurosis in its lower part. In its upper course, the basilic vein is related to it medially.

Ulnar Artery

It is one of the terminal branches of the brachial artery, arises in the cubital fossa at the level of the neck of the radius. It passes downward and medial, deep to the superficial flexor muscles of the forearm. At the wrist, it is quite superficial lies with the ulnar nerve between the tendon of the flexor carpi ulnaris muscle and the tendons of the flexor digitorum superficialis muscle.

The ulnar artery enters the palm after crossing the flexor retinaculum and lies lateral to the pisiform bone. It terminates by joining the superficial palmer branch of the radial artery to form the superficial palmer arch.

It supplies the muscles, bones, and nerves of the forearm.

Radial Artery

It is also one of the terminal branches of the brachial artery, arises in the cubital fossa. It passes downwards and laterally and lies on the lateral side of the tendon of the flexor carpi radialis in the lower part of the forearm. At the wrist, it is covered only by skin and fascia and rests on the radius, where its pulsation may be felt in the living.

The radial artery leaves the forearm by winding around the lateral aspect of the wrist to reach the posterior aspect of the hand and continues in the palm as the deep palmer arch. The arch is completed on the medial side by the deep branch of ulnar artery.

VEINS OF THE UPPER LIMB (FIGS. 5.5A AND B)

Superficial Veins

Most of the superficial veins of the limb join together to form two large veins—(1) a cephalic and (2) a basilic.

Cephalic Vein

It begins from the lateral end of the dorsal venous arch, winds round the lateral border of the forearm in its distal part and continues upwards in front of the elbow. In the arm, it ascends along the lateral border of biceps brachii and pierces clavipectoral fascia and joins the axillary vein below the clavicle. At the elbow, greater part of its blood is drained into the basilic vein through the median cubital vein.

Basilic Vein

It begins from the medial end of the dorsal venous arch, runs upward along the back of medial border of the forearm, and continues upwards in front of the elbow and along the median margin of the biceps brachii up to the middle of the arm where it pierces the deep fascia and continues as the axillary vein at the lower border of the teres major muscle.

Deep Veins

The deep veins of the upper limb follow the course of the arteries and are present in pairs forming the venae comitantes. As the majority of the blood is returned by the superficial veins, the deep veins are small.

Axillary Vein

It is formed by the union of venae comitantes of the brachial artery and the basilic vein at the lower border of the teres major muscle. It runs upward on the medial side of the axillary artery and ends at the outer border of the first rib by becoming the subclavian vein.

The vein receives tributaries, which correspond to the branches of the axillary artery, and in addition, it receives the cephalic vein.

ARTERIES OF THE THORAX (FIG. 5.6)

Aorta

The aorta, the main arterial trunk of the systemic circulation, arises from the left ventricle and is divided for

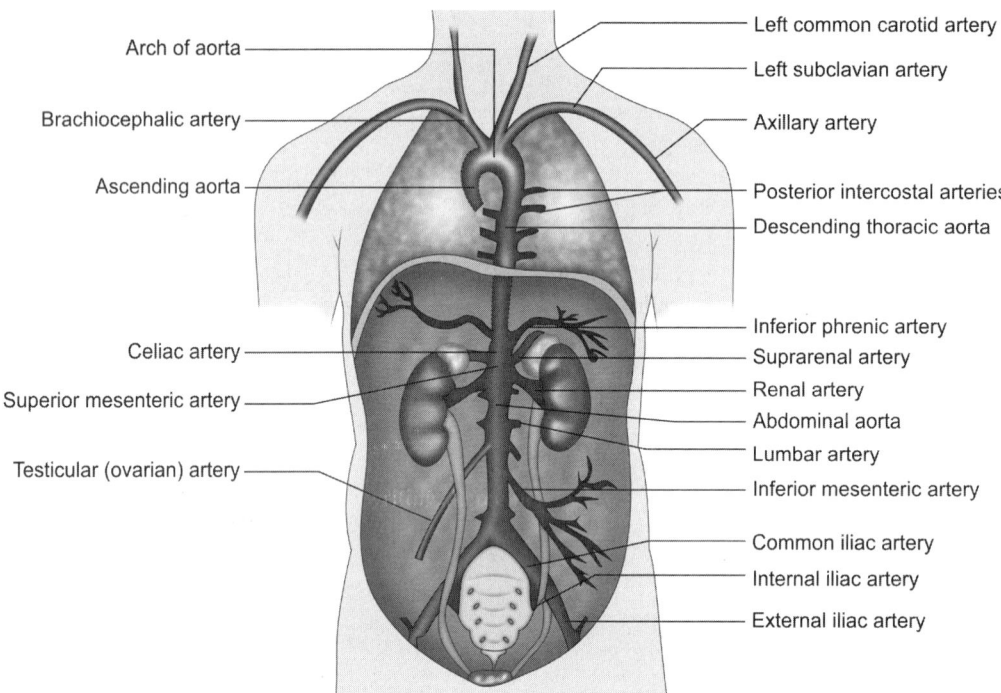

Fig. 5.6: Arteries of the thorax and abdomen.

description into three parts: (1) the ascending aorta, (2) the arch of the aorta, and (3) the descending aorta.

Ascending Aorta

It commences at the base of the left ventricle and runs upward and forward to come to lie behind the right half of the sternal angle, where it becomes continuous with the arch of the aorta.

Branches
- *Right coronary artery*: It arises from the right anterior aortic sinus
- *Left coronary artery*: It arises from the left posterior aortic sinus.

The musculature of heart receives its blood supply from the coronary arteries.

Arch of the Aorta

The arch of the aorta is a continuation of the ascending aorta at the sternal angle. It lies behind the manubrium sterni. It runs upward, backward, and then passes downward to the left of the trachea, and at the level of the sternal angle becomes continuous with the descending aorta.

Branches
- *Brachiocephalic trunk*: It arises from the convex surface of the arch, passes upward to the right of trachea, and divides into the right subclavian and common carotid artery behind the right sternoclavicular joint.
- *Left common carotid artery*: It arises from the aortic arch on the left side of the brachiocephalic trunk. It runs upward on the left of the trachea and enters the neck behind the left sternoclavicular joint.
- *Left subclavian artery*: It arises from the arch behind the left common carotid artery. It ascends upward to enter the root of the neck.

Descending Aorta

The descending aorta begins as a continuation of arch of aorta opposite the sternal angle, on the left side of the body of the fourth thoracic vertebra. It extends downward to the level of the twelfth thoracic vertebra, where it passes through the opening of the diaphragm and becomes continuous with the abdominal aorta.

Branches
- Posterior intercostal arteries are given to the lower nine intercostal spaces on each side.

- Subcostal arteries are given off on each side and run along the lower border of the twelfth rib.
- Pericardial esophageal, bronchial, mediastinal, and superior phrenic arteries are small branches that are distributed to the respective organs.

Pulmonary Trunk

It leaves the upper part of the right ventricle and runs upward and to the left. It is about 5-cm long terminates in the concavity of the arch of the aorta by dividing into right and left pulmonary arteries, which carry deoxygenated blood to the lungs.

Branches

- Right pulmonary artery runs to the right behind the ascending aorta and superior vena cava to enter the root of the right lung.
- Left pulmonary artery runs to the left in front of the descending aorta to enter the root of the left lung.

VEINS OF THE THORAX (FIG. 5.7)

Right Brachiocephalic Vein

It is formed at the root of the neck by the union of the right subclavian and the right internal jugular veins. It is about 2.5 cm long, begins behind the sternal end of the right clavicle and passes vertically downward, and joins the left brachiocephalic vein.

Left Brachiocephalic Vein

It is about 6 cm long and passes obliquely to the right behind the upper half of the manubrium sterni and in front of large branches of the arch of the aorta. Near the sternal end of the first right costal cartilage, it joins the right brachiocephalic vein to form the superior vena cava.

Superior Vena Cava

It is formed by the union of the two brachiocephalic veins and passes downward to end in the right atrium of the heart. It receives all the venous blood from the head and neck and both upper limbs. It is about 7 cm long. It begins behind the lower border of the first right costal cartilage close to the sternum and ends opposite the third right costal cartilage. The vena azygos opens on the posterior aspect of the superior vena cava just before it enters the pericardium.

The tributaries of the vena azygos are—eight right intercostal veins, accessory hemiazygos, hemiazygos, esophageal veins, and mediastinal veins.

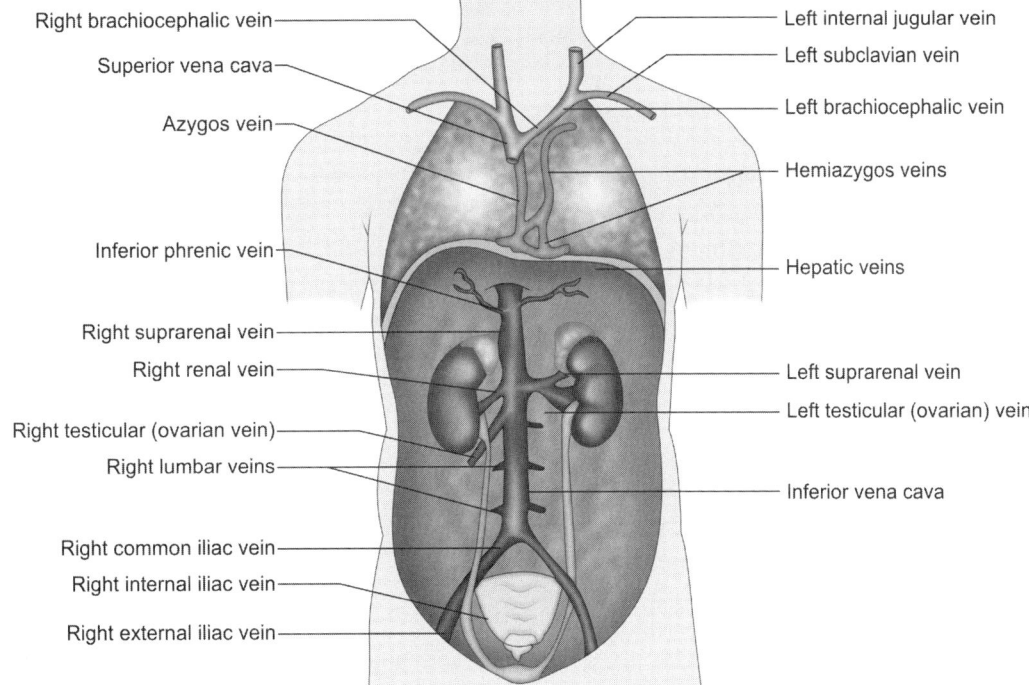

Fig. 5.7: Veins of the thorax and abdomen.

Inferior Vena Cava

It pierces the central tendon of the diaphragm opposite the eighth thoracic vertebra and immediately enters the right atrium.

Pulmonary Veins

There are four pulmonary veins, two from each lung. The pulmonary veins carry oxygenated blood from lungs to the left atrium of the heart.

ARTERIES OF THE ABDOMEN (FIG. 5.6)

Aorta

The descending aorta enters the abdomen through the aortic opening of the diaphragm in front of the twelfth thoracic vertebra. It descends in front of the bodies of the lumbar vertebrae, and divides into terminal common iliac arteries in front of the fourth lumbar vertebra. On its right side, it is related to the inferior vena cava, the cisterna chyli, and the commencement of the azygos vein.

The aorta gives off the following branches.

Anterior Visceral Branches

Celiac trunk: It supplies the structures developing from the foregut, i.e. stomach, liver, gallbladder, pancreas, and a part of the duodenum. It gives off the following branches:
- Left gastric artery
- Splenic artery
- Hepatic artery.

Superior mesenteric artery: It supplies the structures developing from the midgut, i.e. a part of the duodenum, jejunum, ileum, cecum, appendix, ascending colon, right two-thirds of the transverse colon. It gives off the following branches:
- Jejunal and ileal arteries
- Inferior pancreaticoduodenal artery
- Middle colic artery
- Right colic artery
- Ileocolic artery.

Inferior mesenteric artery: It supplies the structures developing from the hindgut, i.e. a part of the transverse colon, descending colon, sigmoid colon, and a part of rectum. It gives off the following branches:
- Superior left colic artery
- Inferior left colic arteries
- Superior rectal artery.

Lateral visceral branches:
- Suprarenal artery
- Renal artery
- Testicular or ovarian artery.
  They are distributed to the organs indicated by their names.

Lateral Abdominal Wall Branches

- Inferior phrenic arteries supply the diaphragm
- Four pairs of lumbar artery—these arteries arise from the abdominal aorta at points opposite the lumbar vertebra. They supply the tissues of the lumbar regions.

Terminal Branches

Median sacral artery: It is considered as a continuation of the abdominal aorta. It arises at the bifurcation of the aorta and takes a vertical course into the pelvis and supplies the tissues surrounding the sacrum and coccyx bones.

Common iliac arteries: The common iliac arteries arise at the bifurcation of the aorta and run downward and laterally along the medial border of the psoas major muscle. Each artery divides into external and internal iliac arteries in front of the sacroiliac joint.

External iliac artery: It runs along the medial border of the psoas major muscle along the pelvic brim. It passes under the inguinal ligament and continues as the moral artery.

Internal iliac artery: It enters the pelvis in front of the sacroiliac joint and at this point, it is crossed anteriorly by the ureter. At the upper border of the greater sciatic foramen, it divides into anterior and posterior divisions, which give off branches that supply the pelvic viscera, perineum, buttock, and sacral canal.

Branches of Anterior Division

- *Umbilical artery*: Its patent part gives off superior vesical artery and artery to vas deferens (in male)
- Obturator artery
- Inferior vesical artery
- Middle rectal artery
- Internal pudendal artery
- Inferior gluteal artery
- Uterine artery (in female)
- Vaginal artery (in female).

Branches of Posterior Division

- Iliolumbar artery
- Lateral sacral artery
- Superior gluteal artery.

VEINS OF THE ABDOMEN (FIG. 5.7)

Inferior Vena Cava

It is formed by the union of the common iliac veins behind the right common iliac artery at the level of fourth lumbar vertebra. It ascends on the right side of the aorta, pierces the central tendon of the diaphragm at the level of the eighth thoracic vertebra, and opens into right atrium of the heart.

The venous blood from the abdominal portion of the gastrointestinal tract is drained to the liver by means of the tributaries of the portal vein. These are:

- *A superior mesenteric vein*: It begins at the ileocecal junction and runs upward on the posterior abdominal wall within the root of the mesentery of the small intestine and on the right side of the superior mesenteric artery. It passes in front of the third part of the duodenum and behind the neck of the pancreas, where it joins the splenic vein to form the portal vein.
- *Splenic vein*: It begins at the hilum of the spleen and is joined by the short gastric and the left gastroepiploic veins. It passes to the right within the lienorenal ligament and runs behind the pancreas below the splenic artery. It joins the superior mesenteric vein behind the neck of the pancreas to form the portal vein.
- *Inferior mesenteric vein*: It begins near the upper part of the anal canal as the superior rectal vein and passes upward on the posterior abdominal wall on the left side of the inferior mesenteric artery. It joins the splenic vein behind the pancreas.
- *Portal veins*: It is about 5 cm long and is formed behind the neck of the pancreas by the union of the superior mesenteric and splenic veins. It runs upward behind the first part of the duodenum and enters the lesser omentum. It then ascends to the porta hepatis, where it divides into right and left terminal branches. It drains blood from gastrointestinal tract, from the lower end of the esophagus to the upper end of the anal canal, from the gallbladder, pancreas, bile duct, and spleen.

Tributaries of the Inferior Vena Cava

Visceral Tributaries

- Hepatic veins—carry the blood from the liver
- Right suprarenal vein
- Renal veins
- Right testicular or ovarian veins.

They drain the organs indicated in their names.

Tributaries from Abdominal Wall

- Inferior phrenic veins drain the tissues of the diaphragm.
- Four lumbar veins drain the tissues of the lumbar region.

Tributaries at Commencement

- Median sacral vein—collects the blood from the tissues surrounding the sacrum and coccyx.
- Two common iliac veins—drain the blood through:
  1. External iliac veins—drain the blood from the lower extremities.
  2. Internal iliac veins—drain the blood from the pelvis, pelvic viscera, and perineum.

ARTERIES OF THE LOWER LIMB (FIGS. 5.8A AND B)

Femoral Artery

The abdominal aorta bifurcates at a point opposite the umbilicus (IA) into the right and left common iliac arteries. Each artery passes downward in a lateral direction and divides into external and internal iliac arteries opposite the disk between fifth lumbar vertebra and sacrum. The external iliac artery descends downwards toward the inguinal ligament, beyond which it is known as femoral artery. Behind the inguinal ligament, it lies midway between the anterior-superior iliac spine and the symphysis pubis. It leaves the femoral triangle at its apex and enters the adductor canal and terminates at the opening in the adductor magnus muscle by entering the popliteal fossa as the popliteal artery. Medially, it is related to the femoral vein in the upper part of its course.

Branches

Superficial

- Superficial circumflex iliac artery
- Superficial epigastric artery
- Superficial external pudendal artery.

Deep

- Deep external pudendal artery
- Profunda femoris artery—it is a large branch that arises from the lateral side of the femoral artery about 4 cm below the inguinal ligament.
- Descending genicular artery.

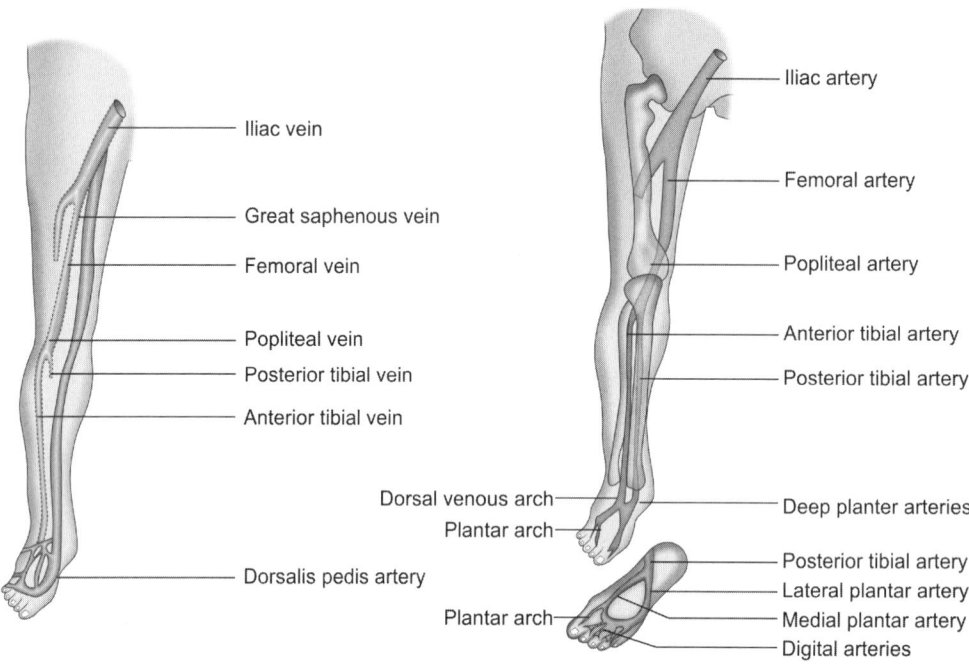

Figs. 5.8A and B: Arteries and veins of the lower limb.

Obturator Artery

It is a branch of the internal mac artery and leaves the pelvis through the upper part of the obturator foramen. On entering the medial side of the thigh, it gives off muscular branches and an articular branch to the hip joint.

Popliteal Artery

It is a continuation of femoral artery in the popliteal fossa. It ends at the level of the lower border of the popliteus muscle by dividing into anterior and posterior tibial arteries. The popliteal vein lies posterior to it.

Branches

- Muscular branches
- Genicular branches to the knee joint.

Anterior Tibial Artery

It is the smaller terminal branch of the popliteal artery. It descends on the anterior surface of the interosseous membrane and supplies the structures in the anterior compartment of the leg. Having p behind the superior extensor retinaculum, it has the tendon of extensor hallucis longus on its medial side and the extensor digitorum longus on its lateral side. It is here that its pulsations can easily be felt in the living. In front of the ankle joint, the artery becomes the dorsalis pedis artery.

Posterior Tibial Artery

It lies on the posterior surface of the tibialis posterior muscle above and on the posterior surface of the tibia below. In the lower part of the leg, the artery lies about 2.5 cm in front of the medial border of the tendocalcaneous and is covered only by skin and fascia. The artery passes behind the medial malleolus deep to the flexor retinaculum and terminates by dividing into medial and lateral planter arteries.

Branches

- Peroneal artery
- Muscular branches to muscles in the posterior compartment of the leg.

VEINS OF THE LOWER LIMB (FIGS. 5.8A AND B)

Superficial Veins

The superficial veins of the leg are the great and small saphenous veins and their tributaries.

Great Saphenous Vein

It is the largest vein in the body. It begins at the medial end of the dorsal venous arch of the foot and passes upward directly in front of the medial malleolus. It ascends in the superficial fascia over the medial side of the leg. It then passes behind the knee and curves forward on the medial side of the thigh. It passes through the lower part of the saphenous opening in the deep fascia and joins the femoral vein about 4 cm below and lateral to the pubic tubercle. The great saphenous vein possesses numerous valves.

Small Saphenous Vein

It arises from the lateral part of the dorsal venous arch of the foot. It ascends behind the lateral malleolus. It follows the lateral border of the tendocalcaneous and then runs up to the middle of the back of the leg. The vein pierces the deep fascia and passes between the two heads of the gastrocnemius muscle terminating in the lower part of the popliteal vein.

Deep Veins

Deep veins of the lower extremity are—the femoral, the popliteal, the venae comitantes of the anterior and posterior tibial arteries, and the profunda femoris vein.

Femoral Vein

It enters the thigh by passing through the opening in the adductor magnus as a continuation of the popliteal vein. It ascends, lying at first on the lateral side of the artery, then posterior to it, and finally on its medial side. It passes behind the inguinal ligament to become the external iliac vein. It ascends to a point opposite the junction of the fifth lumbar vertebra and the sacrum, where it joins the internal iliac vein to form the common iliac vein. The common iliac veins on either side ascend to a point opposite the umbilicus, where they unite to form the inferior vena cava.

Popliteal Vein

It is formed by the union of anterior and posterior tibial veins at the lower border of the popliteus muscle on the medial side of the popliteal artery. It crosses behind the popliteal artery and comes to lie on its lateral side. It passes through the opening in the adductor magnus to become the femoral vein.

CIRCULATION OF BLOOD

Right atrium receives deoxygenated blood from the whole body through the superior and inferior vena cava and coronary sinus of the heart. From right atrium, the blood passes through the tricuspid orifice to the right ventricle. Right ventricle sends the blood into the pulmonary trunk, pulmonary arteries, and finally to the lungs where the blood is oxygenated.

The oxygenated blood is returned to the left atrium through the four pulmonary veins. From the left atrium blood passes through the bicuspid orifice to the left ventricle, which in turn propels it via the ascending aorta to the systemic circulation.

Fetal Circulation

The development of a human begins with fertilization, a process by which the spermatozoon from the male and the oocyte from the female unite to give rise to a new organism, the zygote. From conception to the end of the 3rd month of the pregnancy, it is referred to as an embryo—at the end of the 3rd month of pregnancy to the ultimate birth, the unborn child in the womb is known as the fetus.

During prenatal life, the fetus derives its nutrition from the placenta. There is no pulmonary circulation in the fetus. The arterial blood is conveyed by the umbilical vein from the placenta and venous blood is returned to it by the umbilical arteries. These vessels form part of the umbilical cord, which connects the fetus to the placenta.

On approaching the liver, the main portion of the arterial or oxygenated blood flows through the ductus venosus directly into the inferior vena cava. A small portion enters the liver sinusoids and mixes here with blood from the portal circulation. The inferior vena cava receives blood from three sources:

1. From the umbilical vein directly through the ductus venosus
2. Small amount of the blood returning from portal system via the hepatic veins
3. Deoxygenated blood returning from the lower extremities, pelvis, and kidneys.

During its course from the placenta to the organs of the fetus, the high-oxygen contents of the placental blood gradually decrease by mixing with deoxygenated blood.

From the inferior vena cava, blood enters the right atrium. Here it is guided toward the foramen ovale, and the major amount of the blood passes directly into the left atrium. A small portion remains in the right atrium, which mixes with the deoxygenated blood returning from the head and upper limbs by way of the superior vena cava. In the left atrium, it mixes with a small amount of blood returning from the lungs and then the blood enters the left ventricle and aorta, which carries it to the whole of the tissues of the fetus. The blood is returned to the placenta for oxidation and nourishment by the umbilical arteries.

There are a number of special features present in the fetal blood circulation, which are not apparent in postnatal life, e.g. foramen ovale—a communication between the right and left atria; ductus venosus—a direct link between the umbilical vein and the inferior vena cava; ductus arteriosus—a direct communication between the aorta and the pulmonary artery.

Changes at Birth

During prenatal life, the placental circulation provides oxygen to the fetus, but after birth the lungs become functional and take over the gas exchange. The following changes take place at birth:
- Closure of ductus arteriosus
- Closure of foramen ovale
- Closure of umbilical vein and ductus venosus persisting in adults as ligamentum teres hepatis and ligamentum venosum, respectively
- Closure of umbilical arteries and persistence as medial umbilical ligaments.

It should be noted that there is no direct communication between fetal and maternal blood, which is separated by membranes in the placenta. These membranes prevent the mixing of the fetal blood with the maternal blood.

Chapter 6

Surface Anatomy and Exposure of Blood Vessels

ML Ajmani

INTRODUCTION

This is an important branch of anatomy for an embalmer.

The term surface anatomy means the marking topography of vessels and organs on the surface of the body.

ARTERIES OF THE BODY

Pulmonary Trunk

Draw a line from the sternal end of the third left costal cartilage to second left costal cartilage.

Ascending Aorta

Draw a line from the left margin of the sternum at the level of the third intercostal space to the right half of the sternal angle.

Arch of the Aorta

It lies behind the lower half of the manubrium sterni. It is marked by a line which begins at the right end of the sternal angle, arches upward and to the left and ends at the sternal end of the left second costal cartilage.

Descending Thoracic Aorta

Draw a broad line on the surface of the skin, from a point over the sternal end of the second left costal cartilage, pass downward and medially, to a point in the median plane 2.5 cm above the transpyloric plane or to the lower border of the first lumbar vertebra.

Brachiocephalic Artery

It is marked by a line extending from the center of the manubrium to the right sternocostal articulation.

Common Carotid Artery

The vessel is exposed by an incision on the surface of the skin from a point over the respective sternoclavicular joint to a point on the anterior border of the sternocleidomastoid muscle at the level of the upper border of thyroid cartilage (fourth cervical vertebra) (Fig. 6.1).

Internal Carotid Artery

An incision is given on the anterior border of the sternocleidomastoid muscle at the level of the upper border of thyroid cartilage to a point on the posterior border of the condyle of mandible.

External Carotid Artery

The skin is incised from a point over the anterior border of sternocleidomastoid muscle at the level of the upper

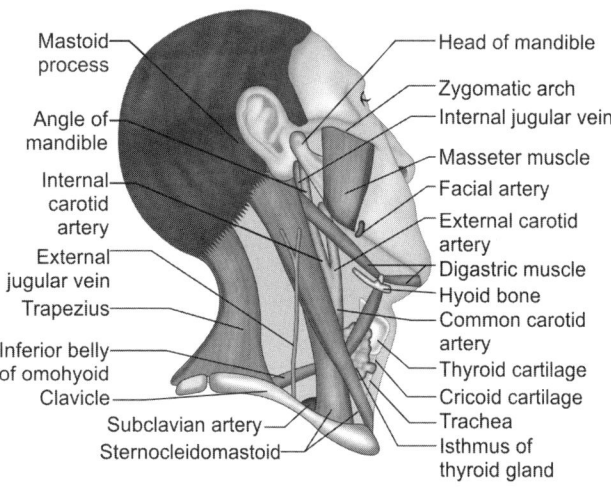

Fig. 6.1: Side of the neck.

border of thyroid cartilage to a point on the posterior border of neck of mandible. The artery is slightly convex forward in its lower half and slightly concave forward in its upper half.

The carotid arteries and the internal jugular vein are enclosed in a fibrous sheath called carotid sheath. It is placed quite deep in the neck. After giving the skin incision, sternocleidomastoid muscle is pushed laterally to carry the deeper dissection. All the small muscles are pushed aside to expose carotid sheath. Cut open the carotid sheath and isolate the vessels.

It is better to inject each common carotid artery separately to ensure equal distribution of the fluid on both sides. Besides this, solutions of different strengths can be used for the head and neck, and the rest of the body. After the completion of the injection, the artery is ligated before the other artery is brought into use. The same artery could be used to embalm the rest of the body by changing the direction of the cannula or needle downward through the aorta. Similarly internal jugular vein should also be drained separately.

Subclavian Artery

It is marked by a broad curved line convex upward rises about 2 cm above the clavicle from a point on the sternoclavicular joint to a point at the middle of the lower border of clavicle. An incision 5 cm long is given in the medial half of the clavicle in the supraclavicular fossa. The vessel is placed quite deep and enclosed in a fascia (cervicoaxillary). The artery and subclavian vein are separated by a muscle called scalenus anterior. The artery lies behind, and the vein in front of the muscle. The nerves of the brachial plexus and scalene muscle have to be pulled apart to expose the vessels.

Axillary and Brachial Arteries

To define this, the arm must be placed at right angle to the trunk with the palm directed upward. Draw a line on the surface of the skin from a point over or through the center of the base of the axilla (or midpoint of the clavicle) to a point through the center of the lateral wall of the axilla, and beyond up to the elbow to a point at the level of the neck of the radius medial to the tendon of biceps brachii muscle, it will be the brachial artery. The former marking will indicate axillary artery (Fig. 6.2).

An incision 5 cm long is made in the floor of the axilla along the line mentioned above in the direction of the artery. Axillary artery is quite deep seated because

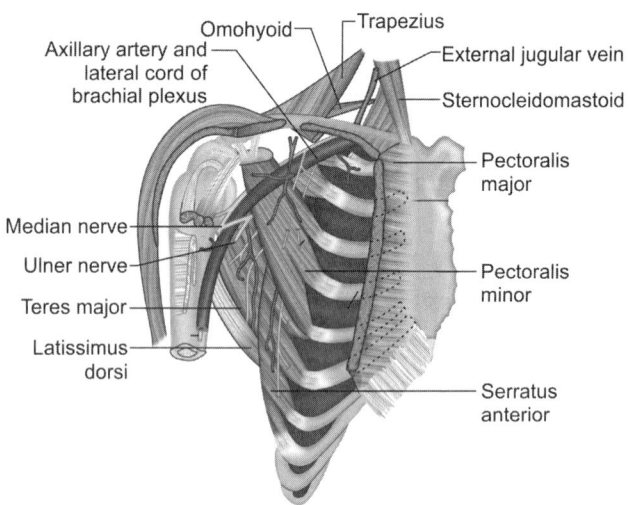

Fig. 6.2: Contents of axilla.

of massive fat in the region. Remove the fat by blunt dissection. Push aside the nerves of the brachial plexus and cut open the axillary sheath to expose the axillary artery. The axillary vein lies anteromedial to the artery and possibly will be engorged with blood.

To expose the brachial artery and basilic vein, give a 4 cm long incision in the middle of the arm along the medial border of the biceps brachii muscle. Basilic vein pierces the deep fascia about 5 cm above the elbow to accompany the brachial artery. Both the structures are superficial.

Radial Artery

It is marked by a line on the surface of the skin from a point in front of the elbow at the level of the neck of the radius medial to the tendon of biceps brachii to a point at the wrist between the anterior border of the radius laterally and the tendon of flexor carpi radialis medially, where the radial pulse is commonly felt.

Ulnar Artery

Draw a line on the surface of the skin from a point in front of the elbow at the level of the neck of the radius medial to the tendon of biceps brachii to a point at the junction of the upper one-third and lower two-thirds of the medial border of the forearm. The third point is taken lateral to the pisiform bone. Thus, the course of the ulnar artery is oblique in its upper one-third, and vertical in its lower two-thirds. The ulnar nerve lies just medial to the artery in its lower two-thirds course.

Abdominal Aorta

It is marked by a broad line extending from a point 2.5 cm above the transpyloric plane (level of first lumbar vertebra) in the median plane to a point 1.2 cm below and to the left of umbilicus.

To expose the aorta, an incision about 8–10 cm long is given in midline of abdomen just below the umbilicus. Push aside the intestine. Aorta and inferior vena cava are seen behind the peritoneum. Aorta is used for injection treatment and inferior vena cava for venous drainage. These vessels are commonly used in embalming the children and autopsied bodies.

Common Iliac Artery

It is represented by the upper one-third of a line drawn from the aortic bifurcation to the midinguinal point.

External Iliac Artery

It is represented by the lower two-thirds of the line drawn from the aortic bifurcation to the midinguinal point.

Celiac Artery

It is marked by a point 1 cm below the beginning of the abdominal aorta.

Superior Mesenteric Artery

It is marked by a curved line extending from the abdominal aorta just above the transpyloric plane to a point of intersection of the transtubercular and right lateral vertical pltanes.

Inferior Mesenteric Artery

It is marked by a curved line extending from the abdominal aorta 4 cm below the transpyloric plane to a point at the level of 4 cm below the umbilicus, and 4 cm to the left of the median plane.

Femoral Artery (Fig. 6.3)

It corresponds to the upper two-thirds of a line drawn from the midinguinal point to the adductor tubercle when the thigh is semiflexed, abducted and laterally rotated (Fig. 6.3).

The femoral artery and the vein are enclosed in a fascial sheath called femoral sheath. The dissection may be little difficult particularly in female because the region is loaded with fat and increases the depth of the dissection. The sheath is cut open and vessels are isolated. Femoral vein lies medial to the artery in the sheath. Expose the vessels to a convenient length and make cut in the anterior wall and cannulate the vessels. Two cannulae in opposite direction are inserted through the cut. The arterial cannula directed upward will embalm the entire body, directed downward will serve to embalm the respective limb only. Similarly the upper cut of the vein will drain the body above the limb, while lower drains the respective limb.

Popliteal Artery (Fig. 6.4)

Draw a line from a point at the junction of the middle and lower third of the thigh, 2.5 cm medial to its posterior midline, to the midpoint between the femoral condyles, continuing inferolaterally to the level of the tibial tuberosity (Fig. 6.4).

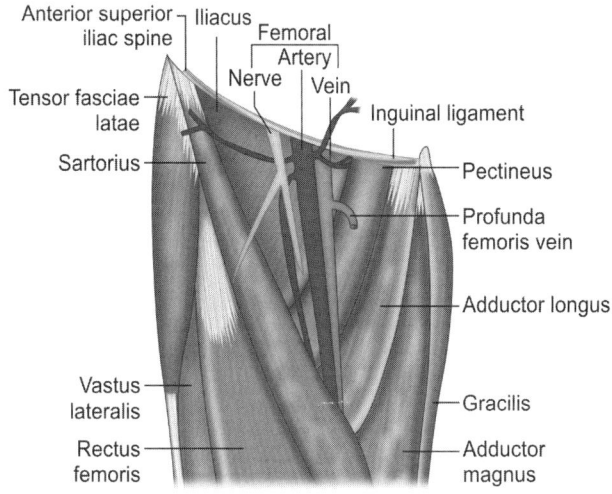

Fig. 6.3: Front of thigh and femoral triangle.

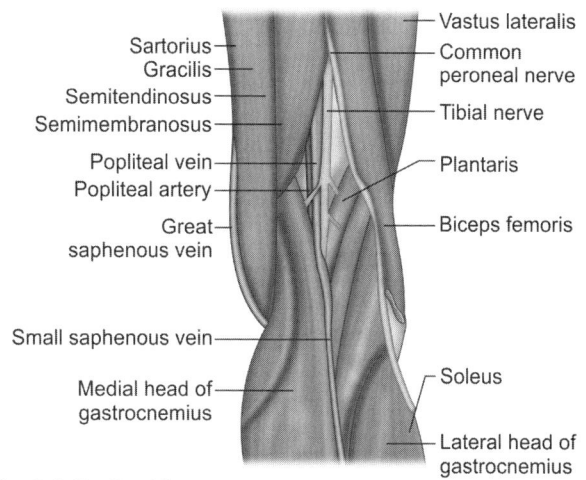

Fig. 6.4: Popliteal fossa.

Anterior Tibial Artery

Draw a line from a point 2.5 cm below and medial side of the fibular head to a point midway between the two malleoli.

Posterior Tibial Artery

It corresponds to a line joining a point 1–2 cm lateral to the calf's midline at the level of neck of fibula, extending downward and medially to the midpoint between the medial malleolus and the medial calcaneal tubercle.

Dorsalis Pedis Artery

It is marked by a line extending from a point midway between the two malleoli to a point at the proximal end of the first intermetatarsal space.

VEINS OF THE BODY

Superior Vena Cava

Draw a broad line from the lower border of the first right costal cartilage to the upper border of the third right costal cartilage, overlapping the right margin of the sternum.

Right Brachiocephalic Vein

It is marked by a line from the sternal end of the right clavicle to the lower border of the first right costal cartilage close to the sternum.

Left Brachiocephalic Vein

Draw a line from the sternal end of the left clavicle to the lower border of the first right costal cartilage. It crosses the left sternoclavicular joint and the upper half of the manubrium.

External Jugular Vein

The vein is usually visible through the skin. It can be marked by joining a point little below and behind the angle of mandible to a point on the clavicle just lateral to the posterior border of sternocleidomastoid muscle.

Internal Jugular Vein

It is marked by a line on the surface of the skin from a point on the neck medial to the lobule of the ear to a point at the medial end of the clavicle. The inferior bulb of the internal jugular vein lies in the lesser supraclavicular fossa between the sternal and clavicular heads of the sternocleidomastoid muscle.

Subclavian Vein

It is represented by a line along the clavicle extending from a little medial to its midpoint to the sternal end of the clavicle.

Inferior Vena Cava

It is marked by a broad line, little to the right of the median plane, from a point just below the transtubercular plane to the sternal end of the right sixth costal cartilage. A band from its lower end to a point on the inguinal ligament 1 cm medial to the midinguinal point indicates the common and external iliac veins on each side.

Femoral Vein

The femoral vein is medial to the femoral artery in the upper part, posterior to it in the middle and lateral to it at the lower end of the thigh. Its marking is same as that of the femoral artery, except that the upper point is taking 1 cm medial to midinguinal point, and the lower point 1 cm lateral to the adductor tubercle.

Great Saphenous Vein

It is marked by joining the following points:
- Medial end of the dorsal venous arch on the dorsum of the foot
- Anterior surface of medial malleolus
- Medial border of tibia at the junction of upper two-thirds and lower one-third of the leg
- Adductor tubercle
- Just below the center of the saphenous opening which lies 4 cm inferior and 4 cm lateral to the pubic tubercle.

Small Saphenous Vein

It is marked by joining the following points:
- Lateral end of the dorsal venous arch on the dorsum of the foot
- Behind the lateral malleolus just lateral to tendocalcaneus above the lateral malleolus
- Center of the popliteal fossa.

Portal Vein

It is marked by a broad line extending from a point on the transpyloric plane 1.2 cm to the right of the median plane upward and to the right for about 8 cm.

VISCERA OF THE BODY (FIG. 6.5)

Trachea

It is marked on the surface by two parallel lines 2 cm apart from the lower border of the cricoid cartilage to the sternal angle, inclining slightly to the right.

Lungs

Apex of the lung is represented by a dome rising 2.5 cm above the medial third of the clavicle. Anterior border is marked by joining a point at sternoclavicular joint, another point in the median plane at the sternal angle and a third point in the median plane just above the xiphisternal joint. The anterior border of the left lung corresponds to the anterior border of the right lung up to the level of the fourth costal cartilage. In the lower part, it presents the cardiac notch of variable size. From the level of the fourth costal cartilage, it passes laterally for 3.5 cm from the sternal margin, and then curves downward and medially to reach the sixth costal cartilage 4 cm from the median plane.

In the cardiac notch, the pericardium is covered only by a double layer of pleura, this is known as the "area of superficial cardiac dullness".

Lower border of each lung corresponds to a line from the anterior border of the sixth rib in the midclavicular line, eighth rib in the midaxillary line, continued medially and slightly up to a point 2 cm lateral to the tenth thoracic spine. Posterior border corresponds to a line from a point about 2 cm lateral to the tenth thoracic spine and upward to a point 2 cm lateral to the seventh cervical spine. It coincides with the posterior margin of the pleural reflexion/reflection.

Heart

Upper border is marked by a line joining a point at the lower border of second left costal cartilage about 1.3 cm from the left sternal border to a point at the upper border of right third costal cartilage 1.3 cm from the right sternal border.

Lower border is marked by a line joining a point at the lower border of the right sixth costal cartilage 2 cm from the right sternal border to a point at the apex of the heart in the fifth intercostal space 9 cm from the midsternal line.

Right border is marked by a convex line to the right, joining the right ends of the upper and lower borders. The maximum convexity is about 4 cm from the median plane in the fourth intercostal space. Left border is marked by a line, convex to the left, joining the left ends of the upper and lower borders.

Apex lies inferomedial to the left male nipple in the fifth intercostal space, slightly medial to the midclavicular line, about 9 cm, from the midline.

Spleen

It is marked on the left side of the back, with its long-axis corresponding with that of the tenth rib. The upper border corresponds to the upper border of the ninth rib, and the lower border to the lower border of the eleventh rib. The medial end lies 4–5 cm from the midline and the lateral end on the midaxillary line.

Stomach

Cardiac orifice is marked by two short parallel lines 2 cm apart, directed downward and to the left on the seventh

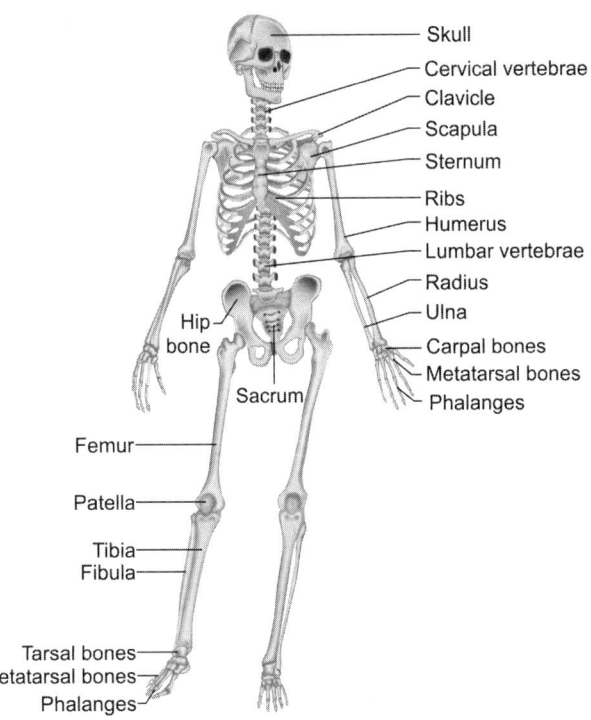

Fig. 6.5: Human skeleton.

costal cartilage, 2.5 cm to the left of the median plane. Pyloric orifice is marked by two short parallel lines 2 cm apart, directed upward and to the right, on the transpyloric plane (at the level of first lumbar vertebra), 1.2 cm to the right of the median plane. Fundus is marked by a convex line drawn from the left margin of the cardiac orifice to the highest point in the left fifth intercostal space just below the nipple.

Liver

The upper most point of the liver lies 6 cm below the right nipple. Its lowest point can be traced on the right, 2.5 cm below the tenth rib. It extends 7.5 cm below the left nipple.

Gallbladder

The fundus of gallbladder is marked at the angle, between the right costal margin and the lateral border of the right rectus muscle.

Pancreas

The head of the pancreas is marked within the duodenal curve. The neck lies in transpyloric plane, behind the pylorus. The body passes obliquely up and left for about 10 cm and lies little above the transpyloric plane. The tail is little above and to the left of intersection of the transpyloric and left lateral planes.

Kidney

It is marked on the back by drawing two horizontal lines, one at the level of eleventh thoracic spine and the other at the level of third lumbar spine. Then two vertical lines are drawn one 2.5 cm and the other 9 cm from the median plane. It forms the Morris parallelogram. The center of the hilum lies opposite the lower border of first lumbar spine.

Cecum

It is marked in the right iliac fossa by drawing two 5 cm long lines. Its axis should be directed downward and slightly medially.

Ascending Colon

It is marked by two parallel lines 5 cm apart, immediately to the right of the right lateral vertical plane, from the level of transtubercular plane (upper end of cecum) to the upper part of the ninth costal cartilage.

Transverse Colon

It is marked by two parallel lines 5 cm apart from a point at the upper part of the ninth costal cartilage, runs downward and medially to the umbilicus and then upward and laterally, crossing the transpyloric plane and left lateral vertical plane, to end at the eighth costal cartilage.

Descending Colon

It is marked by two parallel lines 2.5 cm apart from a point at the eighth costal cartilage, runs downward immediately lateral to the left lateral vertical plane, and ends at the inguinal ligament.

Rectum

It is marked on the back by drawing two lines joining the posterior superior iliac spines (the level of S2 spine) to the anus. The lower parts of these lines 1 cm below the second, sacral spine represents rectum.

Chapter 7

Embalming Chemicals and Fluids

ML Ajmani

INTRODUCTION

Embalming chemicals and fluids should have the following fundamental properties. It should:
- Ensure that there is no risk or fear of infection on contact with the dead body
- Produce without mutilation, a natural color and effect on the body, so that a life-like appearance is produced
- Ensure preservation of the body and the prevention of putrefaction changes and disturbances, which so often results in odious purging and discharge from the various orifices of the body
- Prevent contamination with insects and maggots.

The embalming fluid consists of the following groups of chemicals and their ingredients:
- Preservatives
- Germicides
- Buffers
- Wetting agents
- Anticoagulants
- Dyes
- Vehicle
- Perfuming agents.

These groups of chemicals are combined in various proportions to produce the arterial, cavity and preinjection fluids. In fact, most of these chemicals overcome the adverse effects of the formaldehyde on the tissues of the body.

PRESERVATIVES

Preservatives inactivate saprophytic bacteria and arrest decomposition by altering enzymes and lysins of the body. Formalin, a commercial source of formaldehyde, is the most commonly used chemical for this purpose.

Formaldehyde (Fig. 7.1)

It was discovered in 1856 by the British chemist, August Wilhelm von Hofmann. It is colorless at ordinary temperature and has an irritating pungent odor. It is soluble in water. It is commercially available as formalin containing 37% by weight or 40% by volume of formaldehyde gas in water. Formalin contains an average of 7% methyl alcohol, 37% formaldehyde, and the remaining water. Up to 10% methyl alcohol is added as a stabilizer, because without this the formaldehyde will precipitate and settle to the bottom as a sediment (paraformaldehyde) and lose strength at ordinary temperature. A solution containing 50% or 60% or in 70% formaldehyde in alcohol tends to precipitate the formaldehyde in a fine powdery sediment at the bottom of the container at cool temperature. As a result a weaker concentration of formaldehyde is present in the top layers of the solution than at the bottom.

Formalin may be turbid due to paraformaldehyde production. It can be cleared by filtration. The discoloration by storing in metal container does not impair its potency.

Formalin is an extensively active compound. The carbon atom has three unsaturated bonds and the hydrogen atom taken together with OH with a double bond. This arrangement makes the chemical easy in forming condensation polymers.

It is a biocide and achieves its biocidal effect by coagulation of the bacterial protoplasm. It is a powerful

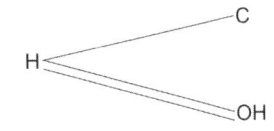

Fig. 7.1: Chemical structure of formaldehyde (CH_2O).

germicide. It preserves tissues by forming new chemical compounds with the tissue protein which is insoluble and unfit as food for organisms. Formalin should not be used in higher concentration as it will dehydrate the tissues and restrict the permeability to deeper tissues. It also constricts capillaries and diminishes the diffusion of fluid. If injected in higher concentration, it will produce excessive hardening of the tissue.

How does embalming work? Pervier in his "Textbook of Chemistry for Embalmers" mentioned the reactions between formaldehyde and body proteins. It states:

"Embalming destroys somewhat the colloidal nature of the proteins, neutralizes the active centers of the molecules and establishes many chemical cross linkages that were not there before between adjacent protein molecules. The net result is the conversion of protein into a high molecular, cross-linked lattice work of inert solid materials that can no longer serve; as food for bacteria as a substrate for enzyme action. The inert structures have lost their ability to retain water and their stability is maintained by the presence of a little uncombined formaldehyde."

It is bactericidal but not an effective fungicidal and insecticidal. Hence embalmed bodies may be affected by molds or maggots infestation.

It has an irritant vapor and can produced sensitization. It has an unpleasant effect on skin and prolonged contact with a mixture greater than 10% should be avoided. Always wear gloves. When working with formalin do not allow it to splash or have contact with your face, it can be extremely painful and also dangerous if it reaches the eyes. Wear eye goggles and protective clothing while working with formalin or any embalming chemicals. If chemicals are splashed or spilled onto the skin, flush the areas with cold running water immediately.

Other Preservative Chemicals

Other preservative chemicals used in combination with formalin include methanol or methyl alcohol and the phenol (carbolic acid). These agents react with tissue protein in a similar manner as formaldehyde, but there is difference in the cost and the rate of penetration.

Methanol (Methyl Alcohol, CH_3OH)

It is volatile, inflammable and poisonous, if consumed it can cause blindness and death. This is the best preservative that precipitates proteins and kills many organisms. The best useful dilution is 75% (v/v) isopropyl alcohol. It is cheaper and more toxic to bacteria than ethyl alcohol or ethanol. It is a good solvent for other chemicals. It stabilizes the formaldehyde in formalin solution. It is unique for its capacity to penetrate and diffuse readily into the tissues and it does not produce excessive hardening. Unfortunately, it tends to bleach the tissues and during dissection will evaporate rapidly therefore the area under dissection requires frequent moistening to prevent damage.

It is highly inflammable; therefore, there should be no smoking or a naked flame near an open container.

Phenol (Carbolic Acid, C_6H_5OH)

Phenol is a coal-tar derivative. It is an extremely poisonous colorless crystalline solid. On exposure to strong light, it turns dark due to oxidation. This change does not affect the potency of phenol. It is very rapidly absorbed by protein contents of the tissue and penetrates the skin readily. It is not soluble in water but is easily soluble in ethanol, chloroform, ether and glycerin. It is a powerful germicide and fungicide. It is a good preservative but tends to produce marked "graying" of tissues. Because of this property, its use is confined to cavity fluids, hypodermic embalming and for external packing. It can be used as a bleaching agent. It is available in percentages ranging from 2% to 90% phenol solution. If splashed on the skin can cause serious burns or if absorbed in large quantity can cause illness even death.

GERMICIDES

The important purpose of the embalming is to sanitize the cavities, surfaces and tissues of the body. Most of the preservative chemicals, incorporated into arterial fluid, cavity fluid or surface disinfectants, act as germicides. Germicides are used in embalming fluids to kill microorganisms. Phenol and phenolic derivatives, Zephiran chloride and glutaraldehyde are good germicides and are used as surface disinfectants and in varieties of embalming fluids.

BUFFERS

The stability of the chemicals in the embalming fluids depends on the pH (hydrogen ion concentration) of the medium. Weak acid or basic salts are used to stabilize the pH and are called "Buffers". Buffers also assist in stabilizing the pH of the tissues and provide good medium for the reaction of preservatives with cellular proteins. Normal body pH is about 7.38–7.4 after death. After death, the tissues of the body pass through varying levels of acids or bases. During rigor mortis, tissue will have an acid pH which becomes basic as it passes off.

Sodium borate (borax) is a good buffer and provides desired degree of alkalinity that rendered formalin stable for long periods without much deterioration in strength.

Sodium bicarbonate, sodium carbonate, magnesium carbonate are good neutralizer for formalin and maintain its pH.

WETTING AGENTS

These agents are used to lower the high surface tension of water and facilitate the penetration and distribution of the embalming fluids through the vascular bed into the tissues. These compounds include glycerin, glycols, sorbitol and sodium lauryl sulfate.

Glycerin

It is a clear colorless syrupy liquid. It is a good solvent for other compounds and itself is freely miscible in all proportions with water and alcohol. It is extensively used in embalming as a wetting agent. It is very hygroscopic and causes dehydration of tissues if used in excess. It increases the capability of embalmed tissues to retain moisture thus prevents drying and helps in keeping muscles soft. It is a good lubricator.

Sorbitol

It is generally available as a 70% aqueous solution. It is better than glycerin because it loses water at a slower rate. It is more efficient than glycerin. The main disadvantage of sorbitol solution is that it tends to drop out of solution at a very low temperature.

Sodium Lauryl Sulfate

It is a substitute for glycerin as a wetting agent without its drying effect.

ANTICOAGULANTS

Clotting of the blood is the main hindrance in embalming procedure. The main component required for clotting of blood is "ionized calcium". Anticoagulants are used to precipitate the calcium to a nonionized state. They maintain blood in a liquid state and thus facilitate the removal of blood and distribution of arterial fluids. Compounds like oxalates or citrates are used in the embalming solution particularly in preinjection fluids and arterial fluid.

Sodium Citrate

It is a white odorless, crystalline substance. It has two-fold action: firstly, if removes the calcium ion, which is essential for blood clotting and secondly, it acts as a buffering agent to stabilize the pH of the fluid. It is soluble in water and used as 2% solution.

Sodium Oxalate

It is a white crystalline material. It is soluble in water and is used as 2% solution to precipitate "ionized calcium" in the blood and arrest coagulation.

DYES

Dyes are mainly used in embalming fluids for the purpose of producing an internal cosmetic effect that closely simulates the natural coloring of the tissues. Dyes will also enable the embalmer to detect "patchy embalming" effects if any.

The following factors may be considered in selecting a suitable dye:
- It should impart a color which closely simulates to the natural living condition.
- It must not be affected by other constituents of embalming fluids.
- It must diffuse readily from circulatory system to the superficial tissues.
- It must be stable in color under pathological conditions.
- It must be water soluble and should have high staining qualities, so that small amount can produce the desired effect.

Eosin (Tetrabromofluorescein)

It is a red crystalline powder. It is soluble in water and is used in 1 in 500 dilutions. This dye group spreads readily and stains the tissues diffusely and thus helps to eliminate the gray color due to death and embalming procedures.

Ponceau

It is a dark-red powder that is soluble in water and forms a cherry-red solution. It does not produce visible tissue staining at the strength which is used in embalming. It stains only in higher concentration.

Other dyes included are erythrosine, amaranth, acid fuchsin, toluidine red and rhodamine.

VEHICLES (DILUENTS)

The vehicle is a solvent or a mixture of solvents that help the ingredients in the solution in a stable and uniform state during transport through the vascular system to different parts of the body. Water is the mainly solvent and forms about 90% of all embalming fluids. Vehicle may include glycerin, sorbitol, alcohols in addition to water.

PERFUMES (DEODORANTS)

Perfumes are of value as masking agents. They convert an unpleasant odor into a more pleasant one. In embalming solution, the harshness of the preservative chemicals is reduced and replaced to some extent by a more pleasant odor. It is not advisable try to ask completely the odor of formaldehyde. This can result in neutralization or destruction of the active ingredients. These agents are generally water soluble or made water soluble by the use of surfactants. Most of the perfumes used are floral compounds, e.g. methyl salicylate (oil of wintergreen) or synthetic compounds, e.g. oil of clove, cinnamon oil, oil of peppermint (menthol) or lavender.

MUSCLE RELAXANTS

It has been suggested that these chemicals relax the smooth muscles in the arterial wall and assist the flow of fluid in the vascular system. Magnesium chloride is used for this purpose.

According to the recent view, the relaxing agents are ineffective in a cadaver.

DISINFECTION

Various methods are used to decontaminate embalming room surfaces, instruments and equipment prior to reuse. Chemical and physical decontamination is a very important weapon to eliminate reservoirs of infectious agents. Certain terms as used in disinfection of the environment are elaborated and defined here.

Disinfectant

An agent used to inanimate objects/surfaces by destroying microbial agents but usually not bacterial spore.

Germicide

An agent used to inanimate objects/surfaces or living tissues by destroying microbial agents but usually not bacterial spores.

Sterilization

It is the most effective method of decontamination. It completely destroys all living microbial agents and their products.

Antimicrobial Activity

Three levels of antimicrobial activities are recognized for proper disinfection of objects and environment, i.e. high, intermediate and low (Block SS, 1983).
- High-level disinfectant is effective against bacterial spores and viruses, e.g. aqueous 2% glutaraldehyde, 8% formaldehyde solution in 70% alcohol, 6–10% stabilized hydrogen peroxide.
- Intermediate-level disinfectants do not kill large numbers of bacterial spores but they do inactivate the tubercle bacillus. They are also effective against fungi and viruses; examples include 0.5% iodine, aqueous formaldehyde 3.0–8.0%, 70–90% ethanol, chlorine compounds (sodium hypochlorite 1,000–5,000 ppm), phenolic compounds (phenol 0.5–3.0%), Betadine, 75–200 ppm.
- Low-level disinfectants do not destroy bacterial spores or tubercle bacillus but they can rapidly kill vegetative forms of bacteria and fungi. They are not effective against all types of viruses; examples include ammonium compounds (Zephiran chloride 0.1–0.2% aqueous solution), mercurial compounds (mercurochrome 0.1–0.2%), phenolic compounds have intermediate to low antimicrobial activity, depending upon the strength of the solution (phenol 0.5–3%) (Block SS, 1983).

EMBALMING FLUIDS

The embalming fluid contains the eight groups of chemicals: (1) preservatives, (2) germicides, (3) anticoagulants, (4) buffers, (5) wetting agents, (6) vehicle, (7) dyes, and (8) perfuming agents.

All the chemicals in the embalming fluid are designed to preserve and sanitize the body. The factors considered in selection and preparation of an embalming fluid are—age, sex, status of the body (autopsied or unautopsied) weather conditions, and type of embalming, i.e. anatomical or funeral embalming. The chemical composition of the embalming fluids used for anatomical purposes varies in most of the medical schools in India.

The following fluids are normally prepared in the practice of embalming:
- Arterial fluid
- Cavity fluid
- Preinjection fluid.

Arterial Fluid

Arterial fluid is injected into the vascular system of the body. The dilution of the arterial fluid varies with the type of bodies, i.e. normal bodies, dehydrated bodies, obese bodies, edematous bodies and in special conditions such as bodies dead for long periods, refrigerated bodies, burnt bodies or of the infants. Dilutions may be increased or decreased to combat the problem.

Arterial Fluid for Obese Subjects

Arterial fluid for obese subjects has been shown in Table 7.1.

Glycerol should be reduced in a fatty body.

In hot countries, formalin should be doubled.

Thymol crystals should be pounded into small particles and then dissolved in a small amount of alcohol before being added to the fluid.

Arterial Fluid for Thin Subjects

Arterial fluid for thin subjects has been shown in Table 7.2.

The formalin strength is increased in autopsied, refrigerated, infected, burnt and decomposed bodies and bodies lying dead for long periods.

Studies have shown that human immunodeficiency virus (HIV) is inactivated rapidly after being exposed to commonly used chemicals at concentrations that are much lower than used in practice (Spire B et al., 1984; Martin LS et al., 1985; McDougal JS et al., 1985; and Spire B et al., 1985). Embalming fluids are similar to the types of chemical germicides that have been tested and found to completely inactivate HIV. A freshly prepared solution of sodium hypochlorite (household bleach) in a concentration ranging from 500 ppm (1:100 dilution) to 5,000 ppm (1:10 dilution) is quite an effective germicide. It is an inexpensive germicide and best suited to clean and disinfect the surfaces. Though most of the organisms may be killed or inactivated at a lower concentration of formalin but to ensure prophylactic and satisfactory results concentrations ranging from approximately 10.0% to 70.0% are used.

Cavity Fluid

The cavity fluid is injected into the body cavities, i.e. thoracic, abdominal and pelvic cavities with a trocar. It is also injected hypodermically into areas of the body that have not received arterial fluid. It may be used as a surface pack in certain pathological conditions and over the surface lesions to dry and disinfect the areas.

For an average body, approximately 2 L of cavity fluid is injected with a trocar over the viscera of the thoracic, abdominal and pelvic cavities.

Cavity fluid preserves and disinfects the walls and parenchyma of the organs, contents of the hollow viscera and the contents of the spaces between the visceral organs. The cavity fluid composition is recommended as shown in Table 7.3.

Table 7.1: Composition of arterial fluid for obese subjects.

Preservative	Formalin	10.0%
	Methanol	55.0%
Buffer	Sodium borate	15.0 g
Anticoagulant	Sodium citrate	15.0 g
Wetting agent	Glycerin	15.0%
Germicide	Phenol	5.0%
Vehicle	Water	15.0%
Fungicide	Thymol	Few crystals
Dye	1% Eosin	5.0 mL
Perfume	Soluble wintergreen	10.0 mL

Note: The above concentration is needed to prepare 1 L of arterial fluid.

Table 7.2: Composition of arterial fluid for thin subjects.

Formalin	10.0%
Methanol	55.0%
Sodium borate	15.0 g
Sodium citrate	15.0 g
Glycerin	20.0%
Phenol	5.0%
Water	10.0%
Thymol	Few crystals
1% Eosin	5.0 mL
Soluble wintergreen	10.0 mL

Table 7.3: Composition of cavity fluid.

Formalin	60.0%
Methanol	25.0%
Glycerin	2.5%
Phenol	10.0%
Mercuric chloride	1.0%
Lavender	1.0%

Table 7.4: Composition of paint mixture.

Glycerin	75.0%
Alcohol	10.0%
Phenol	5.0%
Water	10.0%

Note: Add Teepol to the above with few crystals of thymol.

Table 7.5: Composition of tank (immersion) fluid.

Formalin	15.0%
Glycerin	20.0%
Phenol	5.0%
Water	60.0%

Preinjection Fluid

At death there is contraction of arterial system which forces the greater volume of blood into the capillary bed and venous system. It has been estimated that after death, 85% of the blood is found in the capillaries, 10% in the veins, and 5% in the arteries. Preinjection fluid is injected into the body before the arterial solution. It removes the blood and clears the vascular system and thus also improves drainage. Strong solutions prepared for arterial fluid or cavity fluid cause difficulty in clearing the blood from the capillaries and veins. In fact, preinjection fluid prepares the vascular system for the preservative arterial fluid. Approximately 4–5 L of solution should be injected and a waiting period of about 30 minutes be given before the arterial fluid is injected. This fluid loosens the clots in the venous system and makes them easier to remove and thus improves the drainage. A part of this solution may fill the empty arterial system. The preinjection fluid contains anticoagulants and buffers and rarely small amounts of preservatives. Preinjection treatment is only used in unautopsied bodies. This fluid is not used as a routine in embalming procedures.

Drainage plays an important role in cleaning the vascular system which is brought about by displacement. A 2% arterial solution is recommended for this purpose.

Even milder solution can be used. The purpose of this solution is to displace the contents of the vascular system and make room for preservative arterial solution. The best method to clear the vascular system is to preinject fluid with the drainage kept open.

QUANTITY OF FLUID REQUIRED

There are number of factors which determine the strength and amount of arterial fluids required for effective embalming of a body. These include age, weight of the body, obesity, moisture content of the body (dehydration or nondehydration), time between death and preparation, time between preparation and disposal of bodies that have been refrigerated, bodies with evidence of decomposition, and bodies with edema, etc.

There are 6–7 L of blood in the vascular system of an average body. This accounts for approximately 8.0% of the total body weight. Usually the amount of the arterial fluid injected should be equal to the blood volume of the deceased to ensure effective embalming. It is always better to overembalm than to underembalm a body. Approximately 10 L of arterial fluid is prepared for an average adult weighing 65–70 kg which also includes spillage. It does not include the drained amount. Drainage may involve the removal of 6–7 L of blood and body fluids. To restore the loss of body fluids and to overcome the loss of preservative especially in the use of continuous drainage, it is necessary to prepare the total injection solution volume 15–20 L. Initially sufficient injection pressure is applied to maintain moderate rate of flow (4–5 minutes/L) for prompt diffusion of the fluid. Later the pressure and rate of flow are reduced. It will prevent undesirable tissue distortion and assure uniform distribution of the injection fluid.

The following fluids are used in anatomy dissection laboratories:

Paint Mixture (Table 7.4)

To be used for keeping dissections moist.

Tank (Immersion) Fluid

For immersing cadavers, tank (immersion) fluid is recommended as shown in Table 7.5.

Cloth Fluid (Table 7.6)

To prevent drying of the area under dissection and isolated dissected parts.

Table 7.6: Composition of cloth fluid.	
Formalin	5.0%
Glycerin	50.0%
Phenol	5.0%
Water	40.0%

Note: Add Teepol to the above with few crystals of thymol.

FLUID FOR NERVOUS TISSUE

- Formalin—10.0%
- Do not use a glycerin-based fluid.

Chapter 8

Embalming Fluids and the Safe Levels of Formaldehyde

BS Mitchell, E O'Sullivan

HISTORICAL ASPECTS OF BODY PRESERVATION

The morphology of the human body has intrigued mankind for generations. Indeed, the history of anatomy is inevitably linked to the ability of the dessectors to preserve the body. Whereas the early anatomists dissected fresh corpses, with all the attendant difficulties (!), some preservation of cadavers is nowadays usual. Such preservation is normally achieved through the process of embalming in which a fixative (preservative fluid) is introduced into body tissues in such a way as to maintain, as far as possible, a life-like state, and certainly the normal relationships of, human anatomy. Whilst contemporary fixatives heavily utilize formaldehyde for this purpose, it has not always been the case. Amongst the first attempts at some kind of anatomical preservation was the preparation of Egyptian mummies. Significant advances came once substances which solidified the body tissues were identified. In the 19th century, for example, heavy metal salts were used, however, until the latter part of the nineteenth century.[1] Significantly, nowadays there is a legal requirement for the use of formaldehyde in embalming fluids[2] in the United States of America.

MODERN EMBALMING TECHNIQUES

Little has been written about modern embalming methods for anatomical work aside from the methodology employed by Logan (1983).[3] In the United Kingdom (UK), the use of cadavers for anatomical examination is governed by the Anatomy Act (1984). Under the terms of this act of Parliament, licensed persons may have legal possession of the bodies for examination-periods of up to 3 years, and if permission from relatives is obtained, up to 50% of the body may be retained indefinitely "for further anatomical examination". It is the expectation that all of these cadavers will be subjected to some kind of preservation procedure, though that is not specified by the Act of Parliament. Certain self-imposed controls are placed upon the type of cadavers that are accepted by medical schools. Bodies from persons who have suffered from contagious illness, terminal illness, i.e. cancer, have been subject to a postmortem examination, surgery resulting in organ removal, limb amputation, gross obesity, gross emaciation, and most recently any kind of neurological illness (because of the risk of Creutzfeldt–Jakob disease) are not accepted.

THE RISKS AND PROBLEMS IN THE USE OF FORMALDEHYDE

Prior to the Control of Substances Hazardous to Health Act, 1990,[4] there was variety of formaldehyde-based formulae used for embalming fluids in medical schools in the UK. When the legislation was passed by the UK government, a limit to the concentrations of formaldehyde was set that was permissible in the atmosphere of dissecting rooms, and embalming suites (the occupational exposure levels). This limitation was imposed because it has been shown that formaldehyde is not without its risk to personnel.[5,6] In this work, it was shown that there is significant irritant effect on the eyes and mucosa surfaces by the gas that is emitted from formaldehyde solutions, though no compelling evidence of carcinogenicity was demonstrable. Other suggestions have included an initiation of allergic reactions.[7] In the UK, once this legislation was enacted, the formaldehyde levels in the embalming facilities and dissecting rooms of many medical schools fell short of the safety levels. There are a number of possible reasons for this. For instance, a lack of adequate ventilation in the dissecting room, or embalming suite, poor working practices when embalming causing spillages of fluid, poor condition of cadavers causing embalming fluid to leak out of the cadaver, or using high concentrations of formaldehyde in the embalming fluid. As a consequence in some of these medical schools, students no longer dissect but rely on plastinated specimens,[8] plastic models, or computer-assisted learning programs, either devised in-house, or purchased commercially. The full effects of this on the learning of human anatomy have yet to be realized, but need to be judged in conjunction with the emerging demands of the curriculum changes provoked by the "Tomorrow's Doctors" document published by the General Medical Council in UK, in 1993.[9] In general, the reason that medical schools in the UK are unable to effect the changes required in plant, to improve ventilation, etc. is mainly because of financial strictures imposed by the government, and in relation to possible changes in emphasis in the new curricular patterns developing.

ALTERNATIVES TO FORMALDEHYDE

Attempts to obviate the need for formaldehyde in embalming fluid have been suggested which reduce any potential risks. For example, phenoxyethanol has been employed as a nontoxic substitute for formaldehyde.[10] Although this would appear to meet needs from a safety point of view, its use would prove to be impractical since it requires very large volumes (600 L for each cadaver) of phenoxyethanol and continual immersion in the fluid to prevent mold formation. With large numbers of cadavetic specimens storage for immersion would be problematic. Furthermore, the whole process is said to take 5–10 months to complete which is also not practical. The extraction in dilute ethanol of formaldehyde-fixed dissecting specimens has also been proposed as an efficient method to reduce potential health risks. The methodology employed by Björkman and Christensen (1982)[11] resulted in a significant reduction in the concentration of formaldehyde. A combined perfusion and percolation technique for embalmed animal bodies has been used to remove formaldehyde, again resulting in significant reductions.[12] Glutaraldehyde is an aldehyde related to formaldehyde, with similar fixation qualities. It could be a feasible alternative, but because of the volumes that would be required, it is prohibitively expensive.

Despite all the foregoing attempts to obviate the need for formaldehyde, it remains a very popular fixative. With the current debate on Creutzfeldt–Jakob disease in the UK at present, and in the knowledge that formaldehyde does not kill the agent responsible, there may be a resurgence of interest in nonformaldehyde based "embalming fluids". Nevertheless, despite this, it remains the fixative of choice, because of its undoubted efficiency, and the consistency of results obtained.

USE OF FORMALDEHYDE IN MEDICAL SCHOOLS IN THE UK

In an effort to determine the extent to which formaldehyde figured in the various embalming fluids currently used in the UK, we surveyed the composition of the fluids used in 18 medical schools (Fig. 8.1) by sending out a questionnaire. We ascertained the composition of the fluids, whether formaldehyde vapor levels were monitored, whether the fluid was buffered, whether tap water or distilled water was used, and for details of the embalming procedure utilized. All of the fluids currently in use in the UK claim to preserve the body in an appropriate state for dissection, though whether this is actually the case is not known since no systematic analysis of cadaver quality was undertaken. Indeed, it is difficult to identify criteria which allow comparison. What did emerge from the survey taken by O'Sullivan and Mitchell (1983)[13] was that there was a remarkable variation in the combinations of embalming fluid constituents (Fig. 8.1). Nevertheless, all of the fluids contained formaldehyde, phenol, glycerol, water and industrial methylated spirit. The proportion of formaldehyde was the major variant. As can be seen in Figure 8.1, the highest proportion used was approaching 10% whereas in one institution, there was no formaldehyde

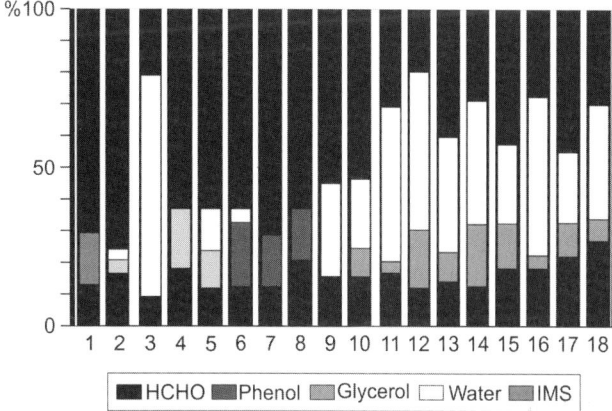

Fig. 8.1: The percentage composition of embalming fluids in 18 medical schools in the United Kingdom.
(HCHO: formaldehyde; IMS: industrial methylated spirit)

at all. The relationship between water and industrial methylated spirit seemed to be inversely related. The spirit was, in fact, the major constituent with water. Next, although phenol was generally the constituent of lowest concentration, it was the most constant, reflecting its disinfectant qualities. The concentration of glycerol in the final embalming fluid appeared to vary without any obvious basis, though the effect of the increased amount of glycerol was to assist in preventing the fat from leaching out of body tissues, and to counter the hardening effects of industrial methylated spirits. The survey did reveal that increasing the quantity of tap water resulted in the development of mold on the specimens. Use of distilled water appears to avoid the problem, presumably because the spores which are contained in tap water are not contained in distilled water, because it is pure. There is always a temptation to increase the water content because it makes the final embalming fluid cheaper!

Medical Schools

The subsequent cadaver storage facilities are also an important factor in avoidance of mold. [If such mold occurs affected parts can be treated by removal and the remaining areas of tissues treated with a 3.0% solution of Everbrite (Chemsearch, UK) applied directly to specimens by spraying on. Bad cases can be immersed in stronger solutions for periods of up to 24 hours or more, if necessary. This treatment appears not to have any deleterious effect on the specimens]. The temperature of storage does not seem to be a factor in mold production, since it is our experience that specimens may be stored at room temperature, although very high temperature (greater than 20°C) may alter the outcome.

EMBALMING PROCEDURES

The embalming procedure used at Southampton involved an initial wash of the cadaver in a disinfectant fluid, and shaving the body of hair before cannulae were inserted into either the femoral or common carotid artery (the latter was the preferred route allowing greater volumes of embalming fluid to be introduced, though the precise route may be dictated by the region of the body required for dissections). A total volume of between 18 L and 30 L of embalming fluid is introduced (depending on the nutritional state of the cadaver; the larger the cadaver, the greater volume required) using a mechanical pump (Dodge Chemical Company) at pressures not exceeding 0.21 kg/cm^2. The use of supplementary local injections of fluid may be required red to effect maximal preservation, since often blockage of blood vessels by clots prevents fluid from reaching all parts of the body. Injections of 50 mls or considerably more, depending upon the area, may be necessary for a large area over a 2 day or 3 day period. After embalming, the body is wrapped in polythene sheet and stored for at least 6 weeks at 10°C. This apparent delay is an important stage to allow fixation to occur which will enhance the quality of dissections. Any attempt to dissect before full fixation has occurred will result in poor preservation and dissections will be subject to greater degrees of wear and tear damage, a factor not to be overlooked in medical schools where student's use of specimens inevitably exacts its toll, especially in anatomy courses where students examine prosected specimens, rather than to dissect for themselves, as is increasingly the case in the UK.

EXPERIMENTS TO MONITOR FORMALDEHYDE LEVELS

To ascertain the levels of formaldehyde vapor arising during embalming or dissecting at Southampton levels were measured by use of the Gastec passive Dosi-tube 91b (Detectawl, UK) of Southampton Safety Office. Each of the Dosi-tube measuring devices is calibrated to indicate parts per million of formaldehyde vapor in air. These measuring devices were attached to the lapels of the personnel involved in dissecting or embalming, as close to the face as possible, and readings taken every 30 minutes throughout any monitored procedure until it was completed.

To investigate the effect of varying the composition of embalming fluids, a number of experiments were undertaken in which cadavers were embalmed using different fluids of various compositions (Tables 8.1 and 8.2). Results indicated that all cadavers appeared to be effectively preserved as judged by inspection; muscles were soft and pink in coloration, whereas the subcutaneous tissues were quite white in appearance. Fascia was strong but easy to remove (an essential in any course in which students dissect), and the bodies generally easy to dissect, even in the deeper compartments, which indicated that fixatives had penetrated these regions, and had been effective. No obvious advantages arose from buffering the embalming fluids. Indeed, in some cases, the concentration of buffer salts was so high that it was not possible to dissolve the fluid and the cannulae became blocked, and the buffering

Table 8.1: The composition of four different embalming fluids, buffered and unbuffered.

Component	Original	Expt 1	Expt 2	Expt 3
Formaldehyde	106 mls/L	53 mls/L	106 mls/L	53 mls/L
IMS	425 mls/L	625 mls/L	625 mls/L	625 mls/L
Tap water	248 mls/L	101 mls/L	48 mls/L	48 mls/L
Phenol	67 g/L	67 g/L	67 g/L	67 g/L
Glycerol	154 mls/L	154 mls/L	154 mls/L	154 mls/L
pH buffered		7.7	7.9	7.7
pH unbuffered		6.7	6.55	6.5

(IMS: industrial methylated spirit)

Table 8.2: Dosi-tube readings for formaldehyde vapor in embalming and subsequent dissection and duration of procedures.

Experiment	Dissect	Embalm	Dissect	Embalm
1	0.67 ppm/15 h	0.53 ppm/4.75 h		
2	1.0 ppm/1.5 h	1.14 ppm/3.5 h		
3	0.2 ppm/2.5 h	0.29 ppm/4 h	0.33 ppm/3 h	0.33 ppm/3 h

(ppm: parts per million; h: hour)

Note: The embalming of three experiments were repeated using different personnel.

was ineffective, as indicated by the change of pH of the fluid before and after embalming. Notwithstanding the lack of effect on fluid composition, there was a measurable effect on the formaldehyde vapor readings. As might be predicted, the embalming fluid with the highest concentration of formaldehyde gave the highest vapor levels. Bearing in mind that the quality of preservation was as good irrespective of formaldehyde concentrations in the embalming fluid, it would appear that the formula with the lowest formaldehyde concentration can be recommended for use in cadaveric preservation.

In this formula, the concentration of glycerol was high to compensate for the higher proportion of industrial methylated spirit, and low proportion of water. The important factor, however, was that the reduction in proportion of formaldehyde resulted in vapor levels that were within the limits set by the government legislation (1 ppm or less over an 8-hour period, or no more than 2 ppm over a 15 minute period).

The embalming experiments were carried out 5 years ago, and the cadaveric material is still in good condition. It may, therefore, be concluded that the reduction in formaldehyde concentration is not deleterious to specimen preservation, but leads to a safer working environment.

REFERENCES

1. Mayer RG. Embalming. History, Theory and Practice, 1st edition. California, US: Appleton and Lange; 1990.
2. Plunkett ER, Barbela T. Are embalmers at risk? Am Ind Hyg Assoc J. 1979;38:61-2.
3. Logan BM The long-term preservation of whole human cadavers destined for anatomical study. Ann R Coll Surg Engl. 1983;65:33.
4. Health and safety executive guidance notes on formaldehyde exposure levels (UK Government) EH 40/90. Control of Substances Hazardous to Health Regulations; 1990.
5. Pabst R. Exposure to formaldehyde in anatomy: an occupational health hazard. Aniat Rec. 19872;19:109-12.
6. Robbins A, Bingham E. Formaldehyde: evidence of carcinogenicity. Joint NIOSH/OSHA Current Intelligence Bulletin No. 34. Cincinnati, US: NIOSH Publications; 1980.
7. Putz R, Poisel S, Tiefenbrunner F. Probleme mit Konservierurigflussigkeiten im anatomischeen Prapariesaalbetrieb. Actn Anat. 1974;90:394-402.
8. O'Sullivan E, Mitchell BS. Plastination for gross anatomy teaching using low cost equipment. Surg Radiol Anat. 1995; 17:277-81.
9. United Kingdom Tomorrow's Doctors. London, UK: General Medical Council; 1993.
10. Frolich KW, Andersen LM, Knutsen A, et al. Phenoxyethanol as a nontoxic substitute for formaldehyde in Jong term preservation of human anatomical specimens for dissection and demonstration purposes. Anat Rec. 1984;208:271-8.
11. Björkman N, Christensen KM. Extraction in dilute ethanol of formaldehyde-fixed dissecting specimens. An efficient method to reduce health hazards. Acta Anat. 1982;112:1-8.
12. Siemiatkowski M, Ploen L, Barkman N. Combined perfusion and percolation of embalmed animal bodies for removing formaldehyde. Acta Anat. 1988;133:251-4.
13. O'Sullivan E, Mitchell BS. An improved composition for embalming fluid to preserve cadavers for anatomy teaching in the United Kingdom. J Anat. 1983;182:295-7.

Chapter 9

Practical Embalming

ML Ajmani

INTRODUCTION

Modem embalming is defined as the study and science of treating a dead human body to achieve an antiseptic condition, a premortem appearance and preservation. Various other terms have been used to describe the treatment of embalming such as sanitary preservation, hygienic treatment, preparation of the body, etc. but the term "modern embalming" is regarded as correct interpretation. It can be defined as follows:

The embalming process acts on the body proteins. It changes the proteins colloidal nature and forms latticework of inert, more stable, longer-lasting, firm substance that can no longer serve as food for bacteria. Moreover, this new protein form cannot be broken down by enzymes from body cells or bacteria.

Body proteins have great affinity to hold water. After embalming, the new protein form no longer has the ability to retain water. As a result, enzymes which break down protein can no longer act on the new form of protein. Therefore, the embalmed tissue becomes drier, as it has lost its ability to hold the moisture, and the body is temporarily preserved.

Embalming solution destroys the pathogenic and nonpathogenic bacteria of the body because their protein bodies are also converted into an inactive state. Therefore, embalming ensures that if death was caused by a communicable disease, the body is no longer a source of that infection.

PRE-EMBALMING CONSIDERATION

No embalmer can really decide what the procedure should be until he has made a thorough study of the case. This study is termed pre-embalming diagnosis. The process of embalming consists fundamentally of an injection of some suitable disinfecting preservative into the vascular system augmented by the relieving of the blood from the veins. There is no ideal vessel that could be used as a standard for arterial injection or venous drainage. Embalming exercise varies from case to case depending upon the diseases suffered during life, sex and general condition of the body. There must be reasons why we should not use any one artery in the treatment of a particular case. It is therefore, essential to become familiar with the use of all possible arteries and veins so that we should be able to select the best possible point for the procedure under different conditions.

Criteria for Selection of a Vessel to be used

- *Size of the vessel:* The vessel should be sufficiently large to afford proper insertion of a cannula for proper embalming and adequate drainage.
- *Depth of the location of the vessel:* The vessel should be superficial enough to avoid unnecessary dissection.
- *Proximity of the vessel to the heart:* In the unautopsied body, the ideal artery for injection is the aorta but its location makes the aorta an impractical choice. Similarly, for the drainage, the right atrium of the heart is the best choice but again its location within the thoracic cavity makes it an impractical choice. Therefore, the vessels used for injection and drainage should be as close as possible to both the aorta and the right atrium.
- *Choice in infants and children:* In infants and children below 5 years of age, the vessels of choice are the abdominal aorta and the inferior vena cava.
- *Choice of artery in nonautopsied bodies:* In selecting a primary injection site, two criteria to be considered are

factors concerning the artery or vein itself, and general body conditions. In the unautopsied body, there is a choice of four primary injection sites: (1) Right common carotid artery; (2) the right femoral (or external iliac) artery; (3) both the right and the left common carotid arteries (in restricted cervical injection); and (4) the right axillary artery. The vessels of the right side of the body are commonly used for embalming.

This is because most of the embalmers are right handed and find much easier to work on the right side of the body. In addition, if internal jugular vein is to be used for drainage, the drainage instrument is much easier and more effective to insert in the right atrium of the heart. It is of the primary importance that the embalmer should be thoroughly acquainted with the surface anatomy of the vessels of the body and their anatomical relationships.

If the selected artery appears to be sclerotic or obstructed, embalmer should try and find out a more suitable artery. Sclerotic arteries are likely to rupture. Sometimes, their outer coats are strong, but the intima may peel off and obstruct the passage. It then becomes extremely difficult to push the cannula further into the artery. If pressure is applied to push the cannula in, the inner walls will rupture, roll inside, and cause obstruction. In such cases, instead of a hard metal cannula, a pliable plastic cannula can be tried and the injection should proceed slowly and at low pressure to avoid damage to the walls. Other factors that may govern the choice of artery are limitations imposed by the disease, surgical operations, tissue damaged by radiation treatment, age of the deceased, obesity, etc.

- *Choice of artery in autopsied bodies:* This depends upon the extent of mutilation and the postmortem carried out. The effects of disease and stage of decomposition will also determine the choice. The embalmer should ascertain that he is not dealing with a dangerous infective or a contagious case. The diseases like jaundice and pseudomonal infections can be diagnosed by the external appearance.

Abdominal aorta is used directly for injection in case of autopsied bodies. If more than one vessel has to be opened for one area, it is better to use multiple injection method. In the autopsied body, there are six primary injection sites—(1 and 2) right and left common carotid; (3 and 4) right and left femoral (external or common iliac); and (5 and 6) right and left subclavian (axillary) arteries. If this method does not produce satisfactory results, the embalmer must evaluate the situation and employ other embalming techniques like surface embalming or hypodermic embalming.

EXPOSURE OF THE VESSELS

Common Carotid Artery and the Internal Jugular Vein

Put a wooden block under the shoulder to elevate the shoulder and lower the head so that the whole length of the neck is exposed. The vessels run vertically from the sternoclavicular joint to the thyroid cartilage and related medially to the trachea and laterally to the sternocleidomastoid muscle. A vertical incision about 1.5–2 inches long is made through the skin at the root of the neck near the sternoclavicular joint. The two vessels are enclosed together in a fascial sheath carotid sheath. The artery occupies a medial position, the vein is lateral one. The vagus nerve lies behind the vessels. Raise the carotid sheath, cut it and dissect out the common carotid artery and internal jugular vein by blunt dissection. Great care should be taken in raising the carotid sheath as the degree of elasticity of both vessels is reduced by their large number of branches.

Axillary Artery and Vein

These vessels are located in the region of armpit or axilla. The arm is placed at right angles to the supine body and forearm, twisted to allow the palm of the hand to face upward. Any rigor mortis in the limbs should be corrected by alternating flexion-extension movements and massage. Hair should be removed and the course of the median nerve which is almost medially situated should be ascertained by touch. An incision about 2 inches long should be made along the course of median nerve through the skin, commencing as near to the trunk of the body as possible. Clean the adipose tissue, and expose the axillary vein. The axillary artery lies lateral and little behind the vein, and median nerve lies medial to the vein.

Brachial Artery and Basilic Vein

The position of the body and limb should be identical to the ones used in exposing the axillary artery and vein. An incision about 2 inches long should be made in a depression in the upper arm between the biceps brachii and triceps brachii muscles. The incision should be made nearer the axilla. The chief guide to the position of the vessels is course of the median nerve. The median nerve and basilic vein are anterior and medial to the brachial artery.

Radial Artery

It is located at the wrist and used for counting the pulse. It is situated on the lateral side of the wrist in the depression between the tendons of the flexor carpi radialis and brachioradialis muscles. The vessel is quite superficial and situated at the lateral side of the wrist in an area about the width of two finger tips from the outer border of the thumb. It is accompanied by small venae comitantes which are impractical for drainage. The radial nerve accompanies the artery on the lateral side.

Femoral Artery and Vein

Femoral vessels are situated in the anteromedial aspect of the upper one-third of thigh in the femoral or Scarpa's triangle. The triangle is formed by inguinal ligament as a base, the sartorius muscle laterally and adductor longus muscle medially. The course of the vessels may be indicated by a line drawn from the midinguinal point to the adductor tubercle of femur. The upper one-third of the line represents the upper half of the artery in the femoral triangle. A vertical incision about 2.5 inches long should be made through the skin along the course of the vessels as indicated. The incision should be made as near the ligament as possible. The femoral vessels are deeply situated in the thigh and this is more so in the obese bodies and in the majority of females. The femoral artery, vein and nerve are usually situated side by side; the femoral artery slightly overlaps nerve and the vein. Care must be taken about the major branches of the artery, particularly profunda femoris.

EXPOSURE AND CANNULATION

Arteries carry blood from the heart to the tissues. They are thick walled, have no valves and are usually empty of blood after death, therefore are best suited to carry embalming fluid to the tissues. They are situated in the deeper plane and are well supported by connective tissue. They do not collapse when cut.

Veins are large and carry blood from the tissues to the heart. They are thin walled, provided with valves, and usually engorged with blood after death. They occur in two planes, subcutaneous and deep with interconnections. Veins are collapsed if empty of blood.

Give a suitable incision; retract the skin; remove the superficial fascia and fat; expose the structures to the same length as the incision; retract the muscles; and cut open the fascial sheath enclosing the vessels. The artery and vein should be isolated by blunt dissection and cleared for about 2 inches. The vessels are brought out separately by a blunt forceps. Ligatures are passed under the vessels, two for each one. To open the artery or vein, a scissor scalpel may be used. Incisions are made on the anterior wall of the vessels. Various types of incisions are used to open artery or vein (Fig. 9.1).

Transverse incision: Make a transverse cut from the edge of the vessel to its center.

Longitudinal incision: This incision is more suitable for vein, as it provides a large opening for the insertion of a drainage instrument.

Combined incision: Combination of transverse and longitudinal incision is preferred especially for opening the veins.

Wedge incision: A wedge can also be cut into an artery or vein. In case the artery is filled with clotted blood, empty it by pulling out the clot through the nick. Check the patency of these cannulae before insertion. The ligatures in relation to the vessels are drawn tight knotted to prevent the slipping out of the cannulae. The other ligature will be used to lift the vessel when needed. Suitable sized arterial and venous tubes can also be used in place of cannulae.

Blood is an excellent culture medium and decomposes rapidly with bacterial contamination. Removal of blood reduces the chance of incomplete preservation and post-embalming complications.

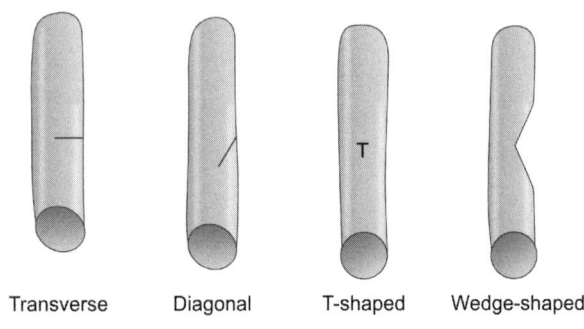

Fig. 9.1: Different incisions.

METHODS OF EMBALMING

Embalming consists of mainly two processes:
1. Arterial embalming
2. Cavity embalming.

Arterial Embalming

In this process, the arterial fluid is injected into the selected artery. Blood is drained simultaneously from the suitable vein to make room for preservative solution. The preservative fluid is distributed from the arch of the aorta and does not flow through the chambers of the heart as blood does in the living. Eventually, the embalming solution passes through the capillaries and enters the tissue spaces. Here it comes in contact with the body cells and changes the proteins colloidal nature by establishing many cross-linkages.

Cavity Embalming

In this process, the organs in the abdominal and thoracic cavities are treated with the preservative solution. The contents of the hollow organs and any liquids or gases that may have accumulated in the body cavities are removed by aspiration. A very strong preservative solution is injected by a trocar or long needle into the abdominal and thoracic cavities through the same openings.

Supplemental Methods of Embalming

These methods are generally used to preserve the local areas of the body that have not received arterial fluid or have received insufficient amounts of preservative fluids. These include:
1. Hypodermic embalming
2. Surface embalming.

Hypodermic Embalming

This method is used to preserve the small local body areas or large areas by subcutaneous injection of a suitable chemical. The solution may be an arterial fluid or cavity fluid and injected by hypodermic syringe and needle ranging from 8 gauge to 19 gauge and of varying lengths.

Surface Embalming

In this method, the local body areas are preserved by application of suitable chemical to the surface of the body. The chemical may be an arterial fluid or cavity fluid. In surface embalming, packs of cotton or gauze are soaked in a suitable chemical and applied to external raw skin areas, for example, burned tissues, bed sores, surface lesions—external or internal in case of autopsied body, within the mouth eyelids.

Hypodermic and surface embalming may be used as a primary method of embalming for the preservation of an infant, fetus, viscera or a mutilated portion of the body.

EMBALMING PROCEDURE

Arterial Embalming

There are several factors which determine the flow of fluid into the tissues. These are capillary resistance, chemical composition of the solution, injection pressure, osmosis, diffusion and gravity. The following methods are common in practice:

Gravity Injection

It is a traditional, simplest, safest and least expensive of the injection methods. It requires a graduated glass bottle or gravity bottle of the capacity of 10 liters with an outlet. The outlet is closed with a cork through which the glass tube is passed which is connected to the transparent rubber tubing with a screw clamp to control the rate of flow; the other end is attached to the cannula or injection needle or the other end of rubber tubing is connected to "T" connection which leads to two rubber tubings connected to two metal cannulae or injection needles separately. The embalming bottle is filled with the arterial fluid and is kept at a height of about 4–6 feet from the embalming table. A rise of one foot gives a fluid pressure of approximately one-half (0.43) pound. More than 6–7 feet of elevation is not practicable. By the pressure of gravity, the embalming fluid starts flowing. Sometimes the pressure is generated in the glass bottle by a simple cycle pump. It overcomes any temporary obstruction and increases the flow of the fluid.

This method is a substitute for mechanical injectors when they are not working or when there is an electrical power failure. This method is commonly practiced for embalming the bodies for dissection purposes in the departments of anatomy in medical schools. This method provides a slow steady and more thorough distribution of fluid. This method is time consuming and needs constant refilling of the bottle.

Electric Pump (Air Pressure Machine)

It is a simple device where pressure is generated to force fluid from an injection tank into the vascular system. Embalming fluid does not flow through the pump. The pump provides only air pressure. A flexible tube from the injection control on the pump is attached to an adopter in the neck of the glass jar containing arterial fluid. Connect a second flexible tube from the adopter to the arterial tube. When the motor is turned on, the pressure is set. The motor forces air into the bottle through one connection on the adopter and forces fluid out through the other connection. The pump provides steady and high pressure. It delivers about 8–10 liters of arterial fluid within 30–45 minutes. Very high pressure should not be used as it can rupture the arterial walls. This method ensures uniformly good embalming results.

Hypodermic Embalming

This method is used to treat small or large body areas that did not receive sufficient embalming fluid by arterial injection. This method is solely used when all arteries are highly atherosed or obstructed due to some reason and it is hard for the minimum diameter cannula or needle to pass through the vessel. In such cases, the whole body is to be embalmed by giving local injections. Hypodermic syringe and needle (ranging from 7 gauge to 19 gauge) is used to inject the embalming fluid locally at a distance of about 15 ems covering the entire body. The release of the embalming fluid should be gradual and from the deep to superficial tissues.

In hypodermic embalming of facial areas, most of the injections can be made from inside the mouth. It reduces the chance of leakage and spilling. The ear can be approached by hypodermic injection from behind the ear. The hands and fingers can be injected from the palmar aspect or from between the fingers.

Hypodermic embalming is a difficult procedure. Generally, embalming fluid gets spilled and formalin fumes irritate the eyes. It takes very long time. Viscera and brain are not properly fixed and embalming is not very effective. Therefore, it is not recommended for routine embalming but may have to be adopted in addition to basic two methods.

Chapter 10

Injection Technique

ML Ajmani

INTRODUCTION

Arteries are used for injection of embalming fluid because they do not have valves. In the unautopsied body, the ideal artery for injection is the largest artery the aorta, but because of its location, the vessel is rarely used in the adult. It is helpful in embalming children. The best choice for drainage is right atrium of the heart, but again, its location within the thoracic cavity makes it an impractical choice. If the use of aorta or right atrium of the heart is impractical then embalmer should select the vessel which should be as close as possible to both Ute aorta and the right atrium. Selection of a vessel as an injection and drainage site depends upon its size, location, position, depth, flexibility and proximity to the arch of the aorta or right atrium of the heart.

Embalming of the unautopsied body begins when the embalmer selects a suitable artery for injection. Various methods have been used for injection and drainage on the basis of pre-embalming considerations. These are described in this chapter.

INJECTION TECHNIQUES

One-point Injection

In this procedure, one site is used for both injection and drainage. The one-point sites are the common carotid artery and internal jugular vein, femoral artery and the femoral vein, the external iliac artery and the external iliac vein, and the axillary artery and the axillary vein. The femoral and the common carotid arteries are the most frequently used one-point injection sites. Most embalmers prefer this procedure because only one incision is required. Moreover, incision would not be seen after the preparation. Mostly right-sided vessels are used. Most embalmers, being right handed, find working on the right side of the body more convenient in pathological conditions; the veins and arteries on the left side can be used.

Split Injection

The injection is given in an artery at one site and the drainage occurs from a vein at another location. This method provides a more even distribution of the arterial fluid but requires two incisions and, therefore, requires more time for suturing and the preparation of vessels. The most frequently used combination of vessels in this method is the internal jugular vein (drainage) and the femoral artery (injection), the common carotid artery (injection) and the femoral vein (drainage), the axillary or subclavian artery (injection) and the internal jugular vein or the femoral vein (drainage).

Multipoint Injection

Any combination of two or more arteries for injection constitutes a multipoint injection on method. It is used after a one-point injection has failed to give satisfactory results. Multipoint injection may also be used in distal parts of the body where fluid fails to reach. This method ensures thorough distribution of fluid throughout the body and allows different fluid strengths to be used in different body regions. In multipoint procedure, several arterial combinations may be used to embalm the various body areas. Drainage is done from each injection site or from one drainage point. For example, if the left common carotid artery is injected and the left arm does not receive fluid, an additional injection can be given into the left axillary, brachial artery, radial artery or ulnar artery.

The multipoint injection is recommended in the following situations:
- When bodies exhibit poor fluid distribution after a one-point injection is completed
- When body areas do not receive arterial fluid
- When a body shows evidence of decomposition
- In bodies with generalized edema
- In bodies dead for long periods of time
- In autopsied bodies
- In bodies dead of highly contagious diseases.

Six-point Injection

In autopsied body, generally a six-point injection is used. Each body extremity is embalmed separately. In this procedure, six arteries are exposed—right and left common carotid arteries, right and left axillary or subclavian arteries, and right and left femoral or external iliac arteries. Drainage can be done from each injection site.

Restricted Cervical Injection

In restricted cervical procedure, the injection is given through both common carotid arteries so that the head, face and neck can be separately injected. It is recommended in bodies with facial trauma, bodies in which eye enucleation has been performed and bodies with distribution problems.

In this method, amount of arterial fluid entering the head and face can be controlled and simultaneously two fluid strengths can be used—one for the trunk and limbs, and another for the head, face and neck. It also allows to use different pressure and rates of flow to inject head and the trunk.

DRAINAGE TECHNIQUE

To obtain excellent embalming results, it is necessary to procure good drainage from all parts of the body. In embalming, the fluid passes from the arteries to the capillary bed and thence into the veins from which the excess of the injected fluid drains from the body. It has been estimated that after death, 85% of the blood is found in the capillaries, 10% in the veins, and 5% in the arteries. In fact, amount of blood in the vascular system varies depending on the cause and manner of death. It is emphasized that if there are parts of the body where the veins have been emptied of blood and other parts where they have not been emptied; the injected fluid will circulate through those parts where the veins have emptied their blood but will lie stagnant in those parts where the veins have not been emptied. As most of the people die in bed with their head elevated, therefore, most of the blood from the head and face has gravitated to more dependent parts before the body is received for embalming. Therefore, the veins of the head and face contain less blood than other parts of the body due to this gravitation; consequently head and face, as a rule, is the first part to indicate the effect of embalming. It is true that there will be less resistance to circulation in the head and face than in any other part of the body, and since fluid flows the path of least resistance, hence there will be larger amount of fluid circulating through the head and face than through any other part of the body. It is important to remember that the appearance of the face is the most important of the embalming results. If the face is over embalmed, there will be over dehydration of the tissues of this area with the tendency toward wrinkling and browning which is certainly not desirable. In fact, weight of the head constitutes about 6–8% of the weight of the entire body and for that reason only 6–8% of the entire volume of embalming fluid injected should circulate through the head.

Contents of Drainage

These are blood, blood clots, arterial fluid and tissue fluid. As the blood in the vascular system is gradually displaced and replaced with embalming fluid, the color of the draining fluid becomes lighter. The initial drainage from the bodies, where the cause of death was blood-borne infection (AIDS, hepatitis or sepsis), should be carefully collected and splashing should be avoided because the bacteria and microbial agents and their products which have entered the blood vascular system before or after death are also removed in the drainage.

The volume of drainage is not equal to the volume of embalming fluid. This is because, a large portion of the blood vascular system, particularly the arteries, remain empty at death. This entire area must be filled with fluid before the start of the drainage. It accounts for the delay between the injection and the start of the drainage.

In certain conditions, there is little to drain, e.g. in esophageal varices and ruptured ulcerations of the gastrointestinal tract in which blood is collected into the lumen of the intestines. Traumatic death may result in loss of large volume of blood outside the body, accidental death may result in the rupture of internal organs leading to collection of blood into the abdominal cavity. It should be noted that if the blood is collected in the digestive tract or abdominal cavity, there will be a gradual swelling of the abdomen as the fluid is injected indicating of accumulation of drainage in the digestive tract or abdominal cavity. This accumulation can be removed with a trocar by aspiration.

Good drainage can be expected only when the interval between the death and embalming is short.

Purpose of Drainage

Fluid is drained for many reasons:
- The main purpose of drainage is to make room for the arterial fluid so that it can be evenly distributed to all tissues of the body with a minimum distension.
- Blood is a liquid tissue that rapidly decomposes after death and results in discoloration, odors and formation of gas. Drainage removes the liquid tissue and prevents decomposition.
- Translocation of the microbes is greatly increased after death. Removal of blood by drainage helps to reduce microbial agents in the body.

Drainage Sites

To procure thorough embalming results, selection of a vein is more important than an artery. Any vein can be used for drainage whether it is large or small, superficial or deep or on the right or left side of the body. In the unautopsied body, the veins commonly used for drainage are the internal jugular, the femoral, and the external iliac. Axillary and basilic veins can be used but for their small size, it is rather impracticable.

Internal Jugular Vein

It is the largest systemic vein which can be used in unautopsied body. The right internal jugular vein leads directly into the right atrium. This is why the right and not the left internal jugular vein is frequently used for drainage. The internal jugular vein is very large and assists direct drainage from the face and head. It is accompanied by the common carotid artery which can be used for injection; therefore, only one incision is necessary for both injection and drainage. Because of the above reasons, it is one of the best possible sites for drainage during arterial injection.

The superior vena cava returns blood from the head, face, neck and upper limb to the right atrium of the heart. The inferior vena cava returns blood from the visceral organs, trunk and lower extremities. After death, blood in the right atrium frequently coagulates. Under such condition, drainage from the right internal jugular is not possible until the coagulum is fragmented. This is done by an angular forceps. It is directly placed into the right atrium and attempt is made to fragment the coagulum.

Femoral Vein

The femoral vein can also be used as a drainage point. The vein is large, easily accessible and because of its location the incision is not visible. It is also assisted by gravity in draining blood from the body. The chief advantage of draining from the femoral vein rather than the internal jugular vein is that only one incision is necessary for both injection and drainage, if femoral artery is selected for arterial injection.

In normal nonautopsied bodies, internal jugular vein is used for drainage and femoral artery for arterial injection. Injection of the femoral would produce a more even distribution of fluid than injection of the carotid. Drainage from the internal jugular vein would give the quickest clearing of the face.

Right Atrium of the Heart

In difficult cases, the right atrium of the heart can be directly drained using a trocar. To drain directly from the right atrium of the heart, inject approximately 2-4 liters of embalming solution to fill the vascular system. To drain from the right side of the heart, the trocar is inserted through the abdominal wall, 2.5 cm to the left and 5 cm above the umbilicus. Draw an imaginary line across the body connecting the left anterior superior iliac spine and the lobule of the right ear. Direct the trocar toward a point where this line crosses the right side of the sternum. This point is approximately at the level where the fourth rib joins the sternum. Drainage starts as soon as the trocar enters the right atrium of the heart.

Inferior Vena Cava

It is used for drainage when autopsy has been performed. The abdominal walls, viscera and the lower limbs can be injected through the abdominal aorta or femoral or external iliac arteries and drainage can be done directly from the remnants of the inferior vena cava. The thoracic walls, viscera, head, neck, face and upper limbs can be injected through the descending aorta or carotid arteries (by damping off the aorta) and the drainage can easily be taken directly from the remnants of the inferior vena cava.

Methods of Drainage

For drainage, an injection with a fluid containing 2% formalin is recommended. The following methods of drainage have been used in relation to injection:

Alternate Drainage

In this method, injection and drainage are alternated until the embalming is completed. The arterial fluid is never injected while drainage is being done. By this method, more thorough distribution of arterial fluid is achieved but the method is time consuming.

Concurrent (Continuous) Drainage

In this method, injection and drainage are allowed to proceed at the same time throughout the embalming. Though this method is less time consuming, but the distribution of the arterial fluid is not complete.

Intermittent Drainage

This method is considered a compromise between the alternate and concurrent methods. In this method, the injection continues throughout the embalming and drainage is stopped for definite period. This method is less time consuming than the alternate method and assists in thorough distribution of the arterial fluid.

Chapter 11

Cavity Embalming

ML Ajmani

NEED OF CAVITY TREATMENT

When the injection treatment has been completed, it is necessary to aspirate the contents of the hollow organs and also body fluids in the trunk cavities. If the cavity treatment is not done, the continued activity of the bacterial flora, already existing in the viscera, will promote putrefaction and ultimately cause failure of the embalming.

Cavity treatment is independent of arterial embalming and demands equal attention for a satisfactory preservation. There are situations in which arterial embalming is not possible. Cavity embalming along with hypodermic and surface embalming would be the chief methods of preserving the remains. These cases include badly burnt and badly decomposed bodies. The cavity treatment is done after a little time gap, after the injection treatment is completed. It will allow the viscera to become hard for further treatment and piercing the viscera with a trocar will be easier if it is not flabby.

Cavity embalming is not a visible process. It is normally a two-step process—(1) aspiration of the cavities and their contents; and (2) injection of a strong preservative chemical. Cavity embalming treats, the contents of the hollow viscera, the walls of the visceral organs which are not embalmed by arterial embalming and the contents of the spaces between the visceral organs. In arterial embalming, it is difficult to determine the level of embalming of the visceral organs. The embalmer cannot see the internal organs for signs of arterial fluid distribution. Therefore, cavity embalming serves to ensure that the walls of the viscera, parenchyma of the solid organs and the contents of the spaces are well preserved. The organs which can be treated by cavity embalming are the spleen, liver, pancreas, kidney, brain and lungs.

INSTRUMENTS REQUIRED FOR CAVITY EMBALMING

- Scalpel
- Electric aspirator
- Rubber tube
- Receptacle jar
- Cavity injector or any other injection device or a simple 100 mL syringe. It is connected with tubing to the trocar to inject the preservative chemicals or disinfectant.
- Needle and ligature.

Pointed trocar: It is a long hollow needle with a removable sharp point. The trocar is attached to the suction device. The trocar is used to withdraw the contents of the organs and residual fluid in the cavities. It is also used to introduce the preservative solution into the internal organs. For an adult body, a 45-cm long, 5/16-inch bore trocar is used. The infant trocar is approximately 30 cm long and about 1/4 inch in diameter.

ABDOMINAL REGIONS TO LOCATE THE INTERNAL ORGANS

The embalmer should have a thorough knowledge of the location of the visceral organs in the body. This understanding is important in the process of cavity embalming. For the location of viscera in clinical practice and cavity embalming, the abdomen is divided into nine regions by two horizontal and two parasagittal or vertical imaginary planes. The upper horizontal, transpyloric plane is indicated by a line encircling the body midway between the suprasternal notch and the pubic symphysis or midway between umbilicus and inferior end of the sternal body or a hand's breadth below the xiphisternal joint; it intersects the lower border of first lumbar vertebra and meets the costal margins at the tips of the ninth costal cartilages. The lower horizontal, transtubercular plane intersects the upper border of the body of fifth lumbar vertebra and intersects the tubercles on the iliac crests. The abdomen is thus divided into three arbitrary zones; each is further subdivided into three by the right and left lateral planes, indicated on the surface by vertical lines through points midway between the anterior superior iliac spines and the symphysis pubis (these lines are also called "midclavicular or mammary" lines) (Fig. 11.1 and Box 11.1).

INSERTION OF THE TROCAR

The topographical system of dividing the abdomen into nine regions gives the embalmer an approximate location of the various abdominal organs. The standard point of trocar entry is located 2 inches to the left and 2 inches superior to the umbilicus. The embalmer can reach all areas of the thoracic, abdominal, and pelvic cavities through this point. The pointed end of the trocar is inserted into the abdomen and kept close to the anterior abdominal wall until the specific organ is reached. The common entry point can be used to aspirate the hollow viscera such as the stomach, heart, urinary bladder, and cecum (Fig. 11.2).

Right side of the heart: Move the trocar along a line from the left anterior superior iliac spine and the right ear lobule.

Stomach: Direct the trocar point toward the intersection of the fifth intercostal space and the left mid-axillary line until the trocar enters the stomach.

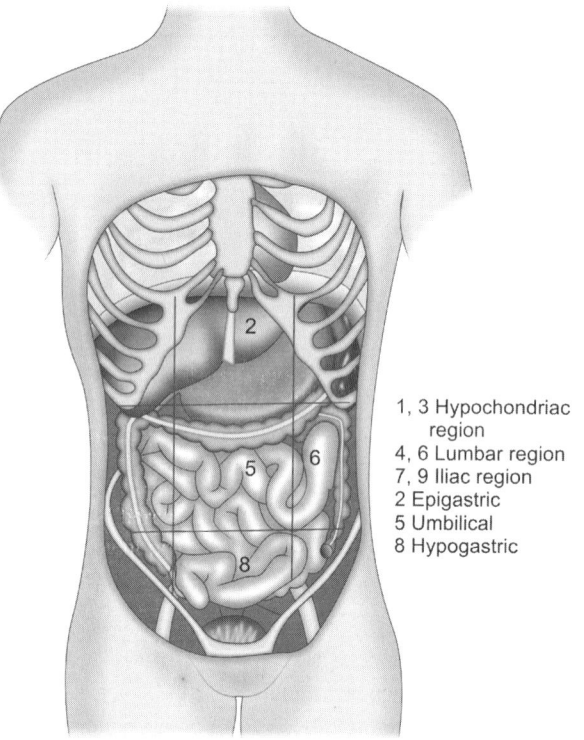

Fig. 11.1: The nine regions in the abdomen.

1, 3 Hypochondriac region
4, 6 Lumbar region
7, 9 Iliac region
2 Epigastric
5 Umbilical
8 Hypogastric

Cecum: The trocar is directed to a point three-fourth of the distance on a line from the pubic symphysis to the right anterior superior iliac spine. When the point of the trocar is approximately 5 cm from the line, the point is depressed 5 cm and then thrust forward to pierce the cecum. In this

Box 11.1: Nine abdominal regions.

Right hypochondriac	Epigastric	Left hypochondriac
Part of the liver, Gallbladder, Part of right kidney, Greater omentum, Coils of small intestine	Part of the liver, Stomach including cardiac and pyloric openings, Duodenum pancreas, Parts of kidneys and suprarenal glands, Greater omentum	Part of the liver, Stomach fundus and cardiac region, Spleen, Tail of pancreas, Left colic flexure, Part of left kidney, Greater omentum
Right lumbar	Umbilicus	Left lumbar
Lower part of the liver, Ascending colon, Right colic flexure, Part of the right kidney, Coils of small intestine, Greater omentum	Transverse colon, Coils of small intestine, Part of both kidneys, Greater omentum, Bifurcation of abdominal aorta and inferior vena cava	Descending colon, Coils of small intestine, Part of left kidney, Greater omentum
Right iliac	Hypogastric	Left iliac
Cecum and appendix, Ascending colon, Coils of small intestine, Greater omentum	Coils of small intestine, Greater omentum, Bladder in adults if distended, Uterus during pregnancy	Part of descending colon, Sigmoid colon, Coils of small intestine, Greater omentum

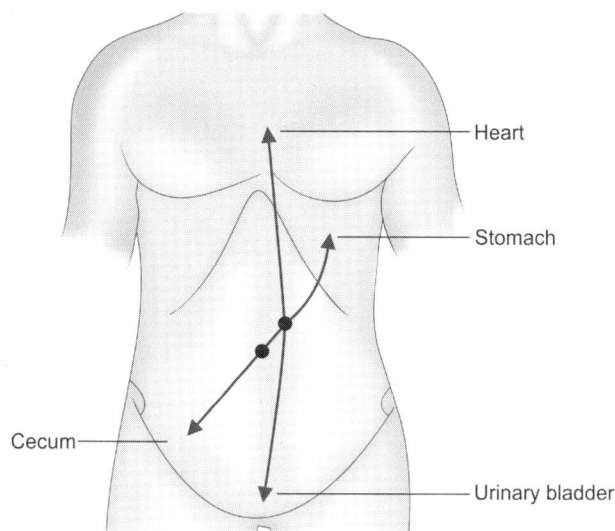

Fig. 11.2: Trocar guides.

position, the cecum is trapped between the pelvis and trocar.

Urinary bladder: The trocar is directed towards the pubic symphysis in the median plane until it touches the bone. Retract the trocar slightly, depress the point slightly, and insert into the urinary bladder.

THE PERIOD FOR CAVITY EMBALMING

The cavity treatment can be given immediately following arterial injection or it can be delayed for several hours. It is suggested that the long time delay, for period of 8–10 hours, will allow the arterial fluid to penetrate into the tissue spaces and help in preserving the walls of the visceral organs. This will then make the work easier to pierce with the trocar when the aspiration is done.

Aspiration of the Thoracic Cavity

Insert the trocar along the imaginary line running from the left anterior superior iliac spine to the lobule of the right ear to aspirate the right side of the heart. Next aspirate the anterior parts of the pleural cavities and lungs. Finally the trocar is directed to either side of the vertebral·column to reach the hilum of the lungs and aspirate the great blood vessels at the root of the bronchial tree leading to trachea.

Aspiration of the Abdominal Cavity

Follow the trocar guide and move the trocar toward a point at the intersection of the fifth intercostal space and left midaxillary line. As the trocar moves toward this point, it should pierce the stomach. Several openings are made through the stomach wall. Aspiration removes the contents of the viscera and also pierces the viscera so that fluid can better penetrate the organs. Next the trocar is withdrawn and moved into the abdomen to make several punctures in the small intestine, large intestine and liver. Cecum and urinary bladder can be aspirated by using the trocar guide as mentioned earlier. Similarly, aspirate the entire abdominal cavity by "fanning" movements (moving the needle in different direction). The trocar is now directed towards the pelvis to make passages in the urinary bladder, the sigmoid colon and the rectum.

Aspiration of the Cranial Cavity

A trocar is introduced into the nostril and pushed through the cribriform plate of the ethmoid bone. The instrument enters the anterior cranial fossa. After aspiration, inject a few ounces of concentrated cavity fluid. After injection, tightly pack the nostril with cotton to prevent leakage.

Some embalmers routinely aspirate and inject the cranial cavity in every case. There is a rich arterial supply to the brain through both the internal carotid arteries and the vertebral arteries. These routes supply sufficient arterial fluid to the brain and even to the cerebrospinal fluids.

At certain occasions such as gunshot wound or recent cranial surgery, aspiration and injection of cavity fluid into the cranial cavity is necessary to prevent the decomposition.

The stillborn or infant brain can decompose very rapidly. In the preparation of such cases, it is necessary to inject the cavity fluid into the cranial cavity with a hypodermic needle.

Injection of Cavity Fluid

After the complete aspiration, the preservative fluid is injected within the cavities and over the viscera. Concentrated cavity fluid is always used because the high moisture content of the viscera, and some residual blood and lymph can dilute it. In cases of hydrothorax and ascites, the fluids—blood and edema further dilute the cavity fluid.

The volume of the fluid is determined by the size of tissues to be treated, which is estimated on the basis of body size and weight. On an average, for a body weighing 70 kg, one liter of cavity fluid is used for each (thoracic and abdominal) cavity. Smaller bodies require less while larger bodies may require more fluid.

The cavity fluid is injected either by 100 mL syringe or lumbar puncture needle, and trocar and cannula may be used for aspiration. The fluid is first sprayed over the anterior surface of the viscera close to the anterior wall of the thoracic and abdominal cavities. The cavity fluid gradually gravitates through the openings in the viscera and is absorbed there.

Cavity fluid is also used to detoxicate those materials that cannot be aspirated through the trocar and thus to assist in the preservation of the viscera. After completion of the cavity treatment, the opening in the body wall is closed. Two sutures are commonly used to close the trocar opening. Nylon thread is commonly used for this purpose. Wound is firmly closed to prevent leak and soiling in the post-embalming period.

Chapter 12

Embalming the Unautopsied Adult Bodies

ML Ajmani

PROCESS OF EMBALMING

A factor that must always be remembered in pre-embalming analysis of a body is age of the cadaver. Other factors are time between death and embalming procedure, progress of decomposition, weight, autopsy, condition of blood vascular system, disease process, trauma, and time between embalming and disposal.

The embalming process begins when the body is transferred on the embalming table. Remove all clothing from the body and check for any valuables. If rings, jewelry, watches, or religious articles are present, make a list and return to the family. Soiled clothing and all contaminated bedding should either be destroyed or stored in a plastic bag.

Disinfect the body with a topical disinfectant solution or spray. The surface disinfectant should be allowed to remain on the body for 15–30 minutes. After topical disinfection, wash the body surface with lukewarm water and a germicidal soap. After thorough washing, the body should be dried with a towel. If the deceased had hepatitis or AIDS infection, add sodium hypochlorite (household bleach) in the washing solution. It is better to use routinely the sodium hypochlorite in the washing of all bodies.

Wash the hair with warm water and a good germicidal soap. Dry the hair and comb it in a life like style. The hair can be washed at the beginning or at the end of the embalming.

The embalmer should ask the family members about moustache or beard pattern on a deceased male. Remove the moustache or beard before the arterial injection, if it has grown excessively. It is easier to remove a moustache or beard before the arterial fluid injection than after the embalming. After shaving, wash the face and apply a thin layer of massage cream. Apply a light coating of massage cream over the neck, hands, and feet. Massage cream protects the face from dehydration, provides a base for cosmetics, and acts as a lubricant.

The position of the body on the embalming table should appear comfortable and restful before the start of the arterial injection. The arterial fluid coagulates and firms the body proteins of the muscles in the position in which the body is placed prior to arterial embalming. Therefore, it is very difficult to repose the body after embalming.

Rigor mortis, if present, may be responsible for any undesirable position of the body. Remove the rigor mortis by firmly manipulating the limbs and muscles. Head, neck, and limbs are flexed, extended, rotated, and massaged to relieve rigor mortis. Repeat this several times. Relief of the rigor mortis results in better arterial fluid distribution and also better drainage. Avoid excessive exercise of the muscles. It can rupture the capillaries and can lead to swelling during arterial injection.

Frozen Cases

It is impossible to embalm the body that is frozen solid. The most effective treatment is to slowly raise the temperature of the tissues by hosing the body with cold water, and wrap blankets soaked in cold water around it or by directing a cool air fan toward the body. When tissues become pliable but still chilled, an arterial injection of embalming fluid can be given at low pressure. In all such cases, there is possibility that frozen deep tissue may not receive adequate embalming fluid. Embalming should not be carried out, if the tissues are not pliable. The use of warm water will cause unequal thawing of the tissues and damage the structure of the skin.

The body should be placed in a supine position on the middle of the embalming table. The elbows should be elevated off the embalming table with a wooden block and the hands should be placed on the lower abdominal wall. An adhesive may be used in keeping the fingers together. The upper limbs may be positioned by the side of the body.

The eyes, nose, and mouth should be cleaned with a mild disinfectant. It should be stressed that the disinfectant used must be mild and not cause any shrinkage of the delicate tissues of the lips and eyelids. The mouth and eyelids should be temporarily closed, as it will be necessary to reopen them on completion of the injection treatment. Failure to close the mouth and eyes may alter the normal appearance of deceased. The action of the embalming fluid is to fix the tissues in the position in which they have been set. If the mouth be left open until completion of the injection, the mouth will wrinkle or bulge outwards when the mouth is finally closed. Failure to close the eyes may result in persistent opening of the lids, which is not desirable.

The expression of the deceased can be one of the most criticized areas of the embalming. Normal muscle tone is lost after death and facial features, which are expressive of an individual, are also lost. To obtain good results, features are set in the pre-embalming period. After the embalming, it may be difficult to align the tissues to obtain the desired expression. The mouth should be closed before embalming. The process involves the raising the mandible and bringing lips into contact to create a pleasant and acceptable appearance. The mouth can be reopened after embalming and checked for fluid leakage into the mouth during injection or purge material and then reclose. The closing of the mouth can be done by the following methods:

- *Needle injector method*: Needle injector resembles an ordinary hypodermic syringe and fits the hand just like a syringe. However, instead of thumb, the two fingers draw the plunger up when operating the needle injector. In this method, a needle injector is used to push a wire into the center of the maxilla, and a similar pin with a wire attached is pushed into the mandible in an opposing position. The two wires are then twisted together to hold the mandible in position. It is a widely used method in the west (Fig. 12.1).
- *Dental tie method*: A strong thread is tied around the base of one tooth in the upper jaw and one tooth in the lower jaw. The ends of the two strings are tied together pulling the jaw in position. Upper and lower incisor teeth are generally used, but any of the front teeth can be utilized.
- *Chin rest method*: The mandible is supported in a closed position with a chin rest. After the embalming, the device is removed.

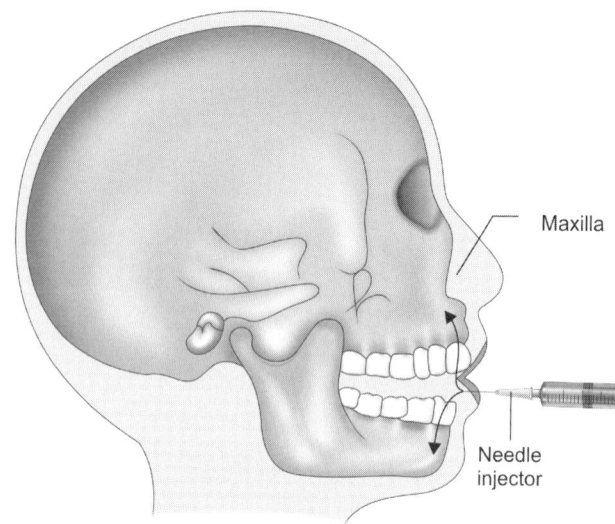

Fig. 12.1: Needle injector method.

- *Close mouth*: The mouth is closed by suturing the lips. Sutures are passed through the lip muscle from within the vestibule of the mouth and the free ends are tied together with the jaws brought together.
- *Gluing the lips*: This method of mouth closure is used in infants and children. It is not recommended for adults. The lips are approximated and sealed prior to arterial injection. After the embalming, the lips can be reopened and checked for any purged material and resealed.

In closing the mouth, attention should be paid to the position of the lips. If there is a denture then closure may be difficult. Place some cotton on the tongue and it helps to hold the dentures in position. When natural teeth are present, place some cotton over the molar teeth to fill out the posterior area of the cheek. Cotton can be used to fill in the missing teeth.

Close Eye Method

The eyes are generally closed prior to arterial injection. Failure to close the eyes may result in persistent opening of the lids. The procedure for eye closure is as follow:

- The eyes are cleaned with moist cotton and disinfected with a topical disinfectant. Cotton wool pads are inserted under the eyelids and the lids are manipulated into a closed position. Lift the upper eyelid and insert the cotton wool under the lid with a forceps. Evert the lower eyelid and insert the cotton behind the lid in the lower fornix. Many embalmers use eyecaps instead

of cotton wool. It is a plastic or metal disk generally perforated and convex in shape. It helps to maintain the convex curvature of the closed eye.
- In establishing the line of eye closure, keep this point in mind that upper eyelid should cover approximately upper two-thirds of the eyeball.

Ears, Throat, and Nasal Cavity

The nasal cavity, throat, and ears should be packed with cotton prior to embalming. If purge develops, all soiled packing should be removed and replaced with dry packing after the body has been embalmed. After arterial and cavity embalming, the vaginal and anal orifices should be tightly packed with cotton saturated with cavity fluid.

Selection of Vessel

The size of the artery, its accessibility, and the possibility of drainage from the accompanying vein are the major factors in selecting an artery for injection. In addition, second group of factors that must be considered in selection of vessel for injection are the age of the body, weight of the body, and the effects of disease. In the unautopsied adult body, the choice is among the common carotid artery, the femoral (external iliac) artery, and the axillary (brachial) artery. Actually, any artery could be used for injection, but the larger arteries such as common carotid and the femoral allow for use of the higher pressure and faster rates of flow, which is necessary for uniform distribution of the arterial fluid.

In the embalming of the normal adult body, the first choice of vessel is "one-point" injection and drainage site, i.e. right common carotid artery and right internal jugular vein or right femoral artery and right femoral vein. In this method, only one incision is required. At death, some blood remains in the arteries, especially in the aorta. After death, this blood can congeal. Arterial injection can loosen and push the coagula into the smaller arteries. If the common carotid arteries are used for injection treatment, this coagula would move toward the legs into the iliac and femoral arteries. In such cases, the femoral arteries can be exposed to embalm the legs or the legs can be treated by hypodermic embalming. On the other hand, if the femoral artery is used for arterial injection, coagula can be moved into the common carotid and stop the flow of fluid into the head and neck region, which is not desirable. If the coagula have moved into the subclavian arteries, expose the axillary or brachial arteries.

Venous coagula does not pose as serious problem as arterial coagula. Venous coagula can block a vein and lead to tissue distension. When this condition occurs in a localized area, massage from distal points toward the heart can dislodge the coagula. Intermittent drainage also helps to increase venous pressure and dislodge coagula from the veins. If the internal jugular vein is used for drainage, coagula can move into the right atrium from where it can be easily removed with an angular spring forceps.

Some embalmers believe that it is better to inject the femoral artery and drain from the internal jugular vein rather than inject the femoral artery and drain from the femoral vein, or inject the common carotid artery and drain from internal jugular vein. In fact, the appearance of the face is the most important of the embalming results. For this reason, drainage from the internal jugular vein would give quickest clearing of the face and it is also believed that the injection of the femoral artery would produce a more even distribution of the embalming fluid than injection of the common carotid arteries.

In obese bodies, the femoral artery is quite deep and difficult to use for arterial injection. Moreover, in obese body, large quantity of embalming fluid is needed to preserve the body. The best choice to embalm the obese body is to expose the common carotid artery and use the internal jugular vein for drainage. This allows the use of higher injection pressure and faster rates of flow. In this manner, large volume of embalming fluid can be injected.

In thin bodies, after considering all the factors, use of the femoral vessels might prove to be the best approach for embalming.

In the elderly person, many times the femoral artery is found to be sclerotic but the common carotid artery rarely exhibits the condition of arteriosclerosis.

Clotting may be suspected in bodies that have been dead for long periods. In such cases, femoral artery should not be used because the clots would be pushed up into the common carotid arteries and the axillary arteries. The best choice is to expose the common carotid artery in such situations.

Injection and Drainage

After selecting the injection site, locate the vessels by the anatomical guide on the surface of the skin. After locating the vessels on the skin surface, make the incision and use blunt dissection to find the vessels. It is well to remember that in the dissection for the vessels, muscles do not have to be cut because arteries, veins, and nerves run in groups between the muscles. The only muscle that may have to be divided for locating vessels is the sternocleidomastoid. Elevate the vessels to the skin surface and give a wedge or "T"-shaped incision on the anterior wall of the vessel. To open the artery or vein, a scissor or scalpel may be used.

Insert the cannulae for arterial fluid injection as well as a drainage device into a selected vein for drainage. Ligate the cannulae at their position. Patency of these cannulae should be checked before insertion. Injection may then be started and continued until the tissues have been emptied of their blood content and are saturated with arterial injection. The pressure and the rate of flow for the injection are determined by the case analysis. If the vessel chosen for arterial injection is patent and regular flow starts, the external elasticity of the skin will go off and the head and face will start getting fixed. The fluid oozes out from nose, mouth, and other orifices. These should be plugged with cotton. The head end may be lowered if need be and so should be the foot end to ensure that the fluid reaches the peripheral parts. Often, no problem is experienced in embalming head and face since the arteries supplying these regions are relatively large. But the hands and feet do suffer. In these cases, the arterial injection is supplemented with hypodermic injection.

Flexing of limbs, changing the position of the body, and massaging intermittently during the procedure enhance the perfusion. Special attention should be paid to areas like the back and distal parts of the limbs. Judging the adequacy of perfusion is a matter of experience. Leakage of embalming fluid does not signify that the entire body is perfused. Each part should be assessed separately by inspection, touching, and tapping. The progress of the injection should be carefully monitored. There is always danger of overfilling tissues and causing swelling, and for this reason, embalmer must continuously observe and be present while injection is in progress.

Local injections are given in the palm, sole, and dorsum of hand and foot till there is rounding up of tips of fingers and toes. Normally, these areas are not completely perfused even on using the gravity or electric pump method because of the hands and feet being the most peripheral parts.

The ideal method of embalming is to puncture the vein or venae comitantes accompanying the selected artery for embalming. A drainage tube is inserted through a nick into the vein and tied in the position. Drain out the blood and flush it with saline solution or weak formalin solution. Then, the embalming fluid should be injected in a routine manner. Though this is the proper method of embalming, yet it takes very long time and may sometime be impractical especially when the body has to be transported immediately.

Reasons for Venous Drainage

When the embalming fluid is injected under pressure into the arteries, the existing blood in the capillaries gets displaced into the already engorged veins and exerts a back pressure thus preventing further entry of embalming fluid. To release the pressure of blood in the veins and to accommodate the embalming fluid, blood has to be drained from the veins.

Aspiration: Aspirate the body cavities and inject the cavity fluid via the trocar. The amount and strength of the fluid vary from body to body. For an average adult body, 2 liters is generally an adequate amount. 1 liter is injected into the thoracic cavity and 1 liter into the abdominal area. After cavity treatment, close the opening in the abdominal wall by suture.

After the completion of the arterial injection, remove the arterial cannula and drainage device. All vessels are securely tied to prevent further leakage. Do not suture the incision until cavity aspiration is done satisfactorily. It relieves pressure on the vascular system and prevents leakage. Dry the incision with cotton and tightly close all sutures.

Cotton or linen thread is used as suturing material. Linen thread is stronger than cotton thread and is recommended for autopsy and vessel incision sutures. A 3/8 inch circle needle is used to suture incisions. The double-curved autopsy needle is used to close autopsy incisions.

Wash the body and dry it thoroughly: Check the mouth for any purge material. If there has been purge in the oral cavity, the existing cotton should be replaced with dry cotton. Now, the mouth and eyes can be closed. The anal and vaginal orifices should be packed with cotton saturated with cavity fluid.

Cosmetic Treatment

The body is now ready for cosmetic treatment and dressing.

Placement of Hands

After embalming hands should be placed on the lower abdomen resting one on top of another or according to the religious dictates. An adhesive may be used in keeping fingers together.

Long Display

If an embalmed body has to be kept exposed for long periods before transportation or final rites, dehydration can be checked by:
- Packing the body in a polythene bag and sealing the ends
- Wrapping the body with bandage soaked in petroleum jelly.

Chapter 13

Preparation of Autopsied Bodies

ML Ajmani

EMBALMING AUTOPSIED BODY

An autopsy is a postmortem examination of the dead body. There are two types of autopsy: (1) the medical (hospital) autopsy and (2) the medicolegal (forensic) autopsy.

The medical autopsy is performed with the permission from the family member who has the authority to take charge of the body after death. Several reasons have been put forward in the performance of the hospital autopsy such as:
- To confirm the diagnosis.
- If death follows the use of an experimental drug or device or a new procedure.
- When environmental or workplace hazards are suspected.

The forensic autopsy is performed to ascertain the cause of death and the manner of death. The following cases should be reported to the forensic expert for medicolegal examination:
- Road side accidents, factory accidents or any other unnatural mishaps.
- Suspected or evident homicides or suicides.
- Suspected or evident poisoning.
- Burn injuries due to any cause.
- Suspected or evident criminal abortions regardless of the length of pregnancy.
- Any fetal death or death of a baby within 24 hours of birth, where mother has not been under the supervision of a physician.
- Unidentified or unclaimed bodies.
- All operative deaths where the death is not explainable on the basis of prior disease.

The forensic autopsy involves the opening of the following cavities and removal of the following organs:
- Cranial cavity and removal of brain and pituitary gland.
- Removal of spinal cord.
- Removal of thyroid gland, larynx, cervical portion of trachea, and esophagus.
- Thoracic cavity and removal of its contents.
- Abdominal cavity and removal of its contents.
- Pelvic cavity and removal of its contents.

Preparation

The initial preparation of the autopsied body is similar to that of the non-autopsied one, but because of the difference in embalming technique, more detailed attention is required.

On the receipt of the body embalmer should wear a suitable apron, disposable skull cap, mask, gloves and shoe covering. All the instruments should be sterilized prior to use to prevent cross infection from body to body.
- The body is placed on the embalming table and remove all clothing and store it in a plastic bag. Remove all surgical dressing if present; wash the body surface with water and soapy solution. If the deceased had hepatitis or HIV infection, add sodium hypochlorite (household bleach) to this washing solution. It is advisable to use sodium hypochlorite routinely in the washing of all bodies. If there is rigor mortis, relieve it by flexing, bending and rotating the body; clean all the body orifices with mild disinfectant solution. Remove the stitches and expose the cranial, thoracic, and abdominal cavities. Spray the cavities with some disinfectant solution.
- Remove the detached calvaria. Remove padding, if placed during medicolegal examination, and brain from the cranial cavity and place in plastic bag for incineration. Swab the cranial cavity with disinfectant solution especially in cases of systemic infection (AIDS, meningitis, and hepatitis).

- All the viscera which have been examined at the autopsy, if are to be returned, should be washed in a cavity fluid and placed in a plastic viscera bag.
- Remove the gut along with its mesentery and place it in plastic viscera bag. If the contents of hollow viscera have been leaked in the trunk cavities, aspiration should be done. The gut can be dangerous and requires special care in handling and washing in 5% phenol or cavity fluid.
- Any blood or liquid contents lying in the trunk cavities should be removed and treated with the cavity fluid prior to disposal. The cavities are washed out with disinfectant solution.
- Add about 500 mL of cavity fluid to the contents of the viscera bag.
- *Preparation of the arterial fluid*: There is always delay between the death and autopsy and between autopsy and release of the body. During this time of delay body is usually refrigerated. There is no fixed volume of fluid or strength to embalm such bodies. Generally a slightly stronger arterial solution is recommended to embalm such bodies. Factors determining the strength of the solution are:
  – Cause of death
  – Size and weight of the body
  – Presence of changes due to decomposition
  – Time between death and preparation
  – Refrigeration.
- *Drainage* with the autopsied body, drainage can be done directly from the cut in vein and the drainage material can flow directly into the body cavities from where it can be aspirated. Intermittent and alternate drainage greatly assist the distribution of the fluid.
- Injection treatment of the head and face is carried out through common carotid, or external and internal carotid arteries. If any of the big vessels or its branches are cut during autopsy, these must be clamped at the cut end and then arterial injection given. After head injection it is essential to "compose" the features and ensures that the fluid does set the tissues in a natural state.

During this operation it is necessary to protect the face from contact with the embalming fluid and prevent dehydration and distortion. Nasal and oral cavities are disinfected with embalming fluid. Nostrils are plugged with a wad of cotton soaked in solution. The cheek may be filled out with cotton soaked in the fluid. The mouth should be closed by needle injector wires or sutures.

Clean the area around the eyes. The position of the eyelids demands special attention to ensure a natural appearance. The eyelids are closed in a manner that the both lids should meet together with the upper eyelid covering approximately two-thirds of the eyeball.

If the eyes have been enucleated, pack the orbit with cotton soaked in the fluid and close the eyelids in a manner that it should give life like appearance.

Apply massage cream to face. The purpose of this is:
- It is a good cleaning agent
- It prevents surface drying, and
- It serves as a base for subsequent cosmetic treatment.

It is well to remember that the features should be composed as far as possible in an autopsied case.

- *Injection treatment of the upper extremities*: If the brachiocephalic trunk is intact, cut it distal to the right common carotid artery and thus clean out the right subclavian artery. The cut end of the left subclavian artery can be located as well. The injection is then given through the subclavian arteries. If there is a flow of blood from the cut ends of the subclavian veins, these should be clamped off. If the venous system of the extremity is distended, cease the injection and release the vein clamp. All blood should be gently massaged from the arm, and thus relieve the venous pressure. Re-apply the vein clamp and repeat procedure until the tissues become saturated with the embalming fluid without causing swelling. The axillary artery can be used by cutting the pectoralis major and minor muscles. It is exposed just as it leaves the cervicoaxillary canal. At this point all its branches can be used to distribute fluid to the trunk walls and shoulder region. Use of the axillary artery avoids many of the leakage problems seen with the subclavian artery.

Drainage can be done from the subclavian vein.

If fluid is not flowing into the hand, lower the hand while injecting, massage the limbs along the arterial route (axillary, brachial, radial, and ulnar arteries), use intermittent drainage, and increase the injection pressure. If above methods are not effective expose the radial and ulnar arteries for injection. If fluid still does not enter the fingers, use hypodermic injection.

- *Injection treatment of lower extremities*: Injection technique is similar to that of upper extremity. Injection is made through the common iliac arteries with clamp on the common iliac veins and severed branches of the internal iliac artery (the vessels were severed when pelvic organs were removed during autopsy). If common iliac arteries have been removed, use external iliac artery to inject each limb. If necessary, expose the femoral artery to inject the lower extremities. The embalming fluid reaches the gluteal region, anal area, and perianal tissues through the branches of internal iliac artery.

If fluid is not flowing into the foot, massage the limb and push strongly along the arterial route (femoral, popliteal, anterior and posterior tibial arteries), use intermittent drainage technique, increase injection pressure similar to the upper extremity. If there are still areas of soft consistency they must be embalmed by hypodermic injection of a preservative fluid. Areas of local putrefaction may require a special local injection of highly concentrated fluid.

- When the injections are completed and all the fluid contents of the trunk cavities have been aspirated, the internal surfaces of the cavities are treated with a sponge soaked in cavity fluid. Absorbent cotton wool soaked in cavity fluid is placed in the pelvic basin to prevent leakage.

Treatment of the viscera: There are two methods:
1. If the viscera are to be returned to the thoracic, abdominal, and pelvic cavities, the viscera should be stored in a viscera plastic bag. Pour and mix about 2 L of cavity fluid over the viscera before the bag is returned to the cavities. Place the viscera bag in the trunk cavity with the sealed end of the bag directed toward the cephalic side.
2. The viscera can be returned to the trunk cavity but not in plastic bag. In this method viscera should be soaked in cavity fluid for several hours and then returned to their normal anatomical position, and covered with absorbent cotton and a piece of plastic sheet as an internal preservative pack. Then the cavities are closed.

If all the viscera have been removed at autopsy, the cavities should be packed and stuffed with absorbent material such as cotton saturated with cavity fluid. It serves as an internal preservative pack.

It is suggested that the paravertebral region should be filled with heavy specially designed sand bags. This will avoid the cracking of the spine on lifting of the body and also avoid the shock to the relatives of lifting a light empty cadaver.

- *Closure of the cavities*: After the cavity treatment, walls of the cavities are treated by hypodermic and surface embalming. To start with approximate the flaps of the incision and tie them together. Use double-curved needle and linen-suture thread or cotton-suture thread. For tightening the stitches, pull the thread and not the needle. Otherwise, the thread may break as it rubs against the eye of the needle. Start the suture from the abdominal cavity at the level of the pubic symphysis and proceed toward the thoracic cavity and neck. If the incision is "Y" shaped, continue the suture up the branch of the "Y" incision which is near the shoulder region.

The cranial cavity is aspirated or sponged to remove the blood and arterial fluid. It is then treated with cavity fluid and filled with absorbent cotton to absorb liquids that may accumulate. Replace the calvaria and stitch the scalp along the line of incision. Begin suturing on the right side of the head and end on the left side. To prevent the calvaria from moving it is sometime necessary to suture through the cut portion of the temporalis muscle attached to the temporal bone and through that portion of the muscle still attached to the calvaria. Care must be taken to prevent the hair being sutured into the incisions. Use hair clamps to keep the hair away from the sutures. The body should be washed thoroughly. It is now ready for the "presentation" treatment.

Chapter 14

Embalming the Infant

ML Ajmani

INTRODUCTION

It is well to remember that age is one of the important factors in the case analysis. Not only does age influence the techniques used in the embalming but also present certain difficulties with respect to selection of injection and drainage sites, strength and volume of embalming fluid, and injection pressure and rate of flow. There are many other factors that influence embalming such as size and weight of the body, cause of death and postmortem changes.

In embalming infants, it is important to note the relationship of body water to body fat. At birth, body water is approximately 75% of total body weight. At the age of 1 year the body water is about 60% of the body weight which is almost equivalent to the normal adult level. Body fat in the newborn is about 12% of total body weight and about 25% at 6 months of the age and then increases to about 30% at the age of 1 year.

Embalming requirement of an infant is not the same as that of an adult. Several important facts should be considered before embalming the infants and children. Infant skin is very delicate and can easily distend and wrinkle after arterial injection. The vessels in the infant are extremely small and delicate. With regard to embalming solutions, use regular arterial fluids of a strength similar to adult or a slightly reduced strength.

PROCEDURE

Disinfect the body with a topical disinfectant solution followed by a soap and water washing of the body. Clean nasal, oral, and orbital areas. Eyecaps or cotton pads may be inserted under the lids to effect eye closure. The mouth is closed prior to embalming either by the use of an adhesive or by suturing. After embalming, the mouth can again be cleaned and reglued.

Selection of Blood Vessels

Common Carotid Artery

It is the largest and easily accessible artery and accompanied by relatively large vein (internal jugular vein) which affords excellent drainage.

Femoral (or External Iliac) Artery

The second largest vessel that can be used is either femoral or external iliac artery; the accompanying veins are relatively large and can be used as points of drainage.

Abdominal Aorta

It is the large artery and is accompanied by the largest vein (inferior vena cava) that could be used for drainage. The vessels are deep seated. To expose the vessels, a 2–3 inches long incision is made just to the left of the midline in the middle of the abdomen. The greater omentum is lifted and loops of the small intestine and large gut are held away to expose the vessels. Aorta can be opened and a cannula is placed in the direction of the legs and another cannula in the direction of the thorax. Inferior vena cava can be opened and the blood allowed to drain in the cavity. Blood can also be drained by the drainage tube.

Ascending Aorta

Exposure of this vessel is complicated. Several incisions are used to reach this vessel. The main advantage to use this vessel is that the entire body can be embalmed from this one point. Right atrium is used for drainage.

Fluid Strengths and Volume

Fluid strength is determined by the condition of the body. Infant body tissues contain a higher percentage of water than adult body tissue. In addition, disease process and drugs may have increased tissue moisture and toxic substances. Therefore, use of the embalming solution containing normal adult dilution is advised. Infants and children require smaller volume of fluid than adults as it depends upon the size and weight of the body.

Pressure and Rate of Flow of Injection

Pressure and rate of flow of injection should be sufficient to overcome the resistance of the body and to distribute the arterial solution without causing tissue distension. The greater the resistance in a body, the greater the pressure required. It must be remembered that sufficient force is necessary to establish good distribution especially in distal parts such as hands and feet. First injection should be slower, to fill the vascular system. Subsequent solutions can be injected at a faster rate. Injection can be given at a faster rate from the very beginning. It will exert great pressure on the arterial side of the capillaries and increases filtration of the embalming fluid through capillaries. With this method, the body must be observed carefully to detect any distension and continuous drainage is used throughout the procedure.

Cavity Treatment

Aspiration and cavity embalming is done by an infant trocar. The infant trocar is about 12 inches in length with an inside diameter of one-fourth inch. Right or left inguinal regions of abdominal cavity may be used as entry point for trocar.

The infant up to 1 year can be treated by wrapping in a thick cotton wad saturated with embalming fluid.

Chapter 15

Delayed Embalming

ML Ajmani

INTRODUCTION

The longer the period between death and preparation of the body, more are the problems generally to be anticipated. The postmortem changes are speeded up by elevation of environmental temperature. The higher temperature speeds the decomposition of the proteins and produces rigor mortis and subsequent decomposition of the body tissues. Though low temperature (refrigeration) affects all chemical reactions but autolysis and bacterial enzymes continue tissue breakdown. Low temperature decreases the fluid diffusion but increases the capillary permeability and thus results in tissue distension during arterial injection.

The postmortem changes include algor mortis, livor mortis, rigor mortis, and decomposition. The longer the time between death and embalming, the more changes will occur and if the delay is more, chemical changes are initiated by the action of bacterial and/or autolytic enzymes resulting in the decomposition of the body tissues. In such cases the embalming process will not be successful. Therefore, the period between death and preparation of the body plays an important role in determining the embalming technique.

Embalming the Bodies in a State of Rigor Mortis

Onset of rigor mortis is within 1-2 hours after death and takes 1-2 hours to develop. It lasts 24-48 hours in winter and 18-36 hours in summer. Depending on cause of death and environmental temperature, the rigor can occur sooner or be delayed beyond the 2 hours. Rigor comprises three stages:
1. *Primary flaccidity*: The period in which the rigor develops and is hardly noticeable.
2. Period of rigor
3. *Secondary flaccidity*: The period in which the rigor passes off from the body.

The most difficult preparation is that when the body is to be embalmed in the intense state of rigor mortis. Embalmer should not wait for the cessation of rigor. Passage of rigor means that the processes of decomposition have already set in due to breakdown of body protein. Therefore, it is not advisable to wait for the rigor mortis to break prior to embalming. The bodies embalmed prior to onset of rigor should be injected with a normal strength of arterial solution. Bodies from which rigor has passed need a stronger than the average arterial solution. Bodies in a state of rigor mortis have very little formalin requirement. After the passage of rigor, requirement for formalin increases greatly. This increased fluid need is brought about by the breakdown of tissues. It is better to overembalm than to underembalm such bodies.

Positioning is a common problem associated with embalming bodies in rigor mortis. Rigor can be relieved by physical manipulations, i.e. flexion and extension of the joints, firm massaging, etc. When rigor sets in early it passes off quickly and vice versa. Rigor passes off early from the muscles of the face and upper extremities, where it first occurs while it is still very intense in the muscles of the leg.

Selection of Vessels

First choice in the embalming of the unautopsied body is to use the right common carotid artery for injection and the right internal jugular vein for drainage. The second choice is to use the femoral artery for injection and femoral or internal jugular vein for drainage.

When injecting, begin at a slow rate of flow. Rate of flow can be increased by manipulating the limbs and firm massage. Initial slow injection minimizes abdominal distension and helps to prevent purge. Once distribution is established, rate of flow can be increased. If any part of the body requires additional treatment, hypodermic embalming can be used. In autopsied bodies, a faster rate of flow may be used, because each area of the body is separately injected.

Swelling of muscles and tissues is common if the arterial injection is given in bodies in the state of rigor mortis. This is because capillary beds are torn while attempting to relieve the rigor by physical manipulation. Tissue also swells because fluid flows to area of least resistance, and not to the deeper tissues which are still in a state of rigor and offer resistance to flow.

EMBALMING OF REFRIGERATED BODIES

Nowadays, almost all dead bodies removed from hospitals have been refrigerated for some period. The cold environment slows down the progress of rigor mortis and decomposition and helps to maintain blood in a liquid state. If the bodies are refrigerated for short period, few problems are encountered. Normally bodies are wrapped in cotton sheets and refrigerated. Surface dehydration occurs easily in such bodies. Dehydration can be avoided by wrapping the bodies in plastic sheet and placing into a large plastic bag. Plastic wrapping traps heat and moisture, and thus, increases the body temperature. Heat speeds up the chemical reactions and produces rigor mortis and decomposition. Moreover during refrigeration, autolysis and bacterial enzymes continue tissue breakdown, which is faster at first while the body is still warm and then slower as the body gradually cools.

It is impossible to embalm a body that in a frozen solid state. In such cases body temperature is raised so that tissues become pliable. The most effective treatment to raise the body temperature is to hose the body with cold water and wrap blankets soaked in cold water around it or direct a cool air fan toward the body. Never use the warm water, it can damage the skin and deeper structures.

Embalming should not be carried out if the tissues are not pliable. When tissues are pliable but still chilled, embalming can be done at low pressure but there is a danger that frozen deep tissue may not receive adequate quantity of embalming fluid. Use of strong arterial solution prepared with slightly warm water produces best result.

The best vessels to use for arterial injection are both common carotid arteries (restricted cervical injection). Right internal jugular vein is the best choice for the drainage. Hypodermic embalming should be used for the areas not receiving sufficient arterial fluid. Approximately one liter of concentrated cavity fluid should be injected into each body cavity. Loose skin should be removed and apply surface embalming over these areas to ensure preservation.

EMBALMING OF DECOMPOSED BODIES

The process of decomposition is speeded by a warm environment. Cool environment slows the chemical reactions. As autolysis and putrefaction occur, foul smelling gases start collecting in the tissues, cavities and intestine causing bloating and swelling of the body and distension of the external genitalia. The pressure resulting from distension of the abdominal cavity causes oral and anal purges. This state of the body is neither desirable nor suitable for embalming. Embalming in decomposed bodies will not be effective. In fact handling and maneuvering of such bodies can prove to be a public health risk. Bodies in advanced stage of decomposition should be wrapped in one or more sheets and placed in a thick polythene bag and sealed air tight. Before wrapping, sprinkle strong embalming solution over the surface of the body. A double polythene bag may be necessary to ensure that the odors are contained in and the bag does not tear when it is lifted.

If the body is in early phase of decomposition, it can be embalmed by arterial injection of a strong embalming fluid or undiluted fluid. The vessels used may be the common carotid or femoral arteries. Do not attempt to drain. In advanced stage of decomposition, if the body has to be embalmed, due to certain unavoidable compulsions, hypodermic embalming is the method of choice. If the embalmer thinks it is feasible, he should raise and inject the right common carotid artery with undiluted fluid. The extremities and trunk walls are treated by hypodermic injection of undiluted fluid. The abdominal and thoracic cavities should be aspirated and filled with two or three liters of undiluted cavity fluid. The more advanced the putrefaction, the stronger the solution to be used. The purpose of using the strong solution is to diminish the odor and slow the progress of decomposition. The cranial cavity may be approached through the roof of the nose. Universal precautions should be observed for embalming and handing over of the decomposed bodies to avoid risk of contracting diseases like tetanus and other saprophytic infections.

Chapter 16

Selected Conditions

ML Ajmani

EMBALMING OF BURNT BODIES

Burns may be caused by heat, electrical shock, and chemical agents. In burnt bodies, effectivity of embalming depends upon the extent and degree of burn. There is likelihood of ulceration and subsequent oozing from it. Clean the skin surface and remove all loose skin. If a body comes in a blistering condition, open and drain the blisters and treat the denuded areas with surface embalming. Extensively, burnt bodies are very difficult to handle as they are covered with various ointments. The skin surface should be thoroughly washed with disinfectant soap and all the debris removed. Expose the body to air to dry the skin surface. Denuded skin areas are treated with surface embalming.

The best vessels to be used for injection and drainage are right common carotid artery and internal jugular vein, respectively. The choice of vessel depends upon the site and degree of burn as well. Very strong arterial solution is used to prepare these bodies. Proper sealing of the ulcer is necessary before injection treatment is given. It will prevent the leakage of embalming fluid from the surface. These bodies also create problems in suturing the incision used for embalming. Application of adhesive or leukoplast may help.

In extensively burnt cases and air crash victims, evisceration, if feasible, is recommended prior to giving the injection. Hypodermic embalming is used for the isolated or fragmented parts of the body.

Other problems arising in such bodies are the leakage and odor. To prevent leakage and to control odor, use double plastic bag for keeping and transferring of bodies.

EMBALMING OF THE BODIES EXPOSED TO RADIATION

Do not attempt to embalm a radiation-treated body unless a radiation expert has certified that the body is safe for handling. The main radioactive isotopes used to treat malignancy are listed below with types of radiation they emit (Table 16.1).

Beta rays are stopped much more readily than the gamma rays, which are similar to X-rays and require lead shielding. 37 millicurie is a safe level of gamma radiation for unautopsied bodies and 5 millicurie is a safe level for autopsied bodies.

Proper protective clothing should be worn, while doing embalming of such cases. The number of people involved in handling the body is kept to minimum thereby reducing the risk of prolonged exposure to more number of people. The body should be washed in water for several hours to reduce the radioactivity level. Discharges from the body should be disposed under the special instructions from the radiation expert.

These bodies are embalmed with highly concentrated arterial fluid.

ASCITES

In this condition, edematous fluid collects within the peritoneal cavity and around the visceral organs. The

Table 16.1: The main radioactive isotopes used to treat malignancy.

Isotope	Type of radiation emitted
Cobalt-60	Beta and gamma rays
Iodine-131	Beta and gamma rays
Phosphorus-32	Mainly beta rays

abdomen can be distended and interfere with the arterial fluid distribution and blood drainage. Ascites also increases the pressure in the abdominal cavity and tenses the abdominal wall. This pressure should be removed prior to arterial injection. Make a small opening in the lower part of the anterior abdominal wall preferably in the right inguinal or left inguinal region or in the hypogastric region. At these lower points, more fluid can be removed from the cavity. Insert the trocar, keeping the point directed downward and drain enough fluid to relieve the pressure. Leave the trocar in its position during the entire embalming.

Though ascites fluid is not mixed with arterial fluid, but it can dilute the cavity fluid. Therefore, it is not necessary to increase the strength of the arterial fluid. Undiluted cavity fluid should be injected.

ARTERIOSCLEROSIS AND ATHEROSCLEROSIS

Most people think that these conditions occur in old age. It is not so. These conditions occur in any age group over the age of 30. There is narrowing/occlusion of the lumen of the arteries up to variable extent and bring about poor and slow distribution of embalming fluid. Most frequently the sclerosis occurs in femoral artery. The common carotid is the artery of choice in such cases. The presence of arteriosclerosis or atherosclerosis is overcome by increasing the strength of the arterial fluid. Use of a stronger solution ensures that even if smaller amount of embalming fluid reaches the tissues, it gives sufficient preservation results.

DECUBITUS ULCERS (BED SORES)

These are the infected necrotic lesions resulted from poor circulation into the areas overlying a bony part of the body against which prolonged pressure has been applied, usually due to the lying supine on the bed. These lesions are most frequently seen over the hips, buttocks, and shoulder. These lesions may emit odor because of the secondary *Staphylococcus* infection.

Remove all bandages and disinfect the surface. Cotton pack soaked in cavity fluid or phenol solution is placed over the ulcers. Embalm the body. Hypodermic embalming is used. Inject the cavity fluid into the areas surrounding the ulcer by hypodermic syringe. After arterial embalming, hypodermic injection, and surface embalming, clothe the body in a sheet and put into plastic bag. When handling these bodies, wear gloves, mask, and gown.

MYCOTIC INFECTION (FUNGAL INFECTION)

The mycotic infections may produce superficial lesions on the skin and mucous membrane or may involve oral cavity, nasal cavity, pharynx, esophagus, larynx, and lungs. Most of the fungi involved are saprophytic and continue to multiply in untreated or poorly embalmed bodies.

Bodies with superficial lesions should never be handled without gloves. A cut in the skin of the embalming personnel may act as a portal of entry for fungal infection, can spread throughout the body and cause serious infection.

Fungal infections give blue, black, or green furry appearance on the surface of the body and the organs. They have been commonly seen on the tissue of the body subjected to dissection over a prolonged period in the anatomy departments. Warm and moist atmosphere is the ideal condition for fungal growth. Most of the fungi form spores. These spores may remain dormant in improperly disinfected articles, rooms, etc. A person may inhale or contract these spores through surface cuts. The personnel handling the body should be properly dressed with protective garments, i.e. gloves, apron, mask, goggles, head and shoe coverings. The body should be thoroughly washed. All superficial lesions should be treated by the use of mycostatic agents and the mouth, nose, and eyes are properly disinfected.

Mercuric chloride (1/1,000 solution) or salicylic or benzoic acid or Lugol's iodine may be helpful in preventing fungal growth.

Once the external disinfection has been completed, embalming procedure is initiated. It is advisable to use the mycostatic agent in the embalming solution and cavity fluid. Oral, nasal, anal, and vaginal cavities are packed with cotton soaked in disinfectant or cavity fluid.

ANATOMICAL EMBALMING

Teaching of anatomy of human body is an integral part of the study of medicine, dentistry, and all paramedical sciences. Dissection of a well-preserved human cadaver is the best method of learning anatomy of different parts of the body. The process of dissection is time consuming and the body remains exposed for several months without dehydration and decomposition. The dissected parts of the body are displayed in the museum for years together. Therefore, proper preservation of the cadaver is necessary to understand the structural integrity and topography of the human body.

There is a difference between anatomical and funeral embalming. The main criterion of anatomical embalming is proper preservation, total sterilization, and suitability for dissection. Venous drainage and cavity treatment is not necessary. The cranial cavity may be approached through the roof of the nose and infiltrated to preserve the brain.

To avoid postembalming dehydration and/or complications, the body is smeared with thin layer of petroleum jelly and wrapped in a sheet. It is then sealed in a polythene bag and stored till required for use. Refrigeration is not necessary for embalmed bodies. Dehydration and hardening is a common complication in the bodies kept in cold storage in a tropical country.

During dissection, body will require periodic moistening and antifungal treatment. The paint solution is applied or sprayed on the dissected body depending on the humidity and temperature of the surroundings. The body is kept covered with cotton sheet soaked in cloth fluid or mackintosh on the dissection table to prevent dehydration particularly in dry season (Tables 16.2 and 16.3).

It is not necessary to transfer the body to the tank periodically provided moisture and antifungal treatment are observed strictly. If an embalmed body is left uncared, it will eventually turn into a mummy because of loss of moisture.

In India, embalming is usually done by the anatomy department of the medical college. Sometime pathology or forensic medicine departments are also involved.

MAGGOTS

There are two types of domestic flies—(1) the house fly (Musca Domestica) and (2) the blow fly (Calliphora Erythrocephala). The former is more common but the later is more responsible for maggots. Fly eggs appear as yellowish clusters in the nose, ears, or corners of the eyes or within the mouth—these eggs can develop into the eating larval stage known as maggots in 24 hours. Maggots eat even embalmed tissue. Plugging the orifices of the body will restrict the entry of fly to the prone areas. Spraying of any common insecticide in the room will prevent the entry of flies.

In the event of maggots invading the body, the orifices should be flushed with the kerosene, concentrated salt water, or warm soapy water. Use the forceps to dislodge the more tenacious insects. DDT (dichlorodiphenyl trichloroethane) and lavender water can be sprayed into the affected areas. These chemical can kill the insects and will bring them to the surface.

To prevent flies from depositing eggs, a piece of cotton can be packed in the nostrils and other openings and keep the body covered.

PACEMAKER

These are normally situated in or near the axilla and can be felt like a big "turnip watch". They are subcutaneous and can be removed by superficial incision. Pacemakers explode under the effects of heat and can be dangerous when the body is cremated or burnt. Therefore, it should be removed before the injection treatment.

OBESITY

It is observed that the arteries in obese bodies are small in size and deeply placed. The restricted cervical injection is the method of choice in these bodies. The internal jugular vein will afford the best drainage. Keep the head high and straight while exposing the vessels. These bodies require large quantities of arterial solution. Fluid strengths can be of an average dilution. In emaciated bodies, fluid strength may be reduced to prevent dehydration. Always place a sheet under the body. It helps in moving and turning the body in a desired position.

Table 16.2: Paint mixture.

Glycerin	75%
Alcohol	10%
Phenol	5%
Water	10%

Table 16.3: Cloth fluid.

Formalin	5%
Phenol	5%
Glycerin	50%
Water	40%

Note: Add teepol and thymol crystals.

PURGE

Purge is defined as the postmortem regurgitation of any substance from any of the orifices of the body as a result of pressure. It can occur prior to during and in postembalming period. In the practice of embalming, the term purge is confined to the regurgitation of the contents of the stomach and the lung through the oral and nasal cavities. The pressure responsible for purge can develop in many ways:

- Gas in the gastrointestinal tract or abdominal cavity can create sufficient pressure on the stomach and force its contents through oral or nasal cavities. The abdominal pressure can push the diaphragm upward and exert sufficient force on lungs, resulting in lung purge through the mouth or nose.
- Arterial injection is given at a faster rate especially in bodies dead for long periods. The hollow visceral organ tends to expand and creates sufficient pressure, resulting in purge.
- Ascites and hydrothorax
- Esophageal varices
- Drowning and asphyxia.

In lung purge, the purging material is clear and frothy; whereas in stomach purge, it is coffee ground (consisting of stomach contents and blood) or brown if it contains acid. The acidity of the stomach purge can damage the face, if allowed to spread.

PRE-EMBALMING TREATMENT

In normal condition, place the body on the embalming table and apply force to remove as much purge material as possible from the body. An aspirator can be used to remove purge from the throat and nasal passages. It decreases the possibility of a postembalming purge. Nasal, oral, anal, and vaginal orifices are tightly packed before the arterial injection.

If a body comes with distended abdomen, introduce a trocar into the upper area of the abdominal cavity and pierce the stomach and transverse colon to relieve gas pressure. If ascites is present, remove fluid from the abdominal cavity to relieve the pressure.

The arterial injection expands the viscera and exerts pressure on the stomach and/or diaphragm, resulting in expulsion of the contents of the stomach and/or respiratory tract. During arterial injection, arterial fluid can be lost in the purge as a result of ruptured capillaries, small arteries, or veins. Therefore, sufficient volume of arterial fluid should be injected to replace the loss.

The ·cavity treatment greatly reduces the possibility of postembalming purge. In case of postembalming purge, replace and tightly repack the nostrils, mouth, rectum, and vagina with cotton soaked with cavity fluid. If anal purge cannot be stopped, tightly close off the anal opening with suture—cover the body with a cotton sheet and put into a plastic bag.

Chapter 17

Effect of Drugs on the Embalming Process

Robert G Mayer

INTRODUCTION

The contemporary professional embalmer practices his art and science in an age that has often been referred to as the chemotherapeutic era *(Chemotherapy is the treatment of disease with chemical agents and drugs)*. The aims of modern medicine are to cure disease and alleviate pain via the long-sought-for "magic bullet" of Dr Paul Ehrlich. Today, there is not a single case that the embalmer works upon that has not been injected, dusted, or made to ingest some type of chemical substance or substances (drugs) prior to death. In many cases, particularly those received from medical facilities and institutions, many different types of drugs were used prior to the patient's death. Although the chemotherapy era began with Ehrlich's "magic bullet" for the treatment of syphilis, today we live in an age of multiagent chemotherapy.

The way antibiotics are used today exemplifies the multidrug approach common to the medical profession. It is very unlikely nowadays that a single antibiotic is prescribed for the treatment of an infection. Usually, two or more antibiotics are administered. In cancer chemotherapy, the multidrug approach is also common. It is not unusual for an oncologist to administer both a cytotoxic drug (one that kills the cancer cell directly) and an antimetabolite (one that slowly "starves" the cancer cell by depriving it of a needed nutrient). One result of this multiagent approach has been an increase in the number and types of embalming problems.

Before the embalming problems caused by chemotherapeutic agents are discussed, "normal" embalming must be defined. There is no "ideal case". It is probably impossible to find a person who has not been treated by one or more doctors with one or more drugs prior to death. So, in addition to the problems caused by the pathological processes resulting in death, the chemotherapeutic agent or agents administered for various intervals prior to death have physiological effects. The longer the drug was taken before death, the more intense are the embalming problems likely to be encountered.

Another problem may arise from the chemical reaction between the administered drugs and the components of the embalming fluid. For example, are there any components of arterial embalming fluid that form insoluble precipitates when they react with antibiotics? If so, the circulatory path may become blocked, thus preventing the preservative component of the arterial fluid from reaching the tissues for preservation.

CHEMISTRY OF PROTEINS

To discuss the chemistry of embalming, it is essential to understand the chemistry of proteins. These materials form the physical structures of the body. They give the body form. The professional embalmer must achieve the absolute preservation of these structures. This means that the proteinaceous materials forming portions of the various tissues and organs of the human body must be rendered chemically inert. Essentially, these structures must be frozen in time and space!

Proteins are labile substances. The molecules breakdown quite rapidly even without bacterial action. There exist proteins that breakdown other proteins. These specialized proteins, called enzymes, are endowed with a physicochemical structure that allows catalytic activity. These enzymes can speed up decomposition reactions. It must be realized that even if a cadaver were completely sterile, the proteolytic enzymes in the cells and tissues of that body would still be fully active and capable of causing the breakdown of tissue proteins.

One goal of embalming must be to render the proteins resistant to attack by catalytic enzymes. There are two ways to do this—(1) the proteins themselves can be treated, so that they are no longer susceptible to the action of proteolytic enzymes. (2) The enzymes themselves can be so changed or inactivated that they cannot exert catalytic action on other proteins. Modem embalming chemicals are formulated to do both.

To determine how both of these goals can be achieved in a so-called "ideal" case, a brief mathematical formula is helpful.

What this means in terms of actual chemicals used to embalm a case should be discussed from a practical standpoint.

For a nonideal case (as practically all cases today are), the conclusion that some of the formaldehyde will be lost in embalming seems obvious. For example, many chemotherapeutic agents are nephrotoxic and, therefore, cause a breakdown of kidney function. As the kidneys are the main organs responsible for elimination of nitrogenous wastes, these waste materials (ammonia, urea, uric acid, etc.) are retained by the body. There is no better way to neutralize formaldehyde than to react it with ammonia, and this is exactly what happens in the body. If there has been a build-up of nitrogenous waste materials as a result of chemotherapy-induced kidney dysfunction, a standard dilution of arterial embalming fluid will not be sufficient. A large proportion of the formaldehyde in the embalming fluid will be neutralized when it encounters the nitrogenous wastes in the body. The remainder is insufficient to preserve the tissues, and the body starts to decay.

Average body protein	The average body = 150 pounds = 65.3 kg. A 65.3 kg body contains 10.7 kg of protein = 10,700 g of protein
Formaldehyde demand	100 g of soluble protein requires 4.4 g of formaldehyde for preservation. The average body contains 10,700 g of protein

Therefore,
$$\frac{10,700 \times 4.4}{100} = 470.8 \text{ g formaldehyde needed}$$

Solution needed given	Standard 30-index arterial fluid contains 16 ounces of 30% formaldehyde = 142.08 g of formaldehyde

Need: 470.80 g of formaldehyde
$$\frac{470.80}{142.08} = 3.31$$

16-ounce bottles of a 30-index fluid needed, or approximately 53 ounces of arterial fluid!

Normally, arterial embalming fluids are supplied as 16-ounce concentrates. These are diluted with water and additives prior to injection into the body. An embalming fluid containing 30% formaldehyde supplies 142 g of formaldehyde per bottle. To embalm the "average" or "ideal" body containing 10.7 kg of protein, 470 g of formaldehyde is needed, that is, a minimum of three bottles of arterial embalming fluid (if the body has been dosed with drugs, more than double this amount of formaldehyde may be necessary!).

CHEMOTHERAPY CASE

All chemotherapeutic agents are toxic. This is the one axiom universally applicable to all drugs. Cellular and tissue changes occur when drugs are used. It does not matter what drug is administered; even the seemingly innocuous aspirin tablet has its effects. Drug-induced changes may be relatively minor in nature, perhaps limited to slight skin discolorations, which, in the deceased, readily respond to cosmetic treatment. When drugs cause major problems, such as acute jaundice, or saturate the body tissues with uremic wastes, the fixative action of the preservative chemicals in the arterial embalming fluid is seriously impaired.

The chemotherapeutic agents common to modem medicine exert their effects in many ways. They may impair function of the liver, the circulatory system (heart and blood vessels), the kidneys, the lungs, and the skin. These drugs can inactivate the embalming fluid by causing the build-up of nitrogenous wastes or decreasing the permeability of the cell membrane.

Because the liver is the main detoxification center, every drug eventually enters the hepatic circulation. While in the liver, the drug may cause profound changes in the liver itself. When the liver is damaged, the embalmer may have to cope with a jaundiced body.

All drugs ultimately pass through the kidneys. Even those that accumulate in other body areas must pass at least once (and often more) through the kidneys. If the drugs cause extensive changes in this organ, renal insufficiency follows, resulting in the buildup of nitrogenous wastes in body tissues. Saturated with urea, uric acid, ammonia, creatinine, and other wastes, the tissues become spongy and difficult to preserve. In such cases, preservation is almost impossible to achieve unless the treatment is modified.

Drugs also change the biochemical constituents of the blood. Some drugs damage even the connecting blood vessels themselves extensively. The circulatory system may become impaired as a result of extensive dot formation, lysis of the blood cells, or extensive damage to the walls of the arteries and veins.

The effects on skin are closely associated with the changes in the circulatory system and may include the formation of widespread areas of discoloration stemming from lysis and release of blood pigments from red blood cells. Lesions on the skin surfaces may also result from use of the nitrogen mustards.

Pharmacologically, the dividing line between the beneficial effects and toxic effects of drugs is very slender. The professional embalmer must learn to cope with these effects.

Inactivation of Preservative Agents by Drugs

The problems likely to be confronted while embalming a body administered chemotherapy do not result from the reactions of formaldehyde or other preservative aldehydes with the drug or drugs. Much too little drug is present, even after aggressive therapy. It is the physiological effect of the drug that is culpable. A drug that causes nephrotoxic changes enhances the accumulation of nitrogenous waste products in the body. These waste products, which result indirectly from the physiological effect of the drug, are responsible for the inactivation or, more specifically, the neutralization of the formaldehyde.

$$4NH_3 + 6CH_2O \rightarrow (CH_2)_6N_4 + 6H_2O$$

This neutralization, whereby formaldehyde is converted into hexamethylene, is probably at the root of at least 90% of the contemporary embalmer's problems.

A change in permeability of the cell membrane is another effect of most systemically administered drugs. It is through this membrane that everything must pass, either to enter or to leave the cell. Preservative chemicals such as formaldehyde must pass through this membrane, if they are going to inactivate the intracellular enzymes that decompose the proteins there.

If a chemotherapeutic agent reduces or destroys membrane permeability, preservative solutions may not be able to enter the cell. The antibiotic tetracycline is a case in point. Although most antibiotics exert their effects on bacteria they also have an effect on the human cell. They are chelating agents and tend to lodge in the cell membrane, causing calcium to form an impenetrable layer around the cell. "Chelating" means they have an affinity for metallic ions, particularly calcium and magnesium. Antibiotics appear to act selectively on cell membranes. After they are entrenched in the membrane, they start chelating or sequestering calcium and magnesium ions [There is generally no shortage of calcium in the body; it is present in all biological fluids (secretions, excretions, etc.)].

Eventually, as more calcium and magnesium ions become lodged in the chelate in the cell membrane, the permeability of the membrane changes; the membrane becomes less permeable. It becomes increasingly more difficult for some chemicals to enter such a cell. As the goal of embalming is to inactivate the intracellular enzymes present, it is essential that the preservative enter the cell. If it does not then the proteolytic enzymes inside the cell can proceed to breakdown the proteinaceous materials in the cell, and the tissue is subject to decomposition and lysis of its structural features. In essence, it turns into a puddle of fluid.

To study these effects, Fredrick has devised a histological method based on a chemical method of Gomori. Gomori observed that if an enzyme were supplied with a substrate, it would release a material (phosphate) that could be precipitated in situ. Using this technique, one is able to determine the location of active enzymes.

There has recently come into use a group of antibiotics that exert their effects in the kidney, hampering its ability to dispose of nitrogenous wastes the aminoglycosides, represented by kanamycin and most recently gentamicin. These antibiotics cause nitrogenous waste products to be retained, and if the so-called standard dilution of arterial fluid is used, embalming will fail.

Combination Antibiotic Chemotherapy

Today, it is routine procedure for physicians to prescribe two or more antibiotics at the same time. This, of course, intensifies the embalming problems. The embalming problems resulting from synergistic combination chemotherapy are not new, only more intense. Use of a combination such as gentamicin and synthetic penicillin (e.g.

methicillin) makes preservation and firming difficult to achieve. These bodies are usually saturated with ammoniacal and other nitrogenous wastes. The arterial fluid in such cases must be very concentrated, if any embalming is to be accomplished.

Corticosteroids and Anti-inflammatory Drugs

If antibiotics are the most widely used drugs then cortisone and its derivatives constitute a close second. The anti-inflammatory drugs have many uses (e.g. itching caused by allergies) and are the drugs of choice for arthritic and rheumatic conditions. Corticosteroids are also widely used in the chemotherapy of cancer.

With regard to specific embalming problems caused by these drugs, the chief effect is blockade of the cell membrane. Corticosteroids decrease the permeability of this membrane and thereby block passage of liquids into the cell. On a gross macroscopic level, liquids are retained by the cells and tissues, resulting in an increase in cell turgor and waterlogging of tissues.

The use of cortisone for the treatment of chronic disease (over long periods) may result in *gastrointestinal ulcerations with possible perforations of the gut*. Prolonged use in the treatment of ulcerative colitis has also resulted in dehydration of the body.

Corticosteroids have been shown to exert a "protective" effect on proteolytic enzymes. This is demonstrated by the difficult task one has in trying to denature these enzymes in cortisone-treated bodies. Even if these enzymes are extracted from such cortisone-treated tissues and are obtained in an almost pure form, they are still difficult to inactivate. They retain the "protective" effect originally conferred by the corticosteroids. This means that more undenatured proteolytic enzymes remain in the body after embalming. Such bodies tend to "go bad" (decompose) very rapidly after an apparently trouble-free embalming.

What has so far been described with respect to corticosteroids can also occur as the result of the use of oral contraceptives by women. Progesterone and its derivatives have chemical structures similar to that of cortisone. It has long been known in pharmacology that similar chemical structures elicit similar biological reactions. Many of the embalming problems observed after use of corticosteroids' are identical to those encountered in bodies of young women who died while taking the oral contraceptive.

Another problem encountered when corticosteroids have been administered for some time prior to death is of a more insidious nature. These persons have been shown to have disseminated tuberculosis. The anti-inflammatory action of the corticosteroids results from their suppression of immunity. If cases of "arrested" (or so-called "cured") tuberculosis in which large doses of cortisone were administered before death, it is not uncommon to find that because immunity was suppressed the Mycobacterium was reactivated and spread throughout the body. Such cases offer hidden hazards to the embalmer's health and sanitation precautions should be observed.

To secure preservation in these bodies, some permeability should be restored to the cell membranes, so that preservatives can enter the cells. This can be done through "the use of adjunct fluids". Preinjecting such a body restores some of the permeability; and the surface active chemicals in such preparations facilitate entry of the preservative components of the arterials into cells. At the same time, a stronger-than-normal arterial injection should be used together with a coinjection fluid (It is also possible to use some coinjection fluid as a preinjection).

Cancer Chemotherapeutic Agents and their Effects

Various drugs are used to treat malignancies, but generally they fall into two main classes. Cytotoxic drugs act directly on the tumor cells to bring about their death. Antimetabolite drugs substitute for an essential metabolite required by the cancer cell for growth. It is not unusual for both types to be given to the cancer patient. This multiagent chemotherapy creates tremendous problems for the professional embalmer.

Cytotoxic drugs (e.g. nitrogen mustards, alkylating agents) kill both malignant and normal cells (A "magic bullet" for cancer has not yet been found). When cells die, proteins breakdown and large amounts of nitrogenous wastes are released. Therefore, the tissues in these bodies, besides containing a small amount of protein as a result of the extreme cachexia associated with cancer, are saturated with nitrogenous waste products. Achievement of preservation under these conditions is a Herculean task in itself, but the embalming problems that arise from the coadministration of antimetabolites must be added. These are sure to cause symptoms of extensive vitamin deficiency. Such bodies may exhibit everything from scurvy to brittle rickets like bone disease. If radiation therapy also been administered, there may be extensive skin and circulatory problems (e.g. purpura and body clots).

Radioactive Isotopes and their Effects

Because radioactive materials are used for cancer therapy, it is not amiss to discuss the radiation-treated body. Do not attempt to embalm a radiation-treated body unless a radiologist has certified the body as safe because of the possibility of gamma radiation (37 millicuries is a safe level for unautopsied bodies; 5 millicuries is a safe level for autopsied bodies). The main radioisotopes used to treat malignancies are listed here with the types of radiation they emit (Table 17.1).

Beta rays are stopped much more rapidly than gamma rays, which are similar to X-rays arid require lead shielding. In addition, tiny needles or "seeds" of gold-198, as well as radon needles, are implanted in tissues to treat metastatic tumors in the abdomen and lungs. These bodies, if declared safe, may be embalmed as would any cancer case, observing the necessity for use of a highly concentrated arterial embalming fluid. It is also a good idea to preinject these bodies before arterial injection.

Tranquilizers and Mood-altering Drugs

It is not easy to discuss prescribed legal drugs without venturing into the field of drug abuse. No matter what the drug is, if it is taken beyond the period of time prescribed, or if more than the dose prescribed is taken, it becomes "abused". For example, if amphetamines are prescribed for dietary or psychiatric reasons and are taken longer than necessary to alleviate the condition, they become illegal or abused drugs. It should be realized that such components of the drug culture as benzedrine, dexedrine, and methedrine were all at one time (and some still are) rigorously and ethically prescribed by physicians to treat specific ills. The same holds true for such tranquilizers as phenothiazine and its derivatives.

There are roughly five classes of tranquilizers and mood-altering drugs. In general, they have one common characteristic—they result in a loss of weight of the abuser. Embalming these bodies is a very frustrating task because of the lack of protein (most of the protein stores have been depleted). A person on a "trip" does not care about nutrition.

- *Sedatives*: Barbiturates (Amytal, Seconal, etc.); meprobamate (Equanil, Miltown, etc.)
- *Stimulants*: Amphetamines (Benzedrine, Dexedrine, etc.); cocaine; Preludin
- *Tranquilizers*: Phenothiazines (Thorazine, Compazine, etc.); reserpine, Librium, Valium
- *Narcotics*: Opiates (opium, heroin, morphine, etc.)
- *Antidepressants*: Ritalin, Tofranil.

The continued use (or abuse) of tranquilizers can also result in such embalming problems as jaundice because of the destructive effect of these drugs on liver cells. In addition, tranquilizers may cause hemolysis of the red blood cells and thereby add to the jaundice problem because pigments are released from these red blood cells. Also common to abusers of all five classes of drugs is the depletion of protein stores resulting from their neglect of nutrition. Protein depletion results in the release of large amounts of nitrogenous waste products. If kidney function is impaired. (Particularly in heroin addicts in whom both constipation and anuresis occur), these waste materials cannot exit the body. They are retained in the tissues and rapidly neutralize formaldehyde (or any aldehyde).

Problems Caused by Oral Drugs that Control

A group of chemotherapeutic agents with broad-spectrum effects comprises those drugs used to control diabetes, and the oral diabetic agents. Use of such drugs as tolbutamide (Orinase) and chlorpropamide (Diabinese) to control adult (type II) diabetes is increasing. These drugs certainly are more convenient (for those who can use them) than the daily (or more frequent) self-injections of insulin.

Orinase was used widely until recently, when it was replaced with another second-generation sulfonylurea called Diabinese. Both may cause jaundice. Most of the sulfonylureas can induce changes in the voluntary muscles (site of glycogen storage and breakdown) and the liver (main glycogen storage organ of the body). Continuous use of oral diabetic agents has been linked with circulatory

Table 17.1: The main radioisotopes used to treat malignancies.	
Isotope	Type of radiation emitted
Cobalt-60	Beta and gamma rays
Iodine-131	Beta and gamma rays
Phosphorus-32	Mainly beta rays

Table 17.2: Problems caused by chemotherapeutic agents.		
Drugs	*Problem*	*Embalming treatment recommended*
Antibiotics (penicillins, synthetic penicillins, aminoglycosides, tetracyclines)	Cotton-like circulatory blockages (fungal overgrowth), jaundice, bleeding, into skin, poor penetration	1, 2, 3, 4
Corticosteroids (cortisone)	Cell membranes less permeable, retention of fluids mild-to-severe waterlogging of tissues, "protects" proteolysis enzymes, resulting in more rapid breakdown of body proteins	1, 2, 3, 4
Cancer chemotherapy (antimetabolites, cytotoxic agents, radioisotopes)	Emaciation and dehydration, extensive purpura jaundice, low protein (because of anorexia and vomiting): perforation of gut, brittleness of bone, nitrogenous waste retention	2, 3, 4, 5
Tranquilizers (phenothiazines)	Dehydration, weight loss and emaciation, low protein, kidney dysfunction and retention of nitrogenous waste products	2, 3, 4, 5
Stimulants (amphetamines, cocaine)	Weight loss, emaciation, low protein, mucous membranes bleed easily, other problems as for tranquilizers	2, 3, 4, 5
Stimulants (amphetamines, cocaine)	Weight loss, emaciation, low protein, mucous membranes bleed easily, other problems as for tranquilizers	2, 3, 4, 5
Sedatives (barbiturates, meprobamate)	Emaciation, dehydration, low protein, difficult of firm	2, 3, 5
Oral antidiabetic agents (tolbutamide)	Muscle atrophy, mild-to-severe jaundice, some emaciation and edema	1, 2, 3, 4
Circulatory drugs (antihypertensives anticlotting agents)	Blood clots, impairment of circulation, poor distribution of fluids, purpura, urine retention, and spongy nitrogenous waste-filled tissues	1, 2, 3, 4

Key to Table: The embalming treatment recommended is designated by a code number interpreted as follows:
- Preinjection required
- Coinjection required
- Increase arterial concentration
- Use less water for total injection
- Use restorative or tissue builder.

Note: The chemicals cited in this table pertain to one particular chemical manufacturer.

Table has been adapted and summarized from many published works it is neither completed nor exhaustive. It is designed to point out categories of chemotherapeutic agents in use now. It is hoped that this Table will stimulate both the student of embalming and the licensed professional to read about the latest developments in journals and trade magazines. As new chemical agents are introduced so frequently by the medical profession, it is impossible to publish up-to-the-minute tables. Keeping up with the literature is of the utmost importance.

problems, which can result in poor distribution of the arterial chemicals (This has been observed to be the result of extensive clot formation in the cadaver). Acidosis sometimes occurs as a result of the altered carbohydrate metabolism and leads to the formation of high concentrations of lactic acid in muscle tissue. Such bodies firm very rapidly unless an alkaline coinjection is used with the arterial embalming fluid.

In general, although oral diabetic agents may cause a large variety of embalming problems, they do not cause as severe embalming problems as do other drugs (Table 17.2).

Neutralizing Chemotherapeutic Agents

It must be understood that chemotherapeutic agents cause embalming problems not through their reactions with embalming chemicals but through their physiological effects on the body prior to death (Table 17.2). No drug, no matter how often, how long, or in what concentration it is used, could ever be administered long enough during life to react significantly with the components of an arterial chemical injected after death. As has previously been stressed, *it is the physiological reaction the drug induces* that causes the problem. For example, the nephrotoxic effect of the aminoglycoside antibiotics is produced not by the reaction between formaldehyde and kanamycin (even if a few grams of the antibiotic are present), but rather by the reaction between formaldehyde and the nitrogenous waste products released into the tissues through the action of the antibiotic.

Once absorbed into the bloodstream, a drug is rapidly diluted. An average body contains about 6 liters (1 liter is equivalent to 2.1 pints) of blood. This volume of blood circulates once per minute. It comes into contact with 35 additional liters of liquid (58% of the body weight of an average 150-pound man is water). Therefore, there is a total of 41 liters of liquid (including blood volume) in the average body. Any drug, usually given in milligram doses, would be so diluted as to have no significant effect in a direct chemical reaction with formaldehyde or any component of embalming fluid.

In the event of a nuclear accident, in addition to the obvious protective equipment required, massive preinjection of the cadaver is necessary (with a chelating agent containing precoinjection fluid). All drainage must be collected in lead-lined containers and disposed per directions of the Nuclear Regulatory Commission.

Possible Solutions to Chemotherapy Problems

The problems arising from chemotherapy vary in severity, but can be divided into a few broad categories. Several preventative and ameliorative treatments are available that have been shown to work in the majority of cases. *The professional embalmer must consider each case as unique.* Just as a physician does not prescribe the same dosage of a medication for all patients, so must the embalmer vary procedures (and preservative fluids) to meet the requirements of the particular case.

In Table 17.2, five different embalming treatments are recommended to combat most chemotherapy-derived problems. Obviously, these cannot solve all the problems the professional embalmer will face. They do, however, serve as a springboard for further research and, therefore, offer the embalmer an opportunity for experimentation and learning both the marks of professionalism.

CONCLUSION

Mistaken ideas about the specificity of a particular chemotherapeutic agent are quite common. For example, one may believe that a drug known to have a pronounced effect on a particular organ will be found only in that organ. This is not so. That a drug shows a more dramatic effect on a particular tissue does not mean that the effect is limited only to that tissue.

In general, no matter what chemotherapeutic agent is used, it is concentrated, metabolized, and detoxified in the liver and excreted via the kidneys (and sometimes, the lungs and skin). But before it reaches these organs, it passes through other tissues of the body, which is contrary to the "magic bullet" concept. Actually, there is no magic bullet! It is impossible for a drug to bring about a single reaction in a single organ or tissue. It should not be surprising then that a single drug can cause a plethora of embalming problems. Simultaneous use of two or more drugs, as is common in medical practice today, intensifies the problems.

In the body, a drug is subject to great dilution. The problems it causes do not result from its direct reaction with components of the embalming fluid, but from the chronic psychological effects it produces.

On the basis of both laboratory studies and field work, five embalming treatments for the problems encountered in bodies that have undergone chemotherapy case have been recommended. It is the responsibility of the embalmer to modify the treatment to suit the particular case.

KEY TERMS AND CONCEPTS FOR STUDY AND DISCUSSION

- It is known that elderly persons present chemotherapy-derived embalming problems because of the ability of the body to circulate, detoxify, and excrete drugs decreases with age. Discuss, on this basis, the possible effects of an aminoglycoside antibiotic such as gentamicin when the "usual" dilution is used.
- If approximately 58% of the human body is composed of water, is it defeating the purpose to embalm the body that has undergone chemotherapy, particularly if there is little protein (as in the drug addict) in that body, by further diluting the embalming fluid with water before it is injected? Discuss how use can be made of this intracellular water as a diluent for concentrated arterial fluid. As this "tissue" water is known to be high in calcium, should it be conditioned with a water softener or conditioner?
- It is a fact that a body treated with antibiotics usually contains all types of fungi. Certain fungi may pose

- a hazard to the embalmer. Discuss the possibility of contracting *Candida*, *Cryptococcus*, and *Histoplasma* infections from cadavers. What can be done to protect the embalmer?
- It has been shown that to embalm an "average" body, at least three to four 16-ounce bottles of a 30% formaldehyde arterial solution are necessary. Discuss whether enough preservative is contained in this amount of arterial fluid to embalm a body treated with corticosteroids. What adjunct embalming chemicals should be added to the arterial injection?
- A young housewife is killed in an automobile accident. The embalmer is told that she has been taking a fertility drug (progesterone) because she was childless and wanted a family. What types of embalming problems can be expected?
- A chronic diabetic is brought to the preparation room. The embalmer discovers that instead of insulin, the man had taken Orinase two times daily for the past 3 years. What embalming fluids should be used on this case, taking into consideration dilution of arterial chemicals, rapidity of firming, and use of preinjection fluid, water conditions, and other fluids?
- After arterial injection, the drainage is observed to contain small wads of greenish "cotton". The patient had been taking massive doses of penicillin prior to death. What could these "cotton wads" be?
- If the professional embalmer knew what medications were used on a case prior to death, he could be better informed as to what embalming problems to expect. Discuss how a funeral director can secure the cooperation of the pathologist and other hospital authorities in obtaining this information.
- Discuss why an embalmer cannot use one type and one concentration of arterial embalming fluid in all cases.
- A particular drug exerts its effect on only one specific organ. Therefore, after a patient treated with cortisone for an arthritic condition dies, high concentrations of cortisone will be found only in the joints. Discuss the fallacy of this type of thinking.

BIBLIOGRAPHY

1. Brozek J. Body Composition. New York: NY Academy of Sciences; 1963.
2. Fredrick JF. An alpha-glucan phosphorylase which requires adenosine-5-phosphate as coenzyme. Phytochemistry. 1963;2:413-5.
3. Fredrick JF. Embalming Problems Caused by Chemotherapeutic Agents. Boston: Dodge Institute for advanced studies; 1968.
4. Goodman L, Gilman A. The Pharmacological Basis of Therapeutics, 4th edition. New York: Macmillan; 1970.
5. Gomori G. Microtechnical demonstration of phosphatase enzymes in tissue sections. Proc Soc Exp Biol Med. 1939; 42:23-6.
6. Goth A. Medical Pharmacology, 6th edition. St. Louis, MO: CV Mosby; 1972.
7. Julian RM. A Primer of Drug Action. San Francisco: WH Freeman; 1975.
8. Long YG. Neuropharmacology and Behavior. San Francisco: WH Freeman; 1972.
9. Medical Economics. Physicians' Desk Reference (PDR), 38th edition. Oradall, NJ: Medical Economics Publishers; 1984.
10. Yessell ES, Braude MC. Interaction of Drugs of Abuse. New York: NY Academy of Sciences; 1976.
11. Windholz M, Budavari S. Merck Index, 10th edition. Rahway, NJ: Merck & Co.; 1983.

Chapter 18

Guidelines for Embalming an Acquired Immunodeficiency Syndrome Body

ML Ajmani

OVERVIEW

Practically, it is almost impossible to know the human immunodeficiency virus (HIV) status of each and every deceased person in any hospital. Moreover, it is quite possible that workers dealing with patients/dead bodies carrying HIV without knowing it. Therefore, we should change our work culture and consider all bodies are potentially infected with HIV and follow "universal work precautions".

To avoid risk to the embalmers, healthcare workers and to the society at large it is prudent to cremate the body at the place of death. Though after death the communicability of virus infection rapidly declines, but this should not form a reason for embalming the body. It is best to avoid embalming of such cases unless it is essential and body has to be transported for funeral service to his or her native place.

The successes of eradicating the risk factors depend on the full national and international cooperation and consciousness that "acquired immunodeficiency syndrome (AIDS) is a global challenge for humans". It will not be overcome anywhere unless it is solved everywhere.

INTRODUCTION

Though much has been said about the risks involved while doing invasive procedures, very little research has been done on the hazards faced by the doctors and paramedical staff involved in embalming of bodies of patient with HIV, hepatitis B virus and other notifiable infections. Scientific investigation has confirmed that with cessation of life, certain bacteria are released which, if allowed to go unchecked, can be a danger to health. Moreover with death, there is neither longer the reticuloendothelial system nor the blood-brain barrier to restrict the translocation of microorganisms within the dead human remains. Organisms were found in brain tissue which is normally sterile during life. It indicates that there is proliferation and translocation of microorganisms in the dead host.[1,2]

Human immunodeficiency virus, the virus that causes AIDS has been isolated in. concentration high enough to become hazardous for transmitting infection from blood, semen, vaginal secretions, saliva, tears, breast milk, cerebrospinal fluid, amniotic fluid, and urine and is likely to be isolated from other body fluids, secretions, and excretions. However, epidemiologic evidence has implicated only blood, semen, vaginal secretions, and possibly breast milk in transmission.[3]

Infection of AIDS can be acquired by transdermal inoculation through cuts and needle punctures. After accidental puncture with needles known to be contaminated with AIDS blood, only 0.5% of individuals will become seropositive.[4] Less than 0.5% of initially seronegative health workers who care for AIDS patients become positive after 2 years.[5] Since, the time AIDS has appeared, thousands of healthcare workers have been caring for AIDS patients with or without their knowledge. Similarly, thousands of medical and paramedical workers are engaged in embalming the bodies of such patients with or without their knowledge. Moreover reports are there to highlight the fact that AIDS does spread through the open wound,[6] infected skin,[7] blood and body fluid. Transmission rates from contaminated needle punctures or dose contact are 10–30 times higher for serum hepatitis than for AIDS.[8,9]

PRE-EMBALMING PREPARATIONS

Workers on duty should be supervised when they remove the IV drip, Ryle's tube, endotracheal tubings urethral catheters, mouth gags, and other such things from the body taking all the precautions for infection control. It should be followed by the plugging the nostrils, mouth, anal, and vaginal orifices to prevent leakage of any fluid. Always put a piece of gauze or cotton and apply leucoplast firmly over the site of IV drip or cut open site. Once this is over, then the body is ready for transportation.

The vehicle transporting the AIDS bodies should have sheets that can be disposed. A plastic bag and rubber gloves should always be present in the vehicle. Wear rubber gloves; cover the body with a sheet before any handling is done. The body should then be placed in a plastic bag and close tightly. The gloves should be put into another thick plastic bag and close tightly. Now if embalming is not required:

Put a label "infection risk-handle with care" on those bodies which are known to carry HIV, hepatitis virus, etc. Viewing of such bodies should not be allowed. Body should be disposed off by burning or burial, depending upon the religion of the deceased. Throwing body in a river should not be allowed at all.

If embalming is required, bring the body to the embalming facility complex. Before removing the body from the plastic bag to the embalming table, the personnel doing the case should be properly garbed in an AIDS suit which consists of:
- A disposable type of scrub suit
- A plastic apron
- Double rubber gloves
- Hair covering
- Shoe covering
- Facemask
- Goggles.

EMBALMING ROOM

A separate room is needed for embalming an AIDS body. No other embalming should be performed along with the AIDS embalming. Access to the embalming room should be limited to a maximum of three persons. Persons preforming autopsies/embalming should not have any external injury.

Once you are dressed with an AIDS suit remove the body from the plastic bag by carefully rolling the body from side-to-side and removing the bag. The sheets and the bag should carefully be rolled and removed then arid place into a double plastic bag. The body should be inspected thoroughly and washed with a disinfectant solution. At this stage, it is better to remove any cotton wool that has been placed in the nostrils, mouth or vagina and any bandage around the face, hands, feet or penis. The oral and nasal orifices should be cleaned and disinfect carefully. Eye comers should be cleaned with great care because any matter in the eye may be a source of contamination.

METHODS OF EMBALMING

The embalming is used because of the following reasons:
- It ensures that there is no risk or fear of infection on contact with the dead body.
- It produces without mutilation, a natural color and effect on the body, so that a life-like appearance is produced.
- It ensures preservation of the body and the prevention of putrefaction changes and disturbances, which so often results in odious purging and discharge from the various orifices of the body.

Embalming Consists Basically of Two Processes

Arterial Embalming

In this method the preservative solution is injected into a large artery of the body. Simultaneously blood is removed from a large vein of the body to make room for the preservative solution. The preservative solution follows the same route as the blood in the living except that the heart is no longer the starting point for the fluid. Fluid does not flow through the chambers of the heart but distributed through the arch of the aorta and its branches.

Cavity Embalming

It is the treatment of the visceras of the thoracic, abdominal and pelvic cavities. The contents of the hollow visceras and the liquid accumulated in the body cavities are removed by aspirations. The left out materials that cannot be aspirated can be preserved by cavity embalming. This treatment detoxicates the materials and assists in the preservation of the viscera. A very strong preservative solution is injected via the trocar and cannula through the anterior abdominal wall. This solution is known as "cavity fluid".

Supplemental Methods of Embalming

These methods are used to preserve local areas of the body that have not received arterial fluid. These methods can be used as the primary methods for embalming an infant, fetus, visceras, burned, and mutilated parts of the body.

Hypodermic Embalming

This method is used to preserve the local body area by subcutaneous injection of the arterial fluid or cavity fluid by hypodermic needle and syringe. It is generally used to preserve the local body areas that have not received arterial fluid or to treat the areas that have received insufficient amount of embalming fluid.

Surface Embalming

It is preservation of the local area by application of a suitable chemical to the surface of the body. The chemical may be an arterial fluid or cavity fluid. A cotton or gauze piece can be used to apply the chemical. Surface embalming can be applied to external skin surfaces (bed sores, wound or local burnt area, etc.) or to internal surfaces, e.g. putting packs under the eyelids, within the mouth or in the autopsied bodies from within the body cavities.

EMBALMING FLUIDS

Normally the strength of the embalming fluids depends upon the age, built and status of the body (i.e. autopsied, autopsied, decomposed, burnt, etc.). The AIDS virus is a very delicate virus and can easily be destroyed. It does not survive for long outside the body. Studies have shown that *HN* is inactivated rapidly after being exposed to commonly used chemical germicides at concentrations that are much lower than used in practice.[10-13] Chemical germicides present in the embalming fluids have been tested and found to completely inactivate HIV. Though a 5% concentration of formalin is quite effective to destroy the *HN*, but a very high concentration of formalin has been recommended especially in the bodies to be transported for funeral service to his/her native place.

If the delay before embalming is considerable, it is advisable to use an even higher concentration of formalin.

The volume of embalming fluid injected depends upon the age and built of the individual. In an average built individual 10–15 L of arterial fluid is required to ensure effective embalming. Obese body will demand large volume of fluid.

Survival of Human Immunodeficiency Virus in the Environment

The most extensive study on the survival of HIV after drying involved greatly concentrated HIV samples, i.e. 10 million tissue culture infectious doses per milliliter.[14] This concentration is at least 100,000 times greater than that typically found in the blood or serum of patients with HIV infection. HIV was detectable by tissue-culture techniques 1–3 days after drying, but the rate of inactivation was rapid. Studies performed at Centers for Disease Control (CDC) have also shown that drying HIV causes a rapid reduction in HIV concentration. In tissue-culture fluid, cell-free HIV could be detected up to 15 days at room temperature, up to 11 days at 31°C (98; 6°C) and up to 1 day if the HIV was cell associated.

PROCEDURE

Normally the arteries are found to be empty in the vast majority of bodies received for embalming. A very considerable quantity of blood or blood clot is always present in the veins. Since two things cannot occupy the same space at the same time and if we expect to get a continuous flow of fluid from the arteries through the capillaries and then out of the veins, the veins must be emptied of blood. Therefore, during the embalming procedure, the vein should be first washed with saline solution containing at least 2% aldehyde. Injection should be given through the selected artery. Selection of vessel depends upon the age and status of the body, i.e. autopsied or non-autopsied. At the completion of the arterial injection, body cavities should be thoroughly aspirated with a trocar and cannula. At least 2 L of cavity fluid should be injected into the thoracic, abdominal, and pelvic cavities. Cavity fluid is used to detoxicate those materials that cannot be aspirated and also assist in the preservation of the viscera. Cavity fluid has high concentration of formalin for quick action. The cavity fluid has the following composition (Table 18.1).

The rectum and vagina should be packed tightly with cotton soaked with cavity fluid. The nasal cavity should be thoroughly cleaned and packed tightly with small amount of cotton. No trace of cotton should be visible on the face. Mouth should be reopened and cleaned. Cotton wool should be put in the throat and mouth should be closed in the same manner as it was prior to embalming. Now cosmetics can be applied and body is dressed according to the appearance of the deceased for public viewing.

Table 18.1: Composition of cavity fluid.	
Formalin	70–60%
Methylated spirit	20–25%
Phenol	5–10%
Sodium lauryl sulfate	1%
Mercuric chloride	1%

Cremation is the best means of disposal of these bodies because all infected materials would be burnt to ashes. For bodies belonging to religions where burial is advocated, it should be ensured that the coffin is well secured.

On completion of the embalming, disinfect the instruments by dipping in 2% glutaraldehyde for 30 minutes, then washed with soap and water and autoclave. Disinfect the sink. After removing the body the table surface should also be thoroughly washed and disinfect the table top. The floor should be mopped with a disinfectant.

Although soiled linen has been identified as a source of large numbers of certain pathogenic microorganisms, the risk of actual disease transmission is negligible. Rather than rigid procedures and specifications, hygienic and common sense storage and processing of clean and soiled linen are recommended.[9] Soiled laundry should be handled as little as possible and with minimum agitation to prevent gross microbial contamination of the air and persons handling the laundry. Put the soiled linen into double plastic bag. Linen soiled with blood or body fluids should be placed in a bag that prevents leakage. At the completion of embalming the personnel involved should carefully remove their AIDS suit and put into double plastic bag, containing the bag, gloves, and sheets used during transportation and tied properly. Label the bag "infectious risk" and send it immediately for incineration.

If the contents cannot be immediately incinerated, it should be treated with disinfectant (i.e. put a disinfectant solution inside the plastic bag). The bag then should be tightly closed and tied shut. The embalmer should then wash thoroughly with soap and water before dressing.

DISINFECTANT

Blood, body fluids and soiled laundry may be treated by sodium hypochlorite, hydrogen peroxide, lysol, etc. In addition to commercially available chemical germicides, a solution of sodium hypochlorite (household bleach) prepared freshly is an inexpensive and effective germicide. Concentrations ranging from approximately 500 ppm (1:100 dilution of household bleach) sodium hypochlorite to 5000 ppm (1:10 dilution of household bleach) are effective depending on the amount of organic material, i.e. blood or mucus, present on the surface to be cleaned and disinfected.

The above method of embalming is used where the cause of death is known, i.e. AIDS or hepatitis B. If the cause of death' is unknown, the body should be treated as dangerous to public health and treated in the same way as an AIDS body. As we know it is almost impossible to know the HIV status of each and every deceased person in any hospital due to practical, financial, ethical or legal reasons, therefore, it is quite possible that workers dealing with patient/dead bodies carrying HIV, etc. without knowing it. Therefore, we should change our work culture and follow universal work precautions. Thus, there is a need to consider all bodies are potentially infected with HIV and adhere rigorously to "universal work precautions" for minimizing the risk of exposure to blood and body fluids. These precautions are based on CDC (Centers for Disease Control) recommendation.[15,16]

Universal Work Precautions or Universal Blood and Body Fluid Precautions

- Entry to the laboratory/work area should be restricted only to persons who are trained to handle infectious material.
- Laboratory door should be closed and should have a "biohazard" "no admission" sign to prevent unauthorized entry.
- Proper protective clothing-staff should wear a fully covered laboratory coat instead of simple surgical gowns, heavy autopsy gloves or double rubber gloves, caps, masks, protective eye-wear or goggles, shoe covers. Cover yourself completely.

Gloves should be worn for all manipulations of infectious material or where there is a possibility of exposure to blood or body fluids.

Gloves should be changed at the least suspicion of damage. Hands and other skin surfaces should be washed immediately and thoroughly if contaminated with blood or other body fluids.

- *Handling sharp instruments*: All workers should take special precautions in handling needles, scalpels and other sharp instruments used during procedure and prevent accidental pricks and cuts.

- *Disposal of used instruments*: After the use, disposable needles and syringes, scalpel blades, and other sharp items should be placed in puncture resistant container for disposal. The puncture resistant container should be located as close as practical to the used area.
- To prevent needle stick injuries, needles should not be recapped, purposely bent or broken by hand, removed from the disposable syringes, or otherwise manipulated by hand.
- Workers who have exudative lesions or weeping dermatitis should refrain to work in those areas until the condition resolves.
- *Clean up procedure*: Wear now intact gloves. Work surfaces should be cleaned and disinfected when procedure is completed at the end of each working day. Small spatters and spills of blood and other body fluids can be wiped up with disposable tissues or towels which are discarded in a special biohazard bag and properly disposed.
- Pregnant workers are not known to be at greater risk of contracting HIV infection then workers who are not pregnant. However, if a pregnant worker develops HIV infection during pregnancy, the infant is at risk of infection resulting from perinatal transmission. Because of this risk, pregnant workers should be especially familiar with and strictly adhere to precautions to minimize the risk of HIV transmission.

In cases of accidental injuries or cut with sharp instruments contaminating with blood or body fluids, while working on a body, the wound should be immediately disinfected and the incident should be reported to the proper authority to get their blood check for HIV seropositivity. Also to minimize exposures, no unauthorized persons should be admitted to the autopsy or embalming rooms.

Universal precautions are meant to apply to blood, semen and vaginal secretions as well as to CSF, synovial fluid, pleural fluid, peritoneal fluid, pericardial fluid, and amniotic fluid. Universal precautions do not apply to feces, nasal secretions, sputum, sweat, tears, urine, and vomitus unless they contain visible blood.[3,17]

REFERENCES

1. Rose GW, Hockett RN. The microbiologic evaluation and enumeration of postmortem specimens from human remains. Springfield, Ohio: Encyclopedia of Mortuary Practice; 1975. pp. 1829-32.
2. Henderson DK, Saah AJ, Zak BJ, et al. Risk of nosocomial infection with human T-cell lymphotropic virus type III/Lymphadenopathy-associated virus in a large cohort of "intensively exposed health care workers". Ann Intern Med. 104:644-47;1986.
3. Centers for Disease Control. Recommendations for prevention of HIV transmission in health-care settings. MMWR. 1987;36:001.
4. Marcus R, CDC Cooperative Needlestick Surveillance Group. Surveillance of health care: workers exposed to blood from patients infected with the human immunodeficiency virus. N Engl J Med. 1988;319:1118-23.
5. Gerberding JL, Bryant-LeBlanc CE, Nelson K, et al. Risk of transmitting the human immunodeficiency virus, cytomegalovirus, and hepatitis B virus to health care workers exposed to patients with AIDS and AIDS-related conditions. J Infect Dis. 1987;156:1-8.
6. Hill DR. I-UV infection following motor vehicle trauma in Central Africa. JAMA. 1989;261:3282-83.
7. McMahon K, Sutterer MG. Safety precautions and hospital practices in dealing with seropositive individuals. In: DeVita VT, Hellman S, Rosenberg SA (Eds.) AIDS. Philadelphia: JB Lippincott; 1988. pp. 397-420.
8. Bernier RH, Sampliner R, Gerety R, et al. Hepatitis B infection in households of chronic carriers of hepatitis B surface antigen: factors associated with prevalence of infection. Am J Epidemiol. 1982;116:199-211.
9. Garner JS, Favero MS. Guideline for hand washing and hospital environmental control. Atlanta: Public Health Service, Centers for Disease Control HHS Pub. No. 99: 1117, 1985.
10. McDougal JS, Martin LS, Cort SP, et al. Thermal inactivation of the acquired immunodeficiency syndrome virus, human T lymphotropic virus-III/lymphadenopathy-associated virus, with special reference to antihemophilic factor. J Clin Invest. 1985;76:875-7.
11. Martin LS, McDougal JS, Loskoski SL Disinfectant and inactivation of the human T lymphotropic virus type III/lymphedenopathy-associated virus. J Infect Dis. 1985; 152:400-3.
12. Spire B, Barre-Sinoussi F, Dormount D, et al. Inactivation of lymphadenopathy-associated virus by heat, gamma rays and ultraviolet light. Lancet. 1985;1:188-9.
13. Spire B, Barre-Sinoussi F, Montagnier L, et al. Inactivation of lymphadenopathy-associated virus by chemical disinfectants. Lancet. 1984;899-901.
14. Resnik L, Veren K, Salahuddin SZ, et al. Stability and inactivation of HTLV III/LAV under clinical and laboratory environments. TAMA. 1986;255:1887-91.
15. Centers for Disease Control. Recommendations for preventing transmission of infection with human T-lymphotropic virus type III/lymphadenopathy-associated virus in the workplace. MMWR. 1985;34:681-6, 691-5.
16. Centers for Disease Control. Recommendations for preventing transmission of infection with human T-lymphotropic virus type III/lymphadenopathy-associated virus during invasive procedures. MMWR. 1986;35: 221-3.
17. Centers for Disease Control (CDC). Update: universal precautions for prevention of transmission of human immunodeficiency virus, hepatitis B virus and other bloodborne pathogens in health-care settings. MMWR Morb Mortal Wkly Rep. 1988;37:377-82, 387-8.

Chapter 19

Cosmetics and Presentation

ML Ajmani

INTRODUCTION

Care should be taken to maintain the pleasant appearance of the face. The eyelids should be gently closed to give an appearance of sleep. Bearing this point in mind the correct appearance is that of both lids meeting together with the upper eyelid covering approximately two-thirds of the eyeball. Nose should be cleaned and a small amount of cotton wool should be pushed through nostrils. No trace of cotton should be visible on the face. Mouth must be reopened and cleaned. Cotton wool should be put in the throat. The upper lip should set in a manner to protrude over the lower lip, and the angles of the mouth should be elevated slightly and the mouth is closed as described earlier.

Shaving of the male subject may be carried out either before or after the embalming process. Shaving must be carried out with great care to avoid causing "razor burns".

The hair must be washed and shampooed following the injection treatment. If a photograph of the deceased be available it should be dressed accordingly to the appearance in life to achieve a natural style.

The ear must be cleaned.

The moustache, eyebrows, and beard, if present, should be combed. A thin application of massage cream should be applied to the face, particularly to lips and eyelids and hands to prevent dehydration by the embalming fluid.

The hands and feet should be cleaned and the nails are trimmed. The anal and vaginal orifices should be cleaned and plugged with cotton wool soaked in cavity fluid.

USE OF COSMETICS

The art of using the cosmetics is mown as cosmetology. It can be:
- *Technical cosmetology*: It is the use of cosmetics on the dead to give a lifelike appearance.
- *Ornamental cosmetology*: It is the use of cosmetics in the living.

Cosmetic consists of semiopaque cream and capable of besides producing a transparent effect on one hand also covering the scars on the surface. Before application, the cosmetic cream is warmed and thinned in the palm by rubbing hands. Thinner the application better the result. It restores the normal characteristic complexion of the deceased which is altered due to the bleaching action of embalming chemicals and blood drainage. The density of the primary application is reduced by using a light brown facial lotion. These colors are carefully blended to match the adjacent skin so that no line of demarcation is visible. The age of the individual is an important factor to be considered while applying any tint on the face.

The deceased is then dressed to give life-like appearance and gently placed in a coffin or casket in a supine position with the upper limbs by the side or according to the deceased religious dictates and then taken to the viewing place.

Chapter 20

Embalmer's Legal Responsibility

TD Dogra, DN Bhardwaj

INTRODUCTION

The act of embalming is essentially a contract between the person requesting for it and the person obliging it (Medical Officer or Embalmer). Once a request for embalming is accepted by the embalmer, onus of certain legal and ethical responsibility is established under common law which predominantly prevails in any criminal or civil justice. The legal responsibilities involved are not only important but at times mandatory to safeguard the interest of society and embalmer. The most important aspect is Legal Documentation before starting to embalm. It should be on the following lines:

IDENTIFICATION OF THE BODY

The identity of the dead body for embalming is required to be established beyond doubt in the presence of a doctor/technician in a prescribed form by a near relative or a person lawfully in possession of the dead bodies. It is to be kept in mind that even close relatives at times avoid looking at the dead body.

CONSENT

A proper consent from a near relative or from the person in lawful possession of the dead body in a prescribed form is necessary as the embalming is a procedure beyond routine and there could be chances of allegations like removal of the organs, eyes, mutilation, discoloration, disfiguration, etc. At times the actual legal heir of the dead body may object on arrival.

DEATH CERTIFICATE

The death certificate issued by a Registered Medical Officer who has attended the deceased during the last illness is extremely necessary. He must write a brief history of the illness and cause of death. Information to concerned authorities is necessary if a dead body of deceased suffering from notifiable diseases is brought for embalming.

FORM OF APPLICATION FOR EMBALMING HUMAN DEAD BODIES

1. Name of the deceased _____
2. Son/daughter/wife of_____
3. Profession of the deceased _____
4. Permanent address of the deceased _____
5. Passport No. (in case of foreigners) _____
6. Time and date of death_____
7. Age_____Years_____Sex_____(M/F)
8. Place of death _____
9. Cause of death _____
10. Status of the body _____
    (autopsied/nonautopsied/mutilated/decomposed/accidental, etc.)
11. The dead body is to be transported to _____
    by air/flight No. _____ Airlines _____
    by road/other _____ in India _____
    Place _____ District _____
12. The applicant is related to the deceased as friend/colleague/relation _____
    any other (specify) _____
13. Name and address of the applicant _____
14. Any specific disease the deceased, suffered from known to the
    Person filling the form _____
    Tuberculosis _____
    Cancer; hepatitis _____
    AIDS _____
    Tetanus; any other (specify)_____

15. Certified that
    a. The body has been identified.
    b. This is a natural death and no foul play is suspected in this case.
    c. The information given here is correct and no relevant fact has been concealed.
    d. Embalming may please be done at our risk and responsibility.
    e. I shall not hold the embalmer responsible for any consequences arising directly or indirectly out of embalming.
    f. The embalmed body will be removed from this department within 24 hours.

*Delete whichever is not applicable.

_____

Signature of witness Signature of applicant
_____ _____
_____ _____

Name Name
_____ _____

_____ _____
Address Address

_____ _____

_____ _____
       Telephone No. _____

CERTIFICATE OF EMBALMING

       Dated _____
This is to certify that the dead body of late _____ S/D/W of Mr _____ an/a _____ national, brought to this Department from _____ _____ Where he/she had died, having been duly embalmed by me and in the present condition, it is not a hazard to public health.

The body after the embalming has been handed over to the claimants, who brought it to this department. Received back the embalmed body of late_____ and 3/5*. Copies of this certificate

Signature of the claimant
With his/her full address
*3 for local transportation/5 for international transit.

       Signature of the
       Faculty Member
       Official Seal
_____ Under Section 297 IPC. "Section 297 states _____

Or as a depository for the remains of the dead or offers any indignity to any human corpse, shall be punished with imprisonment of either description for a term which may extend to one year or with fine or with both". Therefore, it is relevant to mention that any sort of disrespect or unnecessary mutilation of dead body may amount to an offence under Section 297 IPC.

NO OBJECTION CERTIFICATE FROM POLICE

In all the medicolegal cases, "no objection certificate" from the police is necessary. Police Clearance is also needed for embalming the nonautopsied cases.

CLEARANCE FROM EMBASSY, MISSION AND HIGH COMMISSIONS, ETC.

In foreign nationals, such a clearance is necessary to avoid future complications.

Before starting embalming it is advisable to have an external examination of dead body for any marks of violence or other findings suspecting of foul play. If foul play is suspected, police should be informed immediately through the hospital authorities or as per laid procedures. The declaration of the relatives is not enough, that there is no foul play regarding cause of death as per CrPC 39. This is the duty of medical officer to decide whether the case is medicolegal or not. However, such a declaration is a good defense in case of any complications.

Embalming should not be done prior to autopsy as it can destroy the medicolegal evidences.

What Is a Medicolegal Case?

It is a case of injury or ailment where an attending doctor after taking history and clinical examination of the patient, thinks that some investigations by law enforcing agencies are essential so as to fix responsibility regarding the case in accordance with the law of the land.

Following cases are medicolegal:
1. Road side accidents, factory accidents or any other unnatural mishap resulting in death.
2. Suspected or evident homicides or suicides, including attempted.
3. Suspected or evident poisoning.
4. Burn injuries due to any cause.
5. Injury cases where foul play is suspected, if doctor thinks that the patient is an accused or a victim in crime case.
6. Injury cases where there is likelihood of death in near future.
7. Suspected or evident criminal abortions.
8. Unconscious cases, where cause of unconsciousness is not clear.
9. Cases brought dead with improper history.
10. Cases referred by court or otherwise which require age certificate.

On completion of embalming, a certificate is issued by a competent authority (Embalmer). The certificate is a prerequisite for transportation of the dead body. The following format is suggested on the previous page.

Notifiable Diseases

Information to concerned authorities is necessary if a dead body of deceased suffering from notifiable diseases is brought for embalming.

Infectious diseases generally are transmitted by direct contact or contact with infected materials, clothing, discharges, vomits, etc. Necessary precautions must be taken before handling such bodies the following diseases are highly infectious and can be contagious. It is better not to handle these bodies more than necessary. Put the body into a polythene bag and bury or cremate. The diseases are cholera, cerebrospinal meningitis, rabies, poliomyelitis, mumps, Malta fever, plague, septicemia, smallpox, tetanus, typhoid or enteric group of fevers, diphtheria, tuberculosis, hepatitis B, and AIDS. It is advisable not to embalm such bodies unless it is absolutely essential. Always observe "Universal Work Precautions" in handling such bodies.

Refusal on the Ground of Infectious Diseases

Though the doctor is having a right to select patient as a private practitioner but in Government Institution, such a matter may have to be imposed by the Administrative Authority. Ordinarily ethically doctor cannot refuse to handle the infectious dead bodies on the ground of risk involved.

Chapter 21

Soft Embalming

Renu Dhingra, Sanjeev Lalwani

INTRODUCTION

The embalmed cadavers have played an important role in imparting anatomy education to the newly entrant medical students for decades as silent educators and their significance in medical school curriculum cannot be underestimated. However, they also stand out as important learning resource material in training surgeons for sharpening their operative skills that may not be possible on an actual patient as it can have greater chance of misadventure as a result of the relative inexperience. Further, with the evolution of surgical practice over the last few decades with increasing adoption of minimally invasive procedures and newer intervention techniques, improved methods of surgical education become exigent. They can also be used for testing new devices or techniques and provide scope for their improvisation in the early stages.[1] Thus, it becomes absolutely necessary to select the correct preservation method(s) as it will impact the future use of these embalmed cadavers.

Traditionally most of the anatomy departments use formaldehyde-based embalming methods. Though formalin provides a long-term preservation of structures as it is bactericidal, fungicidal, insecticidal (decreasing efficiency) and has an excellent antiseptic properties;[2] however, it causes over hardening, drying, extreme rigidity and has an unpleasant odor. The formalin-based embalming has been in use for more than five decades in spite of the concerns related to its contribution to health hazards. Cost effectiveness, efficiency of preservation and sustainability are the major factors for continued use of this technique. However, this traditional formalin fixation has been found to be unsuitable for the purpose of surgical skills training due to lack of flexibility, suppleness of tissues and low fidelity. The fresh frozen cadavers though offer a good alternative for surgical skills training but they deteriorate faster due to repeated thawing, can be used for short term only and carry a significant risk of infection.[3] Prof Walter Thiel in 1990 developed an embalming technique that produced life like, soft and flexible cadavers and the procedure was since then known as Thiel soft-fix embalming. The Thiel soft-fix embalming method has been refined over the past three decades.[4-6]

PROCEDURE

Soft embalming is an alternative to the traditional formalin-based preservation method consisting of water-based mixtures [propylene glycol, ammonium nitrate, potassium nitrate, sodium sulfite, boric acid, chlorocresol and low amounts of formalin (0.8–3%)] along with alcohol and morpholine.[7,8] The cadavers thus produced are not only soft, pliable, flexible but could also be preserved for longer time and are suitable for the surgical skills training procedures thus offering higher fidelity. The embalming process comprises of an initial perfusion followed by immersion in the immersion fluid for at least 2–3 months. After this, the bodies can be stored in plastic bags and kept in mortuary freezers at –4°C temperature.

The cadavers are embalmed with arterial infusion into the femoral or common carotid artery and venous infusion into the superior sagittal sinus (via a small hole drilled through the skull) or internal jugular vein. The sloughing of keratin layer of skin generally marks the end point of the infusion. An additional intratracheal, intrathecal and intrarectal injection of the fixative has been mentioned in the original Thiel's protocol but it can be performed only if required. After the infusion of fluid, entire body is submerged into tank containing immersion fluid and is ideally kept in tank for 2–3 months. Later the cadavers are

Box 21.1: Chemical constituents of soft embalming solution used for perfusion and immersion.[4]

Solution A
- *Boric acid*: 3 g
- *Ammonium nitrate*: 20 g
- *Potassium nitrate*: 5 g
- *Propylene glycol*: 30 mL
- *Hot tap water*: 100 mL

Solution B
- *Ethylene glycol*: 10 mL
- *4-Chloro-3-methylphenol (chlorocresol)*: 1 mL

Injection solution
- *Solution A*: 14,300 mL
- *Solution B*: 500 mL
- *Formaldehyde*: 300 mL
- *Sodium sulfate*: 700 g

Immersion solution
- *Ethylene glycol*: 10 mL
- *Formaldehyde*: 2 mL
- *Boric acid*: 3 g
- *Ammonium nitrate*: 10 g
- *Potassium nitrate*: 10 g
- *Sodium sulfate*: 7 g
- *Hot water*: 100 mL
- *Solution B*: 2 mL

taken out and tightly wrapped in the plastic bag and kept in the freezer. The chemical constituents of the fluid are shown in Box 21.1.

This preservation is effective in the long term, with estimated viability of 36 months, which allows multiple uses of the cadavers, increasing availability and reducing the cost incurred.

ROLE OF VARIOUS COMPONENTS OF SOFT EMBALMING FLUID

Formaldehyde: It is bactericidal, fungicidal and insecticidal (effectiveness in decreasing grades). It is disinfectant in higher doses (8% formaldehyde in 70% alcohol or 4–8% in water). It destroys putrefactive organisms when dissolved in a vehicle which allows it to permeate the organisms.

Boric acid/sodium borate: It works as insecticide, mild antiseptic or bacteriostatic. The boric acid in soft embalming fluid is responsible for modification of the integrity (cut or ground appearance) and the alignment of muscle fibers.[9]

Phenol or carbolic acid: The phenol and its derivatives are used in resins, general disinfectants and production of organic dyes. It is used as a disinfectant.[10,11] It is bacteriostatic at lower concentrations (0.2%) as it can deactivate intracellular enzymes and affect cell permeability. It acts like bactericidal/fungicidal at concentration of 1.0–1.5% and can destroy the cell walls due to its lipophilic character.[10] Liquefied phenol has been shown to be very effective in preventing molding.[12] Though it is an excellent fungicide and bactericide, it causes discoloration and dryness of tissues.

4-Chloro-3-methylphenol (4-Chloro-m-cresol/PCMC): It is used as an antiseptic and preservative agent. It is highly soluble and remains active over a wide pH range (4–8). PCMC remains sufficiently soluble as compared to other phenol derivatives.[2]

Ethylene glycol: It is used to preserve the moisture and tissue plasticity in the embalmed cadaver, thus being responsible for the haptic properties of the tissues.[7,13-16]

Ammonium nitrate, potassium nitrate and sodium sulfite: The salts used, i.e. ammonium nitrate, potassium nitrate and sodium sulfite absorb the water content of the tissues. The nitrates give red color to the muscles through the action of nitrosomyoglobin formed in the muscle itself.[17,18]

Alcohols: Alcohols have a bactericidal as well as bacteriostatic action against vegetative forms; the specific effect depends on the concentration and the condition. They also have wide range of antiviral, antifungal and antimycosal effects through the action on proteins by their coagulation or denaturation. Ethanol can be used to wash out excess formaldehyde.[19]

The Thiel soft-fix embalmed cadavers have been used for various skills training like laparoscopic procedures in surgery (hernia repair, cricothyroidotomy, chest tube insertion, thoracotomy, vascular repairs, central venous catheterization, etc.) urology (retrograde pyeloureterography, upper and lower urinary tract endoscopy, renal angiography, etc.). They form a useful resource for surgical training in specialties like gynecology, otolaryngology, anesthesia, orthopedics and oral surgery. The consistency, color and tactile feedback has been reported to be almost identical to live procedures.

ALTERNATIVE TO THIEL SOFT EMBALMING

Although the Thiel or modified Thiel soft-fix embalming has the advantage of meeting high standards of

Box 21.2: Advantages and disadvantages of soft-embalmed cadavers.

Advantages
- Excellent flexibility and tissue quality (good haptic properties)
- Increased range of joint movements
- Less dissection time
- Easy identification of individual muscles
- Easy approach toward areas such as axilla
- Manipulation of limbs
- Testing of equipment and devices

Disadvantages
- High cost
- Short-lasting measure (36 months)
- Muscular disintegration
- Difficulty in handling the organs because of increased pliability
- Loss of anatomical impressions and landmarks
- Absence of normal living physiological spaces
- The average age and health of the donated cadavers
- Artifacts caused by the embalming process

Box 21.3: Surgical procedures performed on soft-embalmed cadavers at the All India Institute of Medical Sciences (AIIMS), New Delhi.

1. *Surgery and Obstetrics and Gynecology Department*: Laparoscopic surgical procedures [cholecystectomy, rhinoplasty (repair), appendectomy]
2. Endoscopic thoracic procedures
3. *Anesthesia*: Airway management, ultrasound-guided regional anesthesia and analgesia
4. *Orthopedics*: Arthroplasty, arthroscopy, pelvic surgical approaches, hand surgery
5. *Ear, nose, and throat (ENT)*: Fascioplasty, rhinoplasty, temporal bone dissection, laryngoplasty
6. *Neurosurgery*: Endoscopic procedures, skull base surgical approaches, minimal access spinal surgeries, spinal surgeries
7. *Physical Medicine and Rehabilitation*: Pain management procedures
8. *Emergency medicine*: Tube thoracostomy, cricothyroidotomy
9. *Plastic surgery department*: Skin grafting, vascular repair, nerve and tendon repair, ear reconstruction
10. *Gastrointestinal surgery*: Cadaveric liver harvesting for transplantation
11. *Dental medicine*: Oral and maxillofacial surgeries

preservation without releasing harmful substances into the environment, the method has some drawbacks (Box 21.2) like expensive chemicals, complicated procedure, limited time of preservation, muscular disintegration, absence of normal physiological spaces and lower fidelity of ultrasound images to be used during specific block procedures as compared to live patient.

Logan described a method where he used alcohol, glycerin, phenol and low levels of formaldehyde.[20] Coleman and Kogan modified his protocol by adding high salt component (saturated NaCl solution) and replaced alcohol with isopropyl alcohol.[21] The cadavers preserved by this saturated salt solution (SSS) method were excellently preserved, supple and did not get desiccated.[22]

Although multiple models are being used in teaching and training of surgical skills, e.g. live animals, robotic simulators yet soft-embalmed human cadavers may serve as true anatomical simulator currently available and the only method permitting the practice of entire operation, good tissue fidelity for visceral procedures and providing three-dimensional learning environment.[23,24] By soft embalming the human cadaver, it not only provides flexibility but also improves the learning curve to correctly understand the precise anatomical details and enhances the effectiveness of teaching surgical skills (Box 21.3).

ACKNOWLEDGMENTS

The authors thank Dr Chawi Sahney, Dr Seema Singhal, Dr Hemango Chatterjee for their valuable input regarding the feedback of the soft embalming procedure which enabled them to perform different surgical procedures. We also thank Dr Eisma Roos for her suggestions and guidance all along the journey. We thank the Department of Anatomy and Professor TS Roy, Head, Department of Anatomy, All India Institute of Medical Sciences (AIIMS), New Delhi for his unending streak of generosity and allowing us to soft embalm the valuable donated cadavers, providing the infrastructure for the embalming. The constant support and encouragement by our Ex-Director and Professor MC Misra at every step has helped us a great deal.

REFERENCES

1. Eisma R, Wilkinson T. From "silent teachers" to models. PLoS Biol. 2014;12(10):e1001971.
2. Brenner E. Human body preservation—old and new techniques. J Anat. 2014;224:316-44.
3. Anderson SD. Practical light embalming technique for use in the surgical fresh tissue dissection laboratory. Clin Anat. 2006;19:8-11.
4. Thiel W. Die Konservierung ganzer Leichen in natürlichen Farben. Ann Anat. 1992;174:185-95.
5. Thiel W. Ergànzung für die Konservierung ganzer Leichen nach. Ann Anat. 2002;184:267-9.
6. Ottone NE, Vargas CA, Fuentes R, et al. Walter Thiel's embalming method. Review of solutions and applications in different fields of biomedical research. Int J Morphol. 2016;34(4):1442-54.

7. Eisma R, Lamb C, Soames RW. From formalin to Thiel embalming: what changes? One anatomy department's experiences. Clin Anat. 2013;26(5):564-71.
8. Eisma R, Mahendran S, Majumdar S, et al. A comparison of Thiel and formalin embalmed cadavers for thyroid surgery training. Surgeon. 2011;9(3):142-6.
9. Benkhadra M, Bouchot A, Gerard J, et al. Flexibility of Thiel's embalmed cadavers: the explanation is probably in the muscles. Surg Radiol Anat. 2011;33:365-8.
10. Bedino JH. Phenol exposure in embalming rooms: part 1. Champion Expanding Encyclopedia of Mortuary Practices. 1994;621:2498-2500.
11. Bedino JH. ENIGMA: champion's fourth generation chemostasis infusion chemicals: embalming redefined for the 21st century. Champion Expanding Encyclopedia of Mortuary Practices. 2009;657:2709-17.
12. Bradbury SA, Hoshino K. An improved embalming procedure for long-lasting preservation of the cadaver for anatomical study. Acta Anat (Basel). 1978;101:97-103.
13. Hölzle F, Franz EP, Lehmbrock J, et al. Thiel embalming technique: a valuable method for teaching oral surgery and implantology. Clin Implant Dent Relat Res. 2012;14(1):121-6.
14. Hayashi S, Homma H, Naito M, et al. Saturated salt solution method: a useful cadaver embalming for surgical skills training. Medicine (Baltimore). 2014;93(27):e196.
15. Hammer N, Löffler S, Bechmann I, et al. Comparison of modified Thiel embalming and ethanol-glycerin fixation in an anatomy environment: potentials and limitations of two complementary techniques. Anat Sci Educ. 2015;8(1):74-85.
16. Willaert W, Tozzi F, Van Hoof T, et al. Lifelike vascular reperfusion of a Thiel-embalmed pig model and evaluation as a surgical training tool. Eur Surg Res. 2016;56(3-4):97-108.
17. Janczyk P, Weigner J, Luebke-Becker A, et al. Nitrite pickling salt as an alternative to formaldehyde for embalming in veterinary anatomy: a study based on histo- and microbiological analyses. Ann Anat. 2011;193(1):71-5.
18. Hammer N, Schröder C, Schleifenbaum S. On the suitability of Thiel-fixed samples for biomechanical purposes: critical considerations on the articles of Liao et al. "Elastic properties of Thiel-embalmed human ankle tendon and ligament" and Verstraete et al. "Impact of drying and Thiel embalming on mechanical properties of Achilles tendons". Clin Anat. 2016;29(4):424-5.
19. Bjorkman N, Nielsen P, Moller VH. Removing formaldehyde from embalmed cadavers by percolating the body cavities with dilute ethanol. Acta Anat (Basel). 1986;126:78-83.
20. Logan B. The long-term preservation of whole human cadavers destined for anatomical study. Ann R Coll Surg Engl. 1983;65:333.
21. Coleman R, Kogan I. An improved formaldehyde embalming fluid to preserve cadavers for anatomy teaching. J Anat. 1998;192:443-6.
22. Hayashi S, Naito M, Kawata S, et al. History and future of human cadaver preservation for surgical training: from formalin to saturated salt solution method. Anat Sci Int. 2016;91(1):1-7.
23. Healy SE, Rai BP, Biyani CS, et al. Thiel embalming method for cadaver preservation: a review of new training model for urologic skills training. Urology. 2015;85(3):499-504.
24. Reddy R, Iyer S, Pillay M, et al. Soft embalming of cadavers for training purposes: optimising for long-term use in tropical weather. Indian J Plast Surg. 2017;50:29-34.

Chapter 22

The Law and the Dead

T Jayavelu

THE WESTERN SCENERIO

In the West, the matter of the disposal of the dead is controlled by elaborate statutes and safeguards.
- Embalming is necessary if funeral is delayed by more than 24 hours, whether the body is inhumed or cremated.
- The disposal of the dead is arranged by agencies licensed by the state. The training for the trade and the award for satisfactory completion of the training is rigidly controlled by a National Board, the watchdog of the service.
- The embalming chemicals used should exclude heavy metals like arsenic, mercury, lead, copper, etc. to prevent complication of death due to medicolegal problems.
- Use of cadaver tissue for therapeutic use (transplant) or for teaching in the medical institutions engaged in research and teaching, involves rigid regulations and legal safeguards. "Clinical death" is redefined to this end.
- Where the regulations are not specific the common law (the customary law) of the land prevails.

THE INDIAN PRACTICE

In India it is the common law of the land that is applied in the disposal of the dead. The dictates of the various castes and communities determine the time, interval between death, and disposal. Because of the fear of the dead the disposal is usually quick within 24 hours, and rarely causes any major public health problem.

Cadaver dissection for anatomical study is mentioned in the *Sushruta Samhita*. A surgical treatise, in Sanskrit, on Ayurveda, is the ancient Indian traditional medicine. The author Sushruta, an outstanding surgeon on rhinoplasty in the 6th century BC, tells the method of study and teaching of human anatomy by scraping the decomposing tissue of a corpse kept immersed in a bed of slow flowing stream. Chemical embalming of the human body was unknown till the introduction of modern medicine with the advent of the British rule in India. The teaching medical institutions embalm the bodies to preserve them for anatomical dissection, a part of medical curriculum. The process of embalming is hardly known outside the precincts of such institutions. In the case of death of important personalities who have to be kept in state for public view, or of a decedent for transport to a place outside the country, embalming is done in the anatomy department of medical institutions all of which enjoy statutory protection. Therefore, no separate statutes on embalming by a private individual, or by an institution of undertakers, have been enacted at any time in India.

India was under the imperial rule of Great Britain till 1947, and the rules and regulations were the barest necessary conforming to the British administrative convenience. Except in a gross way, the statutes hardly encroached on the religious beliefs and practices of the population. The people were allowed to follow the customary laws of the land on the disposal of the dead, with minor infringements for sanitary cause. The laws that were enacted were confined to the early part of this century, and death with medical education.

The Indian Medical Degree Act, 1916, to codify the award of medical degree in the modem medical institutions that were organized by the British.

The Indian Medical Council Act, 1933, to create a medical council similar to the British Medical Council for the conduct and control of medical practice and medical education in India. This has been repealed by the Indian Medical Council Act of 1956. With the end of the British rule in India in 1947, i.e. after independence, the Anatomy Act of 1949 was enacted to provide for cadavers required by search purposes. Following this, various acts were passed in the legislatures of the several states of the Republic of India, like (a) Corneal Grafting Act of 1957; (b) Ear Drum and Ear Bones Act of 1982; (c) Kidney Transplantation Act of 1982, etc. These acts provide for the use of donor tissues for therapeutic purpose. The donation should be voluntary and the issues may be removed on the death of the donor by qualified medical men, provided a near relation of deceased does not object to the removal.

While the Anatomy Act has been uniformly adopted in all the States of the Republic of India, the acts on the donation of the tissues for transplant have not been uniform. The Kidney Act is confined to Bombay and Delhi, but the Cornea Act has a wider adoption. The country's human tissue acts are not keeping pace with the advancing transplant surgery and the hunger for tissue for such use. This is likely to lead to exploitation of the people by vulgar and unsavory competition from unscrupulous elements of the society. While the law is indifferent to the donation of blood and skin, which are the easily replaced tissues of the body, it limits the individuals' power to give valid directions regarding the disposal of the body or selected parts thereof after death. A case in point is *Dr Krishnan versus Tamil Nadu State* (1987) on the right to donate his body for anatomical use. The Anatomy Act provides for the collection of a dead body for teaching purpose, only if death occurs in a State hospital or in a public place within the prescribed zone of a medical institution, provided the police have declared after a lapse of 48 hours that there are no claimants for the body and it could be used for medical purpose. The position now is that even if a decedent wills away his body for therapeutic use it could be vetoed by the person having the right to dispose of the body, or by an institution of religio-social character interested in the disposal of the body according to the religious tenets. The court directed that the body of Dr Krishnan shall be accepted provided the next of kin made arrangements for the delivery of the body to the medical institution without contesting the decedents' will. At present the statutes and measure are not conductive to the progressive development of medical science.

The world "transplant" was first used by John Hunter around 1778 when he was experimenting with ovarian and testicular grafts between unrelated animals (xenograft). Early 19th century concentrated on autografts of skin. MacEwen in 1881 successfully allografted (different individuals of the same species) bone; this was followed by the transplant of cornea by Zirm in 1905. This rekindled the interest in transplant surgery, and an allograft of kidney was carried out in Russia in 1933 with poor result. With better methods of harvesting and storage of organs and tissues (cold perfusion and ice storage of kidney up to 36 hours, liver up to 10 hours, and heart up to 4 hours), with matching for blood group and human leukocyte antigen (HLA) including chromosome 6 systems, and with necessary immunosuppressive therapy, renal graft has become the treatment of choice for end-stage renal failure. It is said that about 10,000 renal transplants are carried out in a year throughout the world, half of which are done in the United States of America (USA). There is chronic shortage of donor kidneys to meet the need. The first human heart transplant by Barnard in 17%, because of the publicity attached to it, triggered a spate of transplants in many centers ill-equipped to cope with the problems of rejection and aftercare. The poor survival rate brought in its wake widespread criticism on all transplant surgery. By 1981 over 400 patients had received cardiac transplant. Less than 100 were alive for over a year. The results are not encouraging. Of the 46 patients who received liver transplant before 1981, only 13% survived for 1 year or more. Since then with the introduction of cyclosporin (a fungal therapeutic agent) into the immunosuppressive regimen the survival rate has shown much improvement. Pancreatic transplant as a cure for diabetes mellitus is discouraging. The result of lung transplant has been gloomy. On the whole transplant surgery is mainly concerned with kidney obtained from a living or dead donor. A great majority of organs transplanted in the United Kingdom (UK) and the USA are taken from cadavers certified as brainstem dead. It is estimated that in UK alone about 2,000 patients die annually from end-stage renal failure, from lack of hemodialysis, or a suitable kidney transplant. It is noted that about 4,000 suitable donors die each year but only about 450 are used as organ donors. This is due to the resistance of the society to transplantation, reluctance of the medical community to accept transplant as a method of treatment, antigenic effect of the donor organ on the donee, side effects of the immunosuppressive drugs, and the emotional doubts about the validity of brainstem death. Besides, the community and the state are reluctant to give in for the high cost technology of transplants to benefit a few at the risk of general community health. This is the state of affairs in an advanced country like the UK. Organ transplant is very slow in picking up in India due to multiple handicaps: Lack of trained personnel, equipment, cost structure, and availability of donor. Liberal legalization on obtaining, cadaver tissue should encourage transplant surgery to develop in India on a wider scale. The medical, the theological, and the political personnel should work to this end.

The major medical limitation upon the increase of successful transplants is the problem of incompatibility (antigenicity), i.e. the human body rejects the tissues transplanted from another individual (allograft-genetically different individual of the same species) as a foreign substance, and consequently the body reacts as in a bacterial or viral infection, producing antibodies to reject the implanted tissue. This immunological opposition is greater, the greater the genetic difference between the donor and the recipient. As a result, transplants between twins (isograft) or from the patient himself (autograft) like the skin and bone will not involve rejection. Transplants between blood relations will improve the chances of success considerably. But these are so few and not always practical; ultimately it falls on the nonrelated donors to supply the tissue. Noncritical tissues such as the skin or cornea (within 6–12 hours after death) may be leisurely removed after the donor's death. One of any paired organs, such as the kidneys, can be taken from a living donor without substantial detriment to the health of the donor, the same is not true of the vital organs like the liver, heart, and lungs. For these organs, as well as cornea, blood vessels and bone occasionally, the only practical source is a dead body, a cadaver. Often the donor and the donee should be proximate for the organ removed to be transplanted quickly enough. This will considerably reduce the cost of transplant. Because of the time difference between the somatic and cellular deaths the organ transplants are made possible. The brain is the most sensitive tissue to suffer from oxygen loss, and dies within 3–4 minutes following somatic death. This process of transfer of organs from the dead to the living cells is for better understanding and definition of death. But it is not so easy to define death within the framework of law, religion, and medicine that crowd around the human being in his last minutes.

As far back as 1947, France legislated for the use of cadaver tissue by a group of medical men in an accredited and restricted list of hospitals, obtained from autopsies performed, without the antemortem consent of the deceased or the consent of the relatives, for scientific and therapeutic purposes. Autopsies done on victims of crime, suicides, and accidents, and Moslems for religious reasons were excluded. For the purpose of removal of organs for transplant, a new definition of death was made by the French Government "clinical death is considered to have taken place when a person is affected by lesions incompatible with continued life, though maintained in a state of vegetable existence by various devices, and when an electroencephalogram has shown for a period of at least 10 minutes for lack of function in the higher nervous centers, that is to say when the electroencephalogram tracing is a straight line". The difficulty with accepting irreversible brain damage as the criterion for somatic death (cerebral death) is that a person may die before the heart and lungs have given up functioning, such as in a case of massive cerebral hemorrhage. The individual can continue to exist at a low level carrying on the basic metabolic functions of respiration, circulation, deglutition, and excretion for considerable time by artificial means. Death can be said to have occurred only if the mechanical supports are withdrawn and the patient is unable to maintain the vital functions of circulation and respiration independently. In case where respiratory muscles fail as in a case of poliomyelitis, the patient is maintained in an iron lung though there is no brain damage and cerebral death. Whoever turns off the mechanical means of life support in cases such as these will be exposed to criminal action. Such an act done for the removal of an organ for transplant will be considered as homicide. Because of such possible complications it is now recommended that the medical staff should not prolong the life of an individual who has suffered irreversible brain damage in the hope of benefitting some individual requiring an organ transplant. It is said that the electroencephalogram can only be of great confirmatory value and not the only test to declare an individual dead. To declare a patient dead the following points have been taken into consideration by the German Surgical Society:

- Patient is unconscious for at least 12 hours
- Spontaneous respiration ceases
- Bilateral mydriasis sets in
- Pupils do not react to light, and all reflexes are extinct
- Encephalographic tracing shows an isoelectric line for at least an hour.

It is generally felt that the definition of death is not purely a medical question, but involves the legislative, ecclesiastic, and judicial authorities as a matter of public policy, since the deceased has acquired a new dimension with his value to donate tissues for the medical improvement or health of another. With the living donor there are problems of consent, age of consent, sex, nature of the irreplaceable tissue to be donated, the chance of the donor continuing to be healthy after the loss of the organ, the possibility of a heroic sacrifice of donor to save his alter ego (on the analogy that it is acclaimed as heroism if a person risks his life to save another from drowning), the uncertain legal effect on the competence of a donor to gift an organ, and lastly the civil and criminal liabilities that will involve the medical team or the medical institution. These may not be realities now in India but they definitely loom large in the horizon to threaten the progress of medical science. There is irrefutable evidence that there is exploitation in the assumed voluntary kidney and blood donations. The whole area of tissue replacement is be set with moral and ethical questions in the Western world. Organs such as the test is being transplanted or engrafted upon another may excite hostile reaction from the moralists if it is from a living donor but the hostility may not be so severe if the tissue is got from a cadaver. Implantation of the testis could provide fertile gametes, but the recipient would live all through his life with the knowledge that the child born is by someone else's gamete.

In India there are no proper legislative measures even in the matter of the use of the common transplants of replaceable tissues like blood and skin. The Anatomy Act is not comprehensive enough to encourage bequeathing of human body for medical and scientific advancement. Voluntary donation of tissue by an individual during his life could be revoked by the next of kin or his coreligionists on the death of the donor. Because of this the Kidney Act and the Cornea Act suffer limitations in their applicability, and abbreviate or deny the benefits that they are supposed to confer on the community. The cadaver material for anatomical dissection in the medical institution is based mainly on the presumption that individuals dying in the State hospitals should be declared as destitutes by the police to make them available for medical use. An interval of 48 hours should have lapsed without any claimant for the disposal of the deceased. During this period due to storage defects like improper refrigeration, or exposure to room temperature, putrefaction always sets in the tropical weather conditions of India. Even anatomical embalming sometimes defies such as decomposition with consequent loss of invaluable tissues, and an equal loss of valuable chemicals used in the embalming process. The Anatomy Act of 1949 was made at a time when the demand for cadavers for anatomical dissection was limited. Now with manifold increase in the number of teaching medical institutions and the shrinking in the availability of cadavers due to public consciousness in the care of the destitutes dying in the hospital, or other public places, it has become a common practice to allot, anywhere between 30 students and 40 students to dissect one cadaver, or to conduct one single pathology postmortem in a year to meet the needs of the curriculum. In the years to come with better education, industrialization, and economic improvement the social awareness will further improve, and as in the West will enlighten people to bequeath bodies for medical advancement. The present paucity for cadaver is a setback to the medical education, and it is already apparent in the lack of research in the basic sciences in most of the institutions. The present method of delayed cadaver acquisition is not suited for the surgical use of human tissue. It will be illogical to argue that cadaver tissue is not desirable for transplant since all the critical organs like the heart, liver, and lungs, have to be got only from a cadaver, even a noncritical tissue like an artery can only be obtained from the dead. Even at present cadaver cornea is accepted for transplant by the medical profession, and the society. There is, therefore, an urgent necessity, to legislate on this subject in public interest. The urgency for the legislation is greater now than ever before for the reason that transplant surgery is catching up fast. At present whatever tissue grafting is done in the country, especially the kidney, depends on live donors. This has become a lucrative trade, and before it becomes a festering sore on the social conscience of the Indian Society, proper laws need to be framed by a representative body constituted under the aegis of the Government of India and the Indian Medical Council.

The Indian Medical Council should persuade the Government of India to alter the resent situation and introduce measures similar to the Human Tissue Act of 1961 of Britain, and the Uniform Anatomical Gift Act 1969 (called Uniform Act) of USA to deal effectively with several problems that the piecemeal legislation enacted decades ago, have failed to solve. The committee constituted for this purpose should represent all the interests of the society, political, legal, medical, social, ecclesiastical, scientific, technological, and thanatological groups. They should suggest legal measures acceptable to the majority of the society on:

- The living donor should generally be limited, discouraged, and avoided, especially children and incompetents.
- If organs have to be removed from a case of irreparable brain damage of those in the "twilight zone" of life and death, declaration of the death of the individual should not be left to the attending physician. Death should be defined in the new context, and it should be declared by a team other than the attending physician and the operating team.
- The role of the next of kin or the custodian of the body with rights to dispose of the body, and the power to revoke the will of the donor should be defined.
- The rights of the State to remove whole or part of the body tissues for public good if the cause of death is undiagnosed.
- The rights of the citizen to bequeath his body or part of it for medical and scientific use. It will be an inhuman disrespect for the dead as well as callous indifference to the feelings of the living, if such gifts should not be permitted by the state. There should clear and specific guidance for the decedents body to reach the donee.
- The legislation should not be restricted to state controlled institutions but comprehend the utility of reputed private institutions engaged in the teaching, research, and development of medical and heal sciences.

Chapter 23

Establishment of the Embalming Facilities

ML Ajmani

NEED OF EMBALMING

Embalming is the scientific treatment of the dead human body ensuring that it is free from possible infection to the living. The demand for embalming bodies, for transportation or for preservation when there is delay in performing the funeral ceremony, is increasing in this country. To prevent transmission of certain deadly diseases like HIV infection and hepatitis B, it is necessary to make embalming procedure hazard proof and hygienic. With this view the preparation room should be constructed solely for the purpose of scientific treatment of human remains. It should contain facilities for preventing the diseases and properly disposing of waste material arising out of the embalming process. To summarize, the purpose of embalming would be:
- To prevent spread of infection to the living.
- To arrest process of decomposition and putrefaction
- To pursue scientific studies at leisure
- To allow transportation and delayed funeral service
- To achieve premortem appearance.

The primary purpose of a well-designed embalming area is to provide a safe and comfortable work place. There should be a common layout for the embalming facility area and should be governed by state levels or by local authorities. Authorities are advised to consult experts in the construction fields and to be certain that facilities and plans proposed should conform to all local requirements. Because of the infectious nature of the dead human remains and hazardous effects of the chemicals, planning of the embalming area is a major concern. It is recommended that the embalming facility area should consist of:
- Two embalming rooms
- A preparation room
- A changing room
- A post-embalming room
- A waiting room.

Embalming Room

The ground floor is usually the most ideal and least expensive location for an embalming room. It should be situated at the rear of the premises near to where the deceased is received through a separate entrance. An area of 180–315 ft^2 for this room should be considered an optimum. The room should be built on the same lines as a surgical operation theater. Be sure that site must have adequate space, running water, adequate ventilation, good light, sufficient electrical outlets, and multiple drains. An efficient ventilation system must be maintained in the embalming room so that a constant stream of fresh air remains in circulation and also protect the staff from toxic effects of formalin and other chemicals. There should be two embalming rooms when one room is being fumigated, the other will be in use.

In construction, consideration must be given to the need that all the surfaces should be smooth and even and should be completely washable with disinfectant. Uneven surface can harbor infectious organisms and may need quick repair. Walls must be covered in their entirety by tile or plaster. If plaster is used, it must be finished with enamel, a smooth waterproof material. Floor must be entirely of concrete with glazed surface or tiled of marble so as to be impervious to water. Walls and ceiling may be finished with light colors to give pleasing appearance to the eyes. A central trap drainage system is essential so that all surface wash on the floor will drain into it. A sink with running hot and cold water possessing a two inch capacity drain pipe should be fixed in one corner of the room. The provision of a sluice is necessary for the hygienic disposal of body fluids, aspirated materials, etc.

Doors and corridors leading to the room must be of ample width, if casketing is to be done in the same area.

Equipment and Furniture for Each Room

1. *Embalming table*: The embalming table should be fixed on the well-lit side of the room. The table top should be corrosion resistant-stainless steel with central perforation for good drainage facility is the best choice.
2. Two waste collecting buckets lined with disposable plastic bags should be placed under the table.
3. A waste container with cover.
4. A first aid kit should be placed in a conspicuous place.
5. A marble/granite shelf should be built on the side of the room for keeping the supplies, e.g. embalming solution, cotton, masks, gloves, double plastic bag, viscera bag, and instruments for ready accessibility.
6. Surgical instruments and apparatus for the preparation of embalming of a body. Instruments consisting of:
   - Instrument trolley on wheels
   - Syringes-disposable—10 mL, 50 mL, and 100 mL (Fig. 23.1)
   - Forceps-tissue, straight, and angular (Fig. 23.2)
   - Scalpel with disposable blades (Fig. 23.3)
   - Scissors-curved, straight (Fig. 23.4)
   - Hemostat forceps (Fig. 23.5)
   - Dressing forceps
   - Hypodermic needles of different bores
   - Suture needles—3/8" circle needle with spring eye
   - Half-curved suture needle
   - *Aneurysm needle*: This is used for passing ligature round a vessel
   - Metal cannula of different calibers needle holder
   - Electric aspirator
   - Trocar and cannula
   - Retractor or separator
   - Stopcock
   - Y-tube
   - Arterial tube of different sizes and lengths
   - Suture and cotton
   - Sterilizer.
   - Embalming machine (electric pump or gravity equipment) (Fig. 23.6).

The following articles should also be made available in the embalming room:
- Plastic or rubber sheet
- Dressing material with cosmetic articles
- Double plastic bags
- Plastic viscera bags

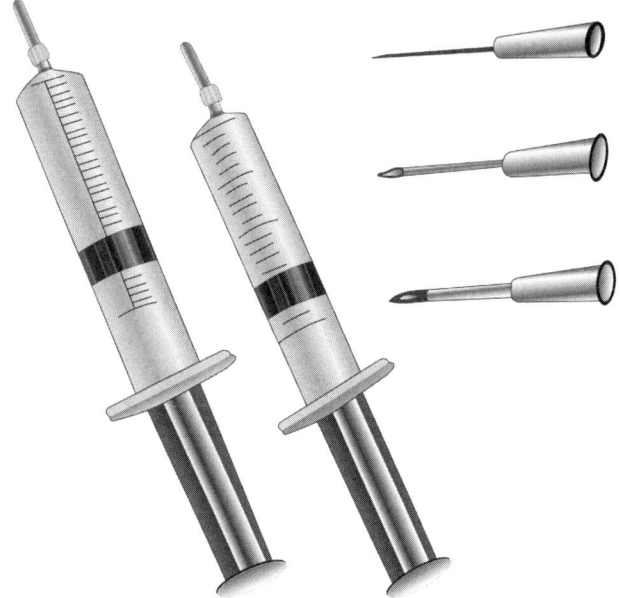

Fig. 23.1: Syringes.

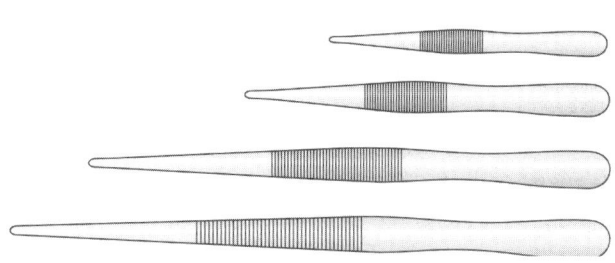

Fig. 23.2: Forceps.

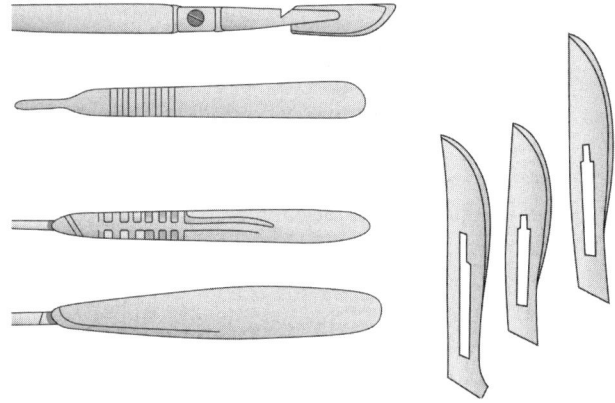

Fig. 23.3: Scalpel and blades.

- Embalming fluid
- Rubber gloves of different sizes
- Bactericidal soap, dressing powder, air freshener, etc.

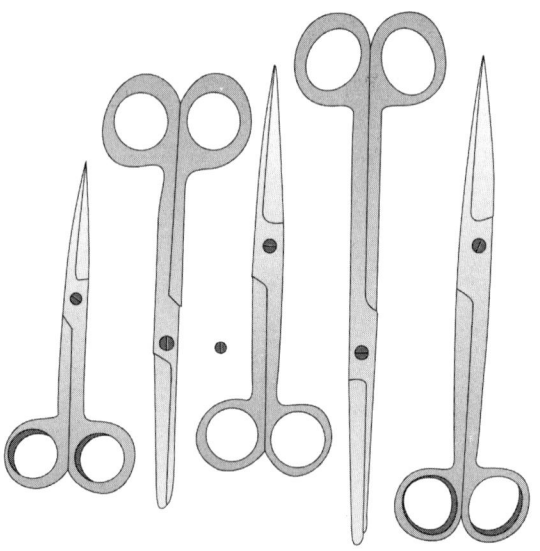

Fig. 23.4: Scissors.

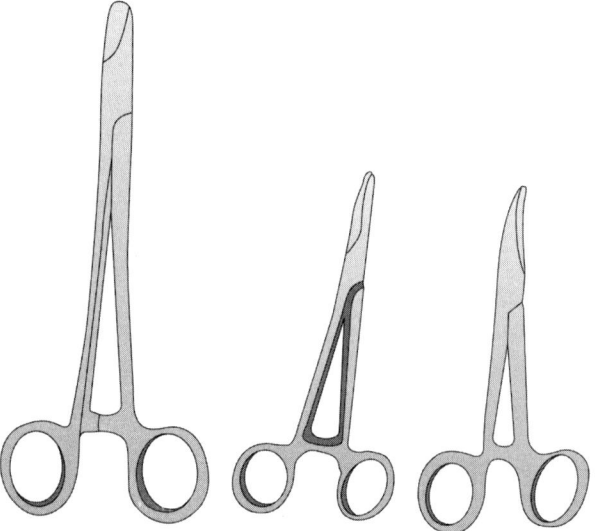

Fig. 23.5: Artery forceps.

The embalming should be strictly private. A "NO ENTRY" sign should be posted on the door of the room. No one should be allowed therein while the body is being embalmed. Access to the room should be from a nonpublic area.

Preparation Room

It should be located adjacent to the embalming room with an interconnection. An area 180 ft² for this room should be considered an optimum. Walls should be covered in their entirety by tile or plastic finished with enamel, which provide smooth, hard, and waterproof surface. Floor must be finished with marble/granite so as to be impervious to water. This room is used for preparing the embalming solutions. It should be well lighted. Odor control and proper exhaust venting must be provided. Room should be equipped with following articles:
- Almirahs to store chemicals
- A waste container with cover
- A sink with running water
- Enamel buckets to prepare embalming fluids
- Work table with stationery and embalming records
- Weighing machine, calibrated jars, and funnels, etc.

Changing Room

It should be located at the rear of the embalming room and should have only one door opening into it. An area 120–150 ft² for this room should be considered an optimum.

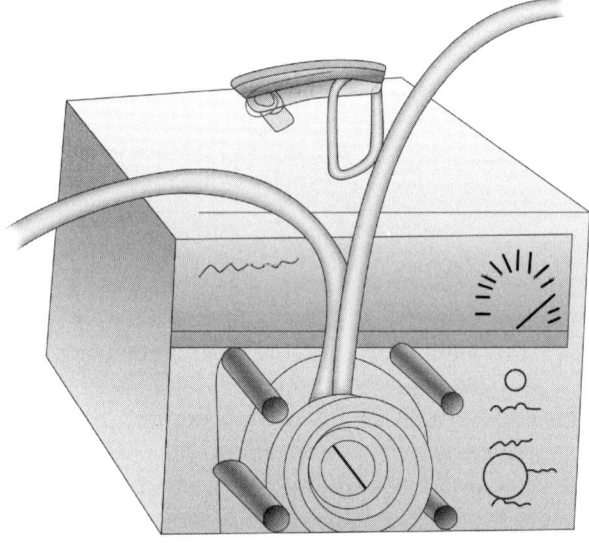

Fig. 23.6: Electric pump.

Walls, floor, and ceiling must be finished on the same lines as the preparation room. This room is used by the medical officer and technical staff for changing the clothes and to wear suitable protective clothing. This room should be equipped with the following facilities:
- Lockers to store goggles, aprons, gloves, caps, masks, shoe covers, and gumboots issued to each individual
- Almirah to store disposable articles
- Movable partition or screen
- A plastic bag to collect disposable articles

- A bin to collect the washable aprons and overalls
- A sink with running hot and cold water
- A bath room should be attached with the changing room where staff can take bath after finishing the embalming. It should be provided with a sink and shower with running hot and cold water.

Post-embalming Room (Mourner's Room)

When death occurs there is often a keen desire on the part of the bereaved to view the remains before the funeral. The post-embalming room is used to perform last religious rites and for display of the casketed body for viewing before final disposal. This room should be located adjacent to the entrance to the embalming facility area where the deceased is received. An area 120 ft^2 is considered enough for the room. This room should be built on the same lines as embalming room. Room should have adequate ventilation and good lightening. It should be provided with the following facilities:
- A 2 ft high platform with marble top. Size of the platform should be 6 ft long and 3 ft wide
- A sink with running water
- A central trap drainage system to drain all water on the floor.

Waiting Room

Death results distressing spiritual and mental effect on the part of the bereaved. In respecting such sentiments, it is essential that the relatives and friends accompanying e body should be provided a well-designed comfortable room. It will help in alleviating their agony state. An area of the room should be between 120–150 ft^2. It should accommodate the following:
- An office table with lockable drawers containing necessary forms, etc.
- Four to six chairs.

THE DOORWAY

Before the construction of the door, an architect is made aware that caskets will be taken through it. A 3 ft width should be absolute minimum but it is always better to have wider doorway as it will permit for free turning of the trolley and the caskets, the passageway from which the embalming room is to be entered, should also be wide. In addition to width, the direction in which the door opens is also very significant.

The staff involved in embalming should be dedicated to their duties. They should be well trained professionally. In fact this is the one field where people need assistance in their saddest moment. Besides embalming the staff should guide and provide all kind of funeral assistance like arrangement of caskets or coffin, securing necessary certificates, arrangement for burial or cremation, etc.
- If a body is fit for embalming, examine the necessary certificates, a prerequisite as laid down in the rules. The embalmer and his assisting staff should handle the body only after they have worn the protective clothing like apron, mask, cap, gloves, gumboots, and shoe cover, etc. The body is then transferred to the embalming room on a stretcher covered with disposable cotton or plastic sheet.
- Remove all clothes and inspect for any labels on forehead, chest, wrist, etc. to indicate any special disease for which extra care has to be taken.
- The body should be thoroughly washed and cleaned.
- Nostrils and mouth should be cleaned, disinfect, and plugged.
- Vaginal orifice and rectum should also be plugged with cotton wool.
- Criteria for selecting the embalming procedure, the vessel, and the strength of the fluid are determined by the needs of the body.
- After embalming is over, the body is cleaned and prepared for cosmetic treatment and then the body is dressed as it was prior to death.
- All the instruments should be properly washed in running water and soap and sterilized before next use.
- Disposable swabs, blades, gloves, masks, needles, and syringes, etc. should be collected in a plastic bag and then incinerated.
- The embalming table should be clean and washed of all blood and fluid stains.
- In case of any contagious disease, the embalming room should be fumigated before next use. After embalming, such bodies should be placed within double plastic bag and its mouth sealed with a clear label stating "health hazard". This is in case the body has to be transported for cremation, etc.

An embalming record must be maintained for reference, research, and even for medicolegal investigations. The format suggested is given here:

Name of the deceased:

Son/daughter/wife of:

Profession of the deceased:

Permanent address:

Date and time of death:

Nationality:

Age: Sex:

Mark of identification (tatoo, scars, mole, birth marks, warts, etc.):

Cause of death:

Status of the body (autopsied/non-autopsied/decomposed/burned/accidental, etc.):

Date and timing of embalming:

Type of embalming (arterial, cavity, hypodermic):

Composition of arterial fluid:

Quantity used:

Arteries used for embalming:

Veins used for drainage:

Cosmetic treatment:

Condition of body after embalming:

Name and address of the applicant:

Date_____

Signature
Name and designation of medical officer

BIBLIOGRAPHY

1. Allen TG. The Book of the Dead. Chicago: University of Chicago Press; 1974.
2. Block SS. Disinfection, Sterilization, and Preservation, 3rd edition. Philadelphia: Lea and Febiger; 1983.
3. Budge EAW. The Mummy. UK: Cambridge University Press, 1893.
4. Calne Roy Yorke. Organ Grafts, Edward Amol 9, 1975.
5. Campus E. Gradwohol's Legal Medicine. Bristol: John Wright and Sons Ltd.; 1976.
6. David WM. The Human Body and the Law. Chicago: Aldine Publishing Co.; 1969.
7. Edwards JES. The Pyramids of Egypt: Pelican Books, 168, 1947.
8. Franklin CA. Modi's Textbook of Medical Jurisprudence and Toxicology, 21st edition. Bombay: NM Tripathy Pvt. Ltd.; 1988.
9. Green Colin. Organ Transplantation: A Review, the Medicine. Publishing company, Oxford; 1983.
10. Guharaj PV. Forensic Medicine. Bombay: Orient Longman; 1982.
11. Haler D. Embalming Theoretical and Practical. Edgbaston Birmingham: The British Institute of Embalmers; 1983.
12. Hamilton WJ. Textbook of Human Anatomy, 2nd edition. London: Macmillan Press Ltd.; 1976.
13. Harrison RJ. Man the Peculiar Animal. London: Pelican Higgins IJ, Bums RG. The Chemistry and Microbiology of Pollution. Cambridge: Academic Press; 1975.
14. History of Herodotus (translated by George H Rawlinson). New York: Dial and Tudor Press; 1928.
15. Hollinshead WH. Textbook of Anatomy, 2nd edition. Delhi: Oxford and IBH Publishers; 1967.
16. Hooton EA. Up from the Ape. Revised edition, Delhi: Motilal Banarsidass; 1946.
17. Jayavelu T. Embalming. New Delhi: BI Churchill Livingstone Pvt. Ltd.; 1991.
18. Journal of the American Funeral Director, 3(9): NY 1988.
19. Mars DD. Bacteriology for Sanitary Engineers. London: Churchill Livingstone; 1974.
20. Martin IS, McDougal JS, Laskoski SL. Disinfection and inactivation of the human T lymphotropic virus type iii/lymphadenopathy-associated virus. J Infect Dis.1985;152: 400-3.
21. Mayer RG. Embalming: History, Theory, and Practice. California, USA: Appleton and Lange; 1990.
22. McDougal JS, Martin IS, Cort SP, et al. Thermal inactivation of the acquired immunodeficiency syndrome virus-iii/lymphodenopathy-associated virus, with special reference to antihemophilic factor. J Clin Invest. 1985;76:875-7.
23. Parikh CK. Medical Jurisprudence and Toxicology. Bombay: CBS Publishers and Distributors; 1990.
24. Pervier NC. A Textbook of Chemistry for Embalmers. Minneapolis: University of Minnesota; 1961.
25. Polson CJ, Green DJ, Knight Bernard. The Essential of Forensic Medicine, 4thedition. Oxford: Pergamon Press; 1985.
26. Polson CJ, Marshal TK. The Disposal of the Dead. London: The English University Press; 1975.
27. Rawling LB. Landmarks and surface markings of the human body, 8th edition. London: HK Lewis; 1940.
28. Reddy KSN. Forensic Medicine and Toxicology, K Suguna Devi, Salim Nagar, Hyderabad; 1990.
29. Spencer AJ. Death in Ancient Egypt. Delhi: Penguin Books; 1982.
30. Spire B, Bane-Sinoussi F, Donnoot D, et al. Inactivation of lymphadenopathy associated virus by heat, gamma rays, and ultraviolet light. Lancet; 1985. pp. ;188-9.
31. Spite B, Montagnier L, Barre-Siniussi F, et al. Inactivation of lymphadenopathy associated virus by chemical Disinfectants. Lancet; 1984. pp. 899-901.
32. Spitz WU, Ftsher RS. Medicolegal Investigation of Death: Guidelines for the Application of Pathology of Crime Investigation: Springfield IL: Charles C Thomas; 1980.
33. Stub Oarense G. Fredrick LG. "Dar/co" The Principles and Practice of Embalming, 4th edition. Texas: Self-publishing; Reprinted; 1986.
34. The American Academy McAllister Institute of Funeral Service. New York, NY Bull 19: 1987-1989.
35. Tompsett DH. Anatomical Techniques. London: E and S Livingstone Ltd.; 1956.
36. Von Hagens G, Klaus T, Wilhelm K. The Current potential of plastination. Anatomy and Embryology. New York: Springer-Verlag, 1987. pp. 411-21.
37. Williams PL, Warwick R, Dyson M, et al. Gray's Anatomy, 38th edition. London: Churchill Livingstone; 1989.

Chapter 24

Formaldehyde and Paraformaldehyde Study in Funeral Homes*

Edward J Kerfoot, Thomas F Mooney

OVERVIEW

Formaldehyde is a toxic gas and classed as an upper respiratory irritant. The gas possesses distinctive physiological properties causing symptoms familiar to many formaldehyde workers, such as burning of the eyes, lacrimation, and general irritation of the upper respiratory passages. To demonstrate this toxic action of formaldehyde, a study was conducted in embalming rooms of funeral homes to determine the concentration and its effect on the embalmers at this level. The control measures in these establishments were also evaluated and found to be inadequate in some respects. Paraformaldehyde powders were sized and found to contain a respirable fraction. The results of the study show that these workers verified the fact that formaldehyde is an irritant at levels that are below the present threshold limit value (TLV).

INTRODUCTION

Most formaldehyde workers are familiar with the physical properties and uses formaldehyde but few are fully aware of its irritant properties. It may be worthwhile here to describe some of the properties of formaldehyde that are important to this study. Formaldehyde is a noxious gas and classed as an upper respiratory irritant because it has a high solubility in water and is therefore held by the moisture covering the respiratory passages.[1] The least detectable odor of formaldehyde is reported, it is 0.05 ppm, and the lowest concentration causing throat irritation is 0.5 ppm.[2] The first symptoms noticed on exposure to small concentration of formaldehyde vapor are burning of the eyes, lacrimation, and general irritation of the upper respiratory passages.[3] Fortunately, these symptoms allow formaldehyde to act as its own warning agent as do certain other gases, such as ammonia. Stronger concentrations produce coughing, constriction in the chest, a sense of pressure in the head, palpitation of the heart, and in some cases, a condition which may appear of similar to alcoholic intoxication.[3] Eye irritation from formaldehyde, a major item of interest currently in air pollution, has been reported to occur in some sensitive individuals at levels which are regarded as "safe" under present recommendations. Morrill[4] states that the threshold of irritant action to be 0.9–1.6 ppm while Bourne and Seferman[5] have established it at 0.13–0.45 ppm. Eye irritation panels have tended to confirm the earlier finding and threshold levels have been recorded by some panel members to be below 0.2 ppm. Elkins claims that some immunity is developed to the lachrymatory action of formaldehyde gas and the exact maximum allowable concentration may be difficult to determine.[1] The previous TLV of 5 ppm was inferred to be low enough to prevent respiratory injury, but not necessarily to prevent subjective evidence of irritation to all exposed individuals. Therefore, the present TLV for formaldehyde has been reduced from 5 ppm to 2 ppm with a ceiling value.

Various incidents have been reported in which formaldehyde workers have experienced the intensely irritating effects of this gas. Specifically, paper-process workers[4] and permanent-press fabric workers[5] have complained of upper respiratory irritation at levels below the present TLV. It may seem that laboratory workers who also use formaldehyde in the form of formalin may be exposed to the same concentrations of this irritant gas. Since this

*American Industrial Hygiene Association Journal. 1975;36(7):533-7.

had not been determined, it seemed apparent that some study was needed in this area to discover these levels of formaldehyde. One of these occupations exposed to this chemical is embalmers. We do not normally like to think of this subject but there are people who must disinfect and preserve dead human bodies in their work. In this respect, these workers must be considered to insure their health and safety.

A study was recently conducted in several Detroit-area funeral homes to establish the formaldehyde concentration to which embalmers are exposed while embalming. This particular study not only determined the formaldehyde concentrations, but also the effectiveness of the control measures (ventilation), and considered some possible adverse effects of this gas and paraformaldehyde powders on the health of the mortician.[6]

METHODS AND MATERIALS

Among the various reagents that can be sued for determination of formaldehyde, the chromotropic acid method is the most useful with regard to sensitivity and overall utility. In general, formaldehyde in the air can be determined by using this method in the concentration range of about 0.01 to at least 200 ppm by a simple and rapid procedure. The method was prepared by Stanley F Sleva of the Air Pollution Training Program, Taft Engineering Center.[7] Along with Altshuller and Miller,[8] Sleva modified the chromotropic acid method which was proposed by West and Sen,[9] and originally, by Eegriwe.[10] Since the interferences are minor, the procedure has been adopted in air pollution work to measure formaldehyde in synthetic atmospheres as well as city atmospheres. For these reasons, the chromotropic acid method was chosen to sample the air in embalming rooms for the formaldehyde vapors emitted.

The only reagent that was needed in the actual sampling experiment was the chromotropic acid, prepared from the disodium salt of 4,5-dihydroxy-2,7-naphthalenedisulfonic acid (Eastman P230).[7] The sampling solution is actually 0.1% chromotropic acid in concentrated sulfuric acid. The sampling train consisted of: Sampling hose, impringer with sampling solution, trap impringer, rotameter, and pump. 10 mL of sampling solution were placed in the fritted midget impringer and air was drawn through at 1.5 L/min until a purple color was obtained. A purple monocationic chromogen is formed when formaldehyde reacts with a chromotropic acid-sulfuric acid solution. The sampling solutions were then read on a DK2 recording spectrophotometer for percent transmission and then converted to absorbance. The absorbance values were plotted on the graph of standards and the concentration of formaldehyde determined in μg/mL. This concentration can be converted to ppm when the volume of solution and volume of air sampled are also known.[7]

In the ventilation study, each funeral home was sketched to scale and the exact measurements taken for the area and volume of each embalming room. Special attention was paid to the location of the windows and fans with respect to the worker and the area where he works. An Alnor velometer was used to measure the velocity of air that was being drawn by the exhaust fan in the embalming room. The ventilation system were evaluated in air changes per hour and compared to the average concentration of formaldehyde in each embalming room.

Air samples containing embalming powders and hardening compounds were taken with a thermal precipitator and then sized microscopically. Since these finely divided particles of paraformaldehyde may have the ability to absorb the toxic formaldehyde vapors, it was important to size these particles retained in the lungs.

A small scale toxicity survey was conducted among the embalmers who worked at the representative funeral homes that were used in the study. Each worker agreed to fill out a detailed questionnaire compiled from the known toxic effects of formaldehyde. It was intended to correlate the findings of the formaldehyde analyses at each funeral home with the irritant effects on the embalmers who worked at that particular funeral home.

RESULTS

Formaldehyde Concentration

The results of the formaldehyde vapor concentrations in this study of embalming rooms consisted of 187 samples with a range from 0.09 ppm to 5.26 ppm and can be observed in Table 24.1. This summary lists the six funeral homes, the concentration range, and the average concentration under normal working conditions. In general, the formaldehyde levels are similar to other situations that also use formaldehyde in their work procedures.[4,5] Some of the values were above the recommended level of the present TLV but the majority were below this level. When the concentrations exceeded 2 ppm there may be a possible health hazard to the workers but below this level the embalmers are probably safe.

Table 24.1: Formaldehyde concentration in the funeral homes.

Funeral home	Concentration range (ppm)	Average concentration (ppm)
#1	0.17–5.26	1.21
#2	0.09–0.89	0.35
#3	0.35–1.22	0.64
#4	0.13–0.45	0.25
#5	0.26–1.23	0.61
#6	0.48–2.10	1.39

Ventilation Systems[11,12]

The ventilation systems were evaluated in two ways. First, samples of formaldehyde concentrations were taken with the ventilation system off (with an average of 1.34 ppm), and then with the ventilation system on (with an average of 0.74 ppm), indicating that the use of a fan reduces the vapors by about half. These values obtained with the fans on were indicative of the efficiency of the ventilation systems with the highest concentration obtained from sampling with the least efficient fan. For example, funeral home #4 expressed 0.25 ppm with the ventilation and 0.92 ppm without ventilation. The other funeral homes displayed an increase of approximately twice that concentration without ventilation with the exception of funeral homes #3 and #6 which only increased slightly without ventilation.

Secondly, the ventilation systems were evaluated in terms of air changes per hour and compared with the average concentration of formaldehyde found in each embalming room. This comparison can be observed in Table 24.2. The large number of air changes did not always correspond to the lower concentration of formaldehyde vapors, indicating the probability that other factors, specifically, the location of the fan and the size of the room were also significant in the efficiency of the ventilation system.[12]

Paraformaldehyde Powders

The air samples containing paraformaldehyde powders were sized and the geometric mean particle size was found to be 1.6 μ, which is optimum for deposition and retention.[13] Since paraformaldehyde is not as soluble in water as formaldehyde, it is therefore not usually held by the moisture coverings the lining of the respiratory tract. Also these particles have the ability to adsorb formaldehyde vapors in the air, so that not only the particles of paraformaldehyde but also the attached formaldehyde vapors may be carried deeper into the lungs and possibly injures the alveolar walls.

Toxicity Survey

The toxicity survey, conducted among the embalmers at the funeral homes sampled, clearly demonstrated that formaldehyde is mainly an upper respiratory irritant causing eye and nose burns, sneezing, coughing, and headaches. The morticians who spent more time in embalming than in general funeral work, also experienced more complaints of irritation. On the other hand, symptoms as sleepiness, weakness, and tightness in the chest were almost never experienced, for these are characteristics of higher, more toxic concentrations. It is interesting to note that three out of seven men's suffered from asthma or sinus problems, which is somewhat higher than the expected population. Also, two workers had experienced a dermatitis with one case being so severe that the worker was forced to discontinue working for a period of time until he recovery and could take more specific safety precautions. Since most of the concentrations rarely exceeded the present TLV under normal conditions, it indicates that anyone working 8 hours per day in formaldehyde concentrations at higher levels could not help but suffer from the irritating

Table 24.2: Comparison of ventilation systems with formaldehyde concentrations.

Funeral home	Formaldehyde ventilation	Concentration: no ventilation (ppm)	Air changes per hour	Fan location to embalmer
#1	1.21	2.50	9.1	Behind
#2	0.35	0.75	88.0	Behind
#3	0.64	0.99	2.7	Opposite
#4	0.25	0.92	54.0	Opposite
#5	0.61	1.10	17.0	Opposite
#6	1.39	1.77	0.8	Opposite
	0.74*	1.34		

*Average concentrations

action of formaldehyde and could very well be affected by its more severe symptoms over a period of many years.

DISCUSSION

The study determined that the formaldehyde vapor concentrations to which embalmers are exposed are generally within the levels of the present TLV of 2 ppm, when the ventilation systems are working effectively. Since these funeral homes were better than average establishments, it may be inferred that concentrations in the smaller, less adequate funeral homes might have been markedly higher than those which were obtained under the more ideal conditions of the funeral homes involved in this project. Under these circumstances, it would seem apparent that some embalmers would be working in concentrations of formaldehyde above the acceptable limit.

This research also showed that there was a great variation in the ventilation systems tested. In this experimental study, three out of the six funeral homes sampled were inadequate in some respects. One embalming room fan showed such small air changes that the embalmers there were never really sure whether the fan was operating. On the other hand, in the embalming room with the very strong fan resulting in concentrations one-fourth that of the concentration with the fan off, the noise from this fan was so loud that many of the workers did not use it. This indicates the need for definite ventilation standards in embalming rooms. Many state mortuary laws require that an embalming room must contain an adequate ventilation system, but it does not specify just exactly what an "adequate" ventilation, system actually is. Definite regulations should be setup regarding the size of the embalming room and the size of the fans and their location in the room to insure good ventilation systems. Some ventilation suggestions for these standards could be stated. The fan should be located on an outside wall opposite the work place of the embalmer so that the fumes do not pass by the workers as they are carried away from him. The fan should be sufficiently powerful to reduce effectively the formaldehyde vapor concentration; specifically, it should cause a minimum of 12–15 air changes per hour according to standards for irritant gases. It must be adequate enough to keep the concentration of formaldehyde vapors at least below the maximum allow able concentration. The fan should also operate quietly, for it so noisy that the embalmer turns it off to avoid a headache, an occurrence which happens all too frequently. When the mortuary state boards realize that this is important to the health and safety of the embalmer, then can establish these standards and enforce them.

Another important fact is the possibility that more serious health problems could occur with the paraformaldehyde powders. This was evident with the determination of the paraformaldehyde particle size because it is evident that they may be deposited into the lungs and be retained. Therefore, these powders and compounds, as well as the attached formaldehyde vapors, can reach an area where they may cause serious lung damage.

The toxicity survey demonstrated the upper respiratory irritation from formaldehyde on the embalmers at rather low levels. It is frequently heard from many experienced embalmers that the formaldehyde fumes do not bother them, for they have become accustomed to the vapors over the years of embalming. Actually, this may be a determinant, for they do not know when the formaldehyde concentrations are high and above a safe level since their olfactory system is "numb" to the irritation effect. This can be exemplified by the fact that another funeral home employee may enter the preparation room during embalming and not be able to open his eyes due to the irritation and began coughing, while the embalmer goes on working after he has become injured to the vapor as the concentrations gradually increased. Over a period of many years of embalming under these conditions, one may wonder if a chronic exposure would contribute to lung disease later in life.

Therefore, this study demonstrated several facts of importance and there is certainly good reason for embalmers to be well educated in the known, and even possible, effects of formaldehyde.

REFERENCES

1. Gross P, Rinehart WE, de Treville RT. The pulmonary reactions to toxic gases. Am Ind Hyg Assoc J. 1967;28: 315-21.
2. Stem AC. Air Pollution. New York: Academic Press; 1968. p. 484.
3. Walker JF. Formaldehyde. New York: Rinehold Publishing Corporation; 1964. p. 99.
4. Morrill EE. Formaldehyde exposure from paper process solved by air sampling and current studies. Air Cond Heat Vent. 1961;58:94-5.
5. Bourne HG, Seferman S. Wrinkle-proofed clothing may liberate toxic quantities of formaldehyde. Indust Med Surg. 1959;28:232.

6. Elkins HB. The Chemistry of Industrial Toxicology. New York: John Wiley & Sons Inc.; 1959. p. 118.
7. US Department of Health, Education and Welfare (Stanley F Slleva: Determination of Formaldehyde Chromotropic Acid Method) Selected Methods for the Measurement of Air Pollutants. 1965:1-5.
8. Altshuller AP, Miller DL, Sleva SF. Determination of formaldehyde in gas mixtures by the chromotropic acid method. Anal Chem. 1961;33:621-5.
9. West PW, Sen B. Spectrophotometric determination of traces of formaldehyde. Z Anal Chem. 1956;153:177-83.
10. Eegriwe E. Z Anal Chem. 1937;110:22.
11. Kerfoot EJ. Formaldehyde vapor emission study in embalming rooms. Tire Director. 1972;42:6.
12. Kerfoot EJ. Evaluation of ventilation systems in funeral homes. Build Sys Design. 1972;96:26.
13. Hatch T, Gross P. Pulmonary Deposition and Retention of Inhaled Aerosols. New York: Academic Press; 1964. p. 68.

Chapter 25

Formaldehyde Vapor Emission Study in Embalming Rooms*

Edward J Kerfoot

INTRODUCTION

Most funeral service licensees are familiar with the physical properties and uses of formaldehyde, but few are fully aware of its toxic properties. Industries that use formaldehyde, as permanent-press fabric and paper processing, show concern about this gas and its effect on their workers. Investigation revealed that no experimentation had ever been done to determine the concentrations of formaldehyde to which funeral licensees are exposed.

It seemed that some study in this was needed—not only to determine if the concentrations of formaldehyde during embalming were within accepted "safe" levels, but also to evaluate the effectiveness of controls on the formaldehyde concentrations and to consider some possible adverse effects of this gas.

PROPERTIES

It may be worthwhile here to describe some of the properties of formaldehyde that are important to this particular study. Formaldehyde is a toxic gas and classified as an upper respiratory irritant because it has high solubility in water and is held by the moisture covering the upper respiratory tract. Gases that dissolve more slowly in water, travel more deeply into the respiratory tract before they are dissolved. So, under ordinary circumstances, formaldehyde, though toxic, does not cause any damage. Formaldehyde possesses distinctive physiological properties causing symptoms very familiar to all funeral licensees such as burning of the eyes, lacrimation, and irritation of the upper respiratory passages. These symptoms allow formaldehyde to act as its own warning agent as other *gases like* ammonia do.

The main purpose of this research was to determine the concentration of formaldehyde vapors that embalmers inhale while embalming. In six Detroit area funeral home preparation rooms the formaldehyde content during embalming procedures was determined chemically. These establishments were not representative of a general cross section of all funeral home but were actually better than average. The concentration of formaldehyde vapors for the total 187 samples taken ranged from 0.09 to 5.26 ppm (parts per million). At the higher levels of this range, the fumes caused such severe upper respiratory distress that the licensees and sampler were unable to remain in the room.

Ventilation systems in the preparation rooms were evaluated in two ways. First, samples of formaldehyde concentrations were taken with the fan off (with an average of 1.34 ppm), then with the fan on (with an average of 0.74 ppm), indicating the use of a fan reduces the vapors by about half. Secondly, the fans were evaluated in terms of air changes per hour. The larger number of air changes did not always correspond to the lower concentration of formaldehyde vapors, indicating the probability that other factors, specifically the location of the fan and size of the room, were also significant in the efficiency of the ventilation systems.

At one funeral home, still another factor was evaluated. A surgical cloth mask was placed in the sample holder and the concentration of formaldehyde after being filtered through the mask again determined. Here the samples showed average values of 2.50 ppm with no ventilation or mask, 1.21 ppm with ventilation but without a mask, and 0.78 ppm using both the ventilation system and mask. This indicated that as the use of the fan reduced the formaldehyde concentrations by half, the further use of masks are not commonly used during embalming but concerned licensees should be aware of the efficiency of a mask in reducing the amount of formaldehyde vapors inhaled.

---
*American Industrial Hygiene Association Journal. 1975;36(7):533-7.

Air samples containing embalming powders and hardening compounds were taken with a thermal precipitator and then sized microscopically; the mean particle size was found to be 1.6 μ. This finding was to definite importance because particles between 1 μ and 2 μ are respirable, deposited, and most importantly, retained in the lung depths. Larger particles could not penetrate as deeply and smaller particles, which could penetrate deeply, are too small to be retained but would be exhaled. Also, the particles of paraformaldehyde powders have the ability to adsorb formaldehyde vapors in the air, so that not only the particles of paraformaldehyde but the attached formaldehyde vapors (which normally affect only the upper respiratory tract) may be carried into the lower respiratory tract of the licensee.

A small-scale toxicity survey was done among the licensees at these funeral homes; they filled out questionnaires concerning the known toxic effects of formaldehyde. This study clearly demonstrated that formaldehyde is mainly an upper respiratory irritant causing eye and nose burns, sneezing, coughing, and headaches. It is interesting that three out of seven men suffered from asthma or sinus problems, which is a somewhat higher proportion than in the general population.

The workers who were bothered more by the irritant action of formaldehyde were exposed to the higher concentrations and those who spent more of their work time in embalming also experienced more severe symptoms. Keep in mind that these symptoms were experienced by workers who spend only part of their work day exposed to formaldehyde and at concentrations well below the present limit.

SAFE LIMIT OF FORMALDEHYDE

This study, then, showed several facts of importance. For one thing, it found the formaldehyde vapor concentrations of which licensees who embalm are exposed to be within the levels of the present threshold limit value (TLV). This means that if the concentrations exceed 5 ppm they pose a possible health hazard to the worker but under this level the worker is "safe". It must be mentioned here that the current TLV of 5 ppm is being challenged and proposals have been made [by Occupational Safety and Health Administration (OSHA)] to lower it to 2 ppm. If this happens it would mean that some licensees would be working in concentrations of formaldehyde far above the accepted "safe" limit.

The results of the toxicity survey verified the fact that formaldehyde is mainly an upper respiratory irritant because all involved experienced, to some degree, the symptoms of upper respiratory irritation. The possibility that more serious damage could occur, however, was evident with the determination of paraformaldehyde particle size. Because it is known that their size makes them able to be carried deep into the lungs and retained there, becomes a finding of much importance. It means that these powders and compounds, as well as the attached formaldehyde vapors, can reach an area where they may cause serious lung damage.

This research also showed that ventilation systems reduce the vapor concentration roughly by half and also showed that great variations in the effectiveness of ventilation system existed. The importance of several factors, namely the size of the fan, the size of the room, and the location of the fan, in influencing the effectiveness of a good ventilation system was shown. Further, it showed that these concentrations can be reduced by almost half again by the use of a mask.

CONCLUSION

From these result some conclusions may be drawn.

There definitely is a need for further study in this area, particularly concerning the paraformaldehyde powders and their ability to penetrate the lung depth.

The need for lowering the TLV to 2 ppm (as has been proposed) seems quite evident. As previously mentioned, when the formaldehyde concentrations approach the present TLV of 5 ppm, the licensee and sampler were too distressed to remain in the embalming room, and the irritating effects experienced by those involved in the toxicity survey at much lower levels seem to back this up.

There certainly is good reason for licensees to be well educated in the known and even possible effects of formaldehyde as well as in the effectiveness of the controls available to them. This knowledge might make more licensees responsible in protecting themselves as well as they can, even to employing the annoyance of a mask, especially when the embalming powders and hardening compounds are used.

Finally, there is a real need for setting up definite standards regarding formaldehyde exposure. Definite regulations should be setup regarding size of embalming rooms, size of fans, and their locations in the embalming room to insure good ventilation systems. Perhaps even the number of hours that one embalmer could be exposed in a given amount of time should be limited. Whether such standards will be determined will depend, in large part, on the interest of funeral service licensees themselves.

Chapter 26

Formaldehyde Study in Preparation Rooms*

Edward J Kerfoot

INTRODUCTION

A study was recently completed in six Detroit-area funeral homes to established the formaldehyde concentration to which embalmers are exposed while embalming. A review of the literature and correspondence with various authorities revealed that no previous experimentation had ever been done to established these values. Consequently, it seemed that some study in this area was needed not only to determine if the concentrations of formaldehyde during embalming were within accepted "safe" levels, but also to evaluate the effectiveness of the controls (ventilation) on the formaldehyde concentrations, and to consider some possible adverse effects of this gas and the embalming powders on the health and safety of the embalmer.

FORMALDEHYDE TOXICITY

Most embalmers are familiar with the physical properties and uses of formaldehyde, but few are fully aware of its irritant properties. It may be worthwhile here to describe some of the properties of formaldehyde that are important to this particular study. Formaldehyde is a noxious gas and classed as an upper respiratory irritant because it has a high solubility in water and is, therefore, held by moisture covering the upper respiratory tract. Formaldehyde possesses distinctive physiologic properties causing symptoms very familiar to all embalmers, such as burning of the eyes, lacrimation, and general irritation of the upper respiratory passages. Fortunately, these symptoms allow formaldehyde to act as its own warning agent, similar to other gases, like ammonia.

A small scale toxicity survey was conducted among the embalmers who worked at the funeral homes that were used in the study; they filled out a questionnaire concerning the known toxic effects of formaldehyde. The results of this survey clearly demonstrated that formaldehyde is mainly an upper respiratory irritant causing eye and nose burns, sneezing, coughing, and headaches. It is interesting to note that 43% of the embalmers in this study suffer from asthma or sinus problems, which is a somewhat higher proportion than in the general population. Two of the workers also suffered from a dermatitis, one of which must take extra precautionary measures. The embalmers who were bothered more by the irritant action of formaldehyde were exposed to the higher concentrations and those who spent more of their work time in embalming also experienced more severe symptoms.

FORMALDEHYDE CONCENTRATIONS

The main purpose of this research was to determine the concentration of formaldehyde vapors that embalmers inhale while embalming. In this study, six of the better funeral establishments in the Detroit-area were evaluated; and consequently, these funeral homes had the more modern, well-equipped embalming rooms.

Air samples were taken as soon as the embalming fluid was mixed in the machine and continued about every 10 minutes from the start of the embalming until the work was

---

*Printed from the Expanding Encyclopedia No. 435, Champion Chemical Company, Springfield, Ohio, 1973.

completed. The samples of formaldehyde were collected in 10 mL of chromotropic acid in a fritted impinger. A purple monocationic chromogen is formed when formaldehyde reacts with a chromotropic acid-sulfuric acid solution. The samples were then taken to the laboratory to be analyzed as soon as possible, and always within 12 hours.

The concentrations of formaldehyde vapors for the total 187 samples were taken, ranged from 0.09 ppm to 5.26 ppm (part per million). At the higher levels of this range, the fumes caused such severe respiratory distress that the embalmer and chemist were forced to leave the room. These higher levels were experienced without the use of the fan, which will be explained later, and thus proved to be unbearable.

EMBALMING POWDERS

Air samples containing embalming powders and hardening compounds were taken with a thermal precipitator and then sized microscopically; the mean particle size was found to be 1.6 µ. This finding was of definite importance because particles between 1 µ and 2 µ and respirable, deposited, and more importantly, retained in the lungs. Larger particles could not penetrate as deeply and smaller particles, which could be respired, are too small to be retained and would be exhaled. Also, the particles of paraformaldehyde powders have the ability to absorb formaldehyde vapors in the air, so that not only the particles of paraformaldehyde but also the attached formaldehyde vapors (which normally affect only the upper respiratory tract) may be carried into the lower respiratory tract of the worker. These properties of the hardening compounds and embalming powders could be the cause of a serious lung disorder to one exposed over a period of years if the ventilation system is not adequate enough to remove these particles.

VENTILATION SYSTEMS

Unfortunately, the embalming room of the modern, spacious, and beautiful funeral home is often the most neglected room of the establishment. Since this is a "behind the scenes" place, not seen by the general public, it is not always given as much consideration as it should. However, the comfort, and more importantly, the health of the embalmer must be given sufficient consideration. The most important control available to the health and protection of the embalmer is a room, placement of windows and fans, and the efficiency of the fans used.

In the ventilation study, each funeral home was sketched to scale and the exact measurements taken for the area and volume of each embalming room. Special attention was paid to the location of the windows and fans with respect of the embalmer and the area where he works. An Alnor Velometer was used to measure the velocity of air that is being drawn by the exhaust fan in the embalming room. The ventilation system was evaluated in air changes per hour and compared to the average concentration of formaldehyde found in each embalming room. This comparison can be observed in Table 26.1. The concentration of formaldehyde was determined by sampling the air with and without the use of the fan or ventilation system. This information related how efficient the fans were by comparing the decrease in formaldehyde vapors when the fans were being used. For example, the ventilation of funeral home #6 has a very poor rating in terms of air changes and this funeral home has the highest concentration of formaldehyde that was sampled. It also shows that there is little difference between concentrations with the ventilation on or off, revealing the inefficiency of the ventilation system. Another factor that must be considered with the ventilation is the location of the fan.

Table 26.1: Comparison of ventilation systems with formaldehyde concentrations.

Funeral home	Formaldehyde concentration		Air changes per hour	Fan location to embalmer
	Ventilation	No ventilation		
#1	1.21 ppm	2.50 ppm	9.1	Behind
#2	0.35 ppm	0.75 ppm	88.0	Behind
#3	0.64 ppm	0.99 ppm	2.7	Opposite
#4	0.25 ppm	0.92 ppm	54.0	Opposite
#5	0.61 ppm	1.10 ppm	17.0	Opposite
#6	1.39 ppm	1.77 ppm	0.8	Opposite

It should not be behind the embalmer, because the fumes are drawn past the worker to be exhausted; instead, the fan should be located opposite the worker so that he is not exposed to the direct vapor emitted. In this experimental study, three out of the six funeral homes sampled were inadequate in some respects. One embalming room showed such small air changes with the use of a fan that the embalmers there were never really sure whether the fan was operating. On the other hand, in the embalming room with the very strong fan where the use of the fan resulted in concentrations one-fourth that of the concentration with the fan off, the noise form this fan was so loud that many of the embalmers did not use it. The fan here was probably off more than it was on. It is very interesting to note that the experiments performed in this study were all done in the better funeral establishments. Suspicion on the part of funeral director-owners of some of the smaller, less adequate funeral homes toward this type of sampling made them rather inaccessible. It may be inferred, however, that concentrations in these small, poorly ventilated rooms would have been markedly higher than what was obtained under the more "ideal" conditions of the funeral homes involved in this experiment. In fairness, however, it should be pointed out that the amount of embalming done in these smaller establishments is far less than in the larger, better equipped funeral homes, yet, one might wonder what effect these vapors might have on the owner-director of the small business where the embalming is done in a poorly ventilated embalming room and the funeral director resides in the same dwelling.

DISCUSSION

This study showed several facts of importance. There is certainly good reason for embalmers to be well educated in the known, and even possible effect of formaldehyde, as well as the effects of the controls available to them. This knowledge might make more embalmers responsible in protecting themselves as well as they can, even to employing the annoyance of a mask, especially when the embalming powders and hardening compounds are used.

This study next found the formaldehyde vapor concentrations to which embalmers are exposed to be within the levels of the present threshold limit value (TLV). This means that if the concentrations exceed 5 ppm, they pose a possible health hazard to the worker. But under this level, the worker is normally "safe", especially if workers only spend part of their work day in embalming and the rest of the time in general funeral work. It must be mentioned here that the current TLV or 5 ppm is being challenged and proposals have been made to lower it to 2 ppm. If this happens, it would seem apparent that some embalmers would be working in concentrations of formaldehyde above the acceptable limit. The need for lowering the TLV to 2 ppm seems quite evident. As previously mentioned, when the formaldehyde concentrations approached the present TLV of 5 ppm without ventilation, the embalmer and chemist were unable to remain in the embalming room, and the irritating effects experienced by those involved in the toxicity survey at much lower levels seems to substantiate this. It is frequently heard by many experienced embalmers that the formaldehyde fumes do not bother them, for they have become accustomed to the vapors over the years of embalming. Actually, this may be a detriment, for they do not know when the formaldehyde concentrations are high and above a safe level for their olfactory system is "numb" to the irritation effect. This can be exemplified by the fact that another funeral employee may enter the preparation room during embalming and not be able to open his eyes due to the fumes and begin coughing while the embalmer goes on working for he has become injured to the vapor as the concentration were gradually increased. Over a period of many years of embalming under these conditions, one may wonder if a chronic exposure will cause serious lung damage later in life.

Another important fact is the possibility that more serious damage could occur with the paraformaldehyde powders. This was evident with the determination of the paraformaldehyde particle size because it is known that these powders can absorb formaldehyde. Their size makes them able to be carried deep into the lungs and remain there which is a finding of much importance. It means that these powders and compounds, as well as the attached formaldehyde vapors, can reach an area where they may cause serious lung damage. There is definitely a need for further study in this area concerning the paraformaldehyde powders and their ability to penetrate the lung depths.

This research also showed that a great variation in ventilation systems tested, even in this small study, indicate the need for definite ventilation standards in embalming rooms. Many mortuary state laws require that an embalming room must contain an adequate ventilation system, but it does not specify just exactly what an "adequate" ventilation system actually is. When the mortuary boards of each state realize that this is important to the health and safety of the embalmer, they can establish standards and enforce them.

Definite regulations should be setup regarding the size of the embalming room and the size of fans and their location in the room to insure good ventilation systems. Some ventilation suggestions for these standards are: The fan should be located on an outside wall opposite the workplace of the embalmer so that fumes do not pass by the embalmer as they are carried away from him. The fan should be sufficiently powerful to reduce effectively the formaldehyde vapor concentration; specifically, it should cause a minimum of 12–15 air changes per hour, according to the standards for irritant gases. It must be adequate enough to keep the concentration of formaldehyde vapors at least below the maximum allowable concentration. The fan should also operate quietly; it is of little value to have a powerful fan if it is so noisy that the embalmer turns it off to "avoid a headache", an occurrence which happens all too frequently, unfortunately.

Whether such standards will be determined will depend, in large part, on the interest of the embalmers themselves. When the irritant formaldehyde vapors and possibly more serious paraformaldehyde powders are exhausted properly, better protection and health of the embalmer can be insured.

BIBLIOGRAPHY

1. Altshuller AP, Miller DL, Sleva SF. Determination of formaldehyde in gas mixtures by the chromotropic acid method. Anal Chem. 1961;33:621-5.
2. Edward KJ. Evaluation of ventilation systems in funeral homes. Build Syst Design. 1972.
3. Edward KJ. Formaldehyde vapor emission study in embalming rooms. NFDA. 1972.
4. Hatch TF, Gross P, Clayton GD. Pulmonary Deposition and Retention of Inhaled Aerosols. New York: Academic Press; 1964. p. 68.

Chapter 27

Reported Studies on Effects of Formaldehyde Exposure*

Leandro Rendon

EFFECTS OF EXPOSURE

The general effects related to human exposure to formaldehyde appear to included many different symptoms and conditions. Perhaps, the most frequently mentioned effects are those associated with the pungent, irritating properties of formaldehyde involving the eyes, nose, and throat. The degree of response will vary depending upon the amount of formaldehyde present and from individual to individual.

It has long been known that high concentrations of formaldehyde are irritating to man and that it can cause skin sensitization. Because of formaldehyde's importance, the Chemical Industry Institute of Toxicology (CIIT) sponsored a conference in November 1980, in which current research on formaldehyde was presented. The event brought scientists and government regulators together to hear and discuss the wide variety of then-current research.

Issue No. 517, May 1981, of the Expanding Encyclopedia discussed some of the available data regarding "health risk from formaldehyde". Since then more information has become available and it is the purpose of this discussion to update what is known regarding effects of formaldehyde exposure.

In his presentation at the November 1980 conference, Richard J Levine et al.[1] distinguished between two important categories of embalming practice in relation to exposure: (1) The embalming of "normal" (nonautopsied) and (2) Of autopsied remains. In their studies, the group found time-weighed-average formaldehyde concentration to be 0.3 ppm during the embalming of nonautopsied cases and 0.9 ppm for autopsied remains. The highest concentrations were 0.4 ppm and 2.1 ppm, respectively. The investigator commented that while exposure found in embalming autopsied bodies are more intense, autopsied bodies usually comprise only a minority of total bodies embalmed. He further stated:

In a summary, pulmonary function of West Virginia (where the study was performed) morticians compared favorably to that of residential populations in Oregon and Michigan. Among morticians, high exposure was linked neither to chronic bronchitis nor to pulmonary function deficits. The results suggest that intermittent exposure to low levels of formaldehyde gas over the long term exerts no meaningful chronic effect on respiratory health.

All the same CIIT conference on November 1980, Walrath et al.[1,2] presented a preliminary study that investigated whether embalmers, compared with the general population, have a greater proportion of cancer deaths that might be associated with exposure to formaldehyde. The study group consisted of deceased embalmers licensed to practice embalming in New York State between 1902 and 1979. The death certificates revealed data indicating that the embalmers in that group experienced a slightly elevated mortality from cancer, a significant excess of arteriosclerotic heart disease, and a very low incidence of pneumonia deaths. Skin cancer mortality was significantly elevated as well as kidney and brain cancers. On the other hand, there was no excess mortality from cancers of the respiratory tract, including the nasal passages. The

---

*Printed from the Expanding Encyclopedia No. 542, Champion Chemical Company, Springfield, Ohio, 1983.

investigators point out, however, "that embalming fluids contain a mixture of other chemicals that are partly intended to offset the adverse reactions of formaldehyde".

It should be pointed out that commercially available fluid from 1902 to approximately the late 1930s tended to be rather harsh and astringent compositions. The embalmer did not often use or wear gloves when working with embalming compositions as happens today. It is possible to assume that prolonged contact of the embalming fluids with the skin could produce adverse effects. Also, it is possible that adequate ventilation and exhaust systems were not available in preparation rooms in the "early" days.

On November 3, 1982 the formaldehyde Institute sponsored a formaldehyde toxicology conference as a means of continuing the open dialog between interested parties that was initiated at the November 1980 meeting. Another important paper was presented at the meeting by Dr Richard J Levine et al.[3] The investigators made a study of the mortality of Ontario undertakers during the period between 1928 and 1957 as was the purpose in the study among West Virginia funeral licensees. Dr Levine was interested in learning more about possible effects of formaldehyde among groups of workers who are known to work with the compound possibly to a greater extent than others and over a longer period of time.

The sites felt to be of particular interest as being of special risk for cancer from exposure to formaldehyde were skin, nasal passages, buccal cavity, pharynx, and larynx. Among the Canadian funeral licensees no deaths due to nasal cancer were observed. Mortality attributed to cancers of the buccal cavity, pharynx, and respiratory system exclusive of trachea, bronchus, and lung was less than expected.

Cirrhosis of the liver was the only cause of death found to be significantly in excess. The investigators felt that perhaps this might be due to a higher consumption of alcoholic beverages by this group than the general population. They believed this might account for the increase in mortality from liver cancer, disease of the circulatory system, and acute respiratory diseases, which are characteristically elevated among alcoholics. The preliminary conclusion is that formaldehyde exposure among Ontario's funeral licensees had no effect on cancer mortality.

A new British epidemiology study released in August 1983 contains some interesting information. Dr EA Acheson, Director of the British Medical Research Council's Environmental Epidemiology Unit, Southampton General Hospital, in the United Kingdom, presented a report based on a study of more than 7,700 chemical workers from six factories among the country's chemical industry where formaldehyde has been manufactured or used for more than 15 years. The study sought to find an increase in the incidence of cancer types among long-term employees exposed to formaldehyde. The levels workers were exposed to over the period studied were as much as three times higher than those allowed under present regulations.

Results of the Acheson study show no excessive risk for formaldehyde workers of contracting nasal, lung, prostrate, brain, skin, kidney, or bladder cancers. The report, according to the Formaldehyde Institute, brings the total number of epidemiology studies performed to 12, all revealing no excess cancer types in persons exposed to formaldehyde. In this country, the major manufacturers of formaldehyde have accomplished similar studies among their workers and report data similar to those of Acheson.

In Iowa, a study was accomplished jointly by the Iowa State Department of Health and the University Hygienic Laboratory. The study was carried out with the endorsement of the Board of Mortuary Science Examiners and the Iowa Funeral Directors Association. The first phase of the two-part study determined formaldehyde exposure during embalming's. The second part examined cancer death rates among funeral directors as compared to the general population.

During the study, personnel from the Iowa State Department of Health visited 44 funeral homes that had been randomly selected throughout the state. At each place, two samples of formaldehyde gas were collected during embalming procedures—(1) One at the operator's breathing zone and (2) One ambient room air sample. According to the Iowa State Department of Health, the following determinations were found as a result of the study, June 1983.

Formaldehyde concentrations measured in breathing zone samples ranged from nondetectable to 3.5 ppm. The average detectable level of formaldehyde in the breathing zone was 0.84 ppm. Ambient room sample concentrations ranged from nondetectable to 1.99 ppm, with an average reading of 0.23 ppm determined.

The Iowa State Department of Health reported its findings to the Iowa Funeral Directors Association and listed the following measures that should be followed to reduce exposure whenever practicable although none of the reported levels were in excess of federal standards:

- Local exhaust ventilation should be used whenever persons are working in the preparation room, particularly during embalming procedures. Significantly higher concentrations of formaldehyde would be expected when no local exhaust ventilation is used during embalming procedures. Ventilation systems should be properly designed with consideration for room volume, embalming workload, and avoidance of dead air spaces.
- During embalming procedures, personnel should avoid working in locations between the exhaust vent and sources of formaldehyde (for example, embalming tank, mixing tank, etc.).
- Situations in which formaldehyde is exposed to room air (for example, spills, open tanks, *open* bottles, etc.) should be minimized. In situations where opportunities for volatilizing formaldehyde into the room air cannot be avoided, the length of exposure should be maintained at as short an interval as is practicable.
- Direct skin contact with formaldehyde should be avoided. Use of protective equipment, such as rubber gloves and aprons, will reduce the chances of skin exposure.

In this study, at least one instance of contact dermatitis was reported to occur from embalming fluid.

ACKNOWLEDGMENTS

Acknowledgment is hereby extended to the Iowa Funeral Directors Association for making available the preceding information which should be of immense interest to all funeral licensees.

REFERENCES

1. Levine RJ, DalCorso RD, Blunden PB, et al. The effects of occupational exposure on the respiratory health of West Virginia morticians. In: Gibson JE (Ed). Formaldehyde Toxicity. New York: Hemisphere Publishing Corporation; 1983. pp. 212-26.
2. Walrath J, Fraumeni JF. Proportionate mortality among New York embalmers. In: Gibson JE (Ed). Formaldehyde Toxicity. New York: Hemisphere Publishing Corporation; 1983. pp. 227-36.
3. Levine RJ, Andjelkovich DA, Shaw LK, et al. Mortality of Ontario undertakers: A first report. In: Clary JJ, Gibson JE, Waritz RS (Eds). Formaldehyde: Toxicology, Epidemiology and Mechanisms. New York: Marcel Dekker; 1983. pp. 127-40.

Chapter 28

Recommendations for Prevention of HIV Transmission in Healthcare Settings*

INTRODUCTION

Human immunodeficiency virus (HIV), the virus that causes acquired immunodeficiency syndrome (AIDS), is transmitted through sexual contact and exposure to infected blood or blood components and perinatally from mother to neonate. HIV has been isolated from milk, cerebrospinal fluid, amniotic fluid, and urine and is likely to be isolated from other body fluids, secretions, and excretions. However, epidemiologic evidence has implicated only blood, semen, vaginal secretions, and possibly breast milk in transmission.

The increasing prevalence of HIV increases the risk that healthcare workers will be exposed to blood from patients infected with HIV, especially when blood and body fluid precautions are not followed for all patients. Thus, this document emphasizes the need for healthcare workers to consider all patients as potentially infected with HIV and/or other blood-borne pathogens and to adhere rigorously to infection control precautions for minimizing the risk of exposure to blood and body fluids of all patients.

The recommendations contained in this document consolidate and update the Centers for Disease Control and Prevention (CDC) recommendations published earlier for preventing HIV transmission in health care settings: precautions for clinical and laboratory staffs[1] and precautions for healthcare workers and allied professionals;[2] recommendations for preventing HIV transmission in the workplace[3] and during invasive procedures;[4] recommendations for preventing possible transmission of HIV from tears;[5] and recommendations for providing dialysis treatment for HIV-infected patients.[6] These recommendations also update portions of the "Guideline for Isolation Precautions in Hospitals"[7] and re-emphasize some of the recommendations contained in "Infection Control Practices for Dentistry".[8] The recommendations contained in this document have been developed for use in healthcare settings and emphasize the need to treat blood and other body fluids from all patients as potentially infective. These same prudent precautions also should be taken in other settings in which persons may be exposed to blood or other body fluids.

DEFINITION OF HEALTHCARE WORKERS

Healthcare workers are defined as persons, including students and trainees, whose activities involve contact with patients or with blood or other body fluids from patients in a healthcare setting.

HEALTHCARE WORKERS WITH AIDS

As of July 10, 1987, a total of 1,875 (5.5%) of 32,395 adults with AIDS, who had been reported to the CDC national surveillance system and for whom occupational information was available, reported being employed in a health care or clinical laboratory setting. In comparison,

---

*Printed from the Centers for Disease Control. Recommendations for Prevention of HIV Transmission in Health-Care Settings. MMWR Suppl. 1987;36(2):1S-18S.

6.8 million persons—representing 5.6% of the US labor force—were employed in health services. Of the health care workers with AIDS, 95% have been reported to exhibit high-risk behavior; for the remaining 5%, the means of HIV acquisition was undetermined. Health care workers with AIDS were significantly more likely than other workers to have an undetermined risk (5% vs 3%, respectively). For both healthcare workers and non-healthcare workers with AIDS, the proportion with an undetermined risk has not increased since 1982.

The AIDS patients initially reported as not belonging to recognized risk groups are investigated by state and local health departments to determine whether possible risk factors exist. Of all healthcare workers with AIDS reported to CDC who were initially characterized as not having an identified risk and for whom follow-up information was available, 66% have been reclassified because risk factors were identified or because the patient was found not to meet the surveillance case definition for AIDS.

Of the 87 healthcare workers currently categorized as having no identifiable risk, information is incomplete on 16 (18%) because of death or refusal to be interviewed; 38 (44%) are still being investigated. The remaining 33 (38%) healthcare workers were interviewed or had other follow-up information available. The occupations of these 33 were as follows: 5 physicians (15%), 3 of whom were surgeons; 1 dentist (3%); 3 nurses (9%); 9 nursing assistants (27%); 7 housekeeping or maintenance workers (21%); 3 clinical laboratory technician (9%); 1 therapist (3%); and 4 others who did not have contact with patients (12%).

Although 15 of these 33 healthcare workers reported parenteral and/or other non-needlestick exposure to blood or body fluids from patients in the 10 years preceding their diagnosis of AIDS, none of these exposures involved a patient with AIDS or known HIV infection.

RISK TO HEALTHCARE WORKERS OF ACQUIRING HIV IN HEALTHCARE SETTINGS

Healthcare workers with documented percutaneous or mucous membrane exposures to blood or body fluids of HIV-infected patients have been prospectively evaluated to determine the risk of infection after such exposures. As of June 30, 1987, 883 healthcare workers have been tested for antibody to HIV in an ongoing surveillance project conducted by CDC.[9] Of these, 708 (80%) had percutaneous exposures to blood, and 175 (20%) had a mucous membrane or an open wound contaminated by blood or body fluid. Of 396 healthcare workers, each of whom had only a convalescent-phase serum sample obtained and tested less than 90 days postexposure, one—for whom heterosexual transmission could not be ruled out—was seropositive for HIV antibody. For 425 additional healthcare workers, both acute and convalescent-phase serum samples were obtained and tested; none of 74 healthcare workers with nonpercutaneous exposures seroconverted, and three (0.9%) of 351 with percutaneous exposures seroconverted. None of these three healthcare workers had other documented risk factors for infection.

Two other prospective studies to assess the risk of nosocomial acquisition of HIV infection for healthcare workers are going in the United States. As of April 30, 1987, 332 healthcare workers with a total of 453 needlestick or mucous membrane exposures to the blood or other body fluids of HIV-infected patients were tested for HIV antibody at the National Institutes of Health.[10] These exposed workers included 103 with needlestick injuries and 229 with mucous membrane exposures; none had seroconverted. A similar study at the University of California of 129 healthcare workers with documented needlestick injuries or mucous membrane exposures to blood or other body fluids from patients with HIV infection has not identified any seroconversions.[11] Results of a prospective in the United Kingdom identified no evidence of transmission among 150 healthcare workers with parenteral or mucous membrane exposures to blood or other body fluids, secretions, or excretions from patients with HIV infection.[12]

In addition to healthcare workers enrolled in prospective studies, eight persons who provided care to infected patients and denied other risk factors have been reported to have acquired HIV infection. Three of these healthcare workers had needlestick exposures to blood from infected patients.[13-15] Two were persons who provided nursing care to infected persons; although neither sustained a needlestick, both had extensive contact with blood or other body fluids, and neither observed recommended barrier precautions.[16,17] The other three were healthcare workers with non-needlestick to blood from infected patients.[18] Although the exact route of transmission for these last three infections is not known, all the three persons had direct contact of their skin with blood from infected patients, all had skin lesions that may have been contaminated by blood, and one also had a mucous membrane exposure.

A total of 1,231 dentists and hygienists, many of whom practiced in areas with many AIDS cases, participated in a study to determine the prevalence of antibody to HIV; one dentist (0.1%) had HIV antibody. Although no exposure to a known HIV-infected person could be documented, epidemiologic investigation did not identify any other risk factor for infection. The infected dentist, who also had a history of sustaining needlestick injuries and trauma to his hands, did not routinely wear gloves when providing dental care.[19]

PRECAUTIONS TO PREVENT TRANSMISSION OF HIV

Universal Precautions

Since medical history and examination cannot reliably identify all patient infected with HIV or other blood-borne pathogens, blood and body fluid precautions should be consistently used for all patients. This approach, previously recommended by CDC[3,4] and referred to as "universal blood and body fluid precautions" or "universal precautions", should be used in the care of all patients, especially including those in emergency care settings in which the risk of blood exposure is increased and the infection status of the patient is usually unknown.[20]

1. All healthcare workers should routinely use appropriate barrier precautions to prevent skin and mucous membrane exposure when contacted with blood or other body fluids of any patient is anticipated. Gloves should be worn for touching blood and body fluids, mucous membranes, or nonintact skin of all patients, for handling items or surfaces soiled with blood or body fluids, and for performing venipuncture and other vascular access procedures. Gloves should be changed after contact with each patient. Masks and protective eyewear or face shields should be worn during procedures that are likely to generate droplets of blood or other body fluids to prevent exposure of mucous membranes of the mouth, nose, and eyes. Gowns or aprons should be worn during procedures that are likely to generate splashes of blood or other body fluids.

2. Hand and other skin surfaces should be washed immediately and thoroughly if contaminated with blood or other body fluids. Hands should be washed immediately after gloves are removed.

3. All healthcare workers should take precautions to prevent injuries caused by needles, scalpels, and other sharp instruments or devices during procedures; when cleaning used instruments; during disposal of used needles; and when handling sharp instruments after procedures. To prevent needlestick injuries, needles should not be recapped, purposely bent or broken by hand, removed from disposable syringes, or otherwise manipulated by hand. After they are used, disposable syringes and needles, scalpel blades, and other sharp items should be placed in puncture-resistant containers for disposal; the puncture-resistant containers should be located as close as practical to the use area. Large-bore reusable needles should be placed in a puncture-resistant container for transport to the reprocessing area.

4. Although saliva has not been implicated in HIV transmission, to minimize the need for emergency mouth-to-mouth resuscitation, mouthpieces, resuscitation bags, or other ventilation devices should be available for use in areas in which the need for resuscitation is predictable.

5. Healthcare workers who have exudative lesions or weeping dermatitis should refrain from all direct patient care and from handling patient care equipment until the condition resolves.

6. Pregnant healthcare workers are not known to be at greater risk of contracting HIV infection than healthcare workers who are not pregnant; however, if a healthcare worker develops HIV infection during pregnancy, the infant is at risk of infection resulting from perinatal transmission. Because of this risk, pregnant healthcare workers should be especially familiar with the strictly adhere to precautions to minimize the risk of HIV transmission.

Implementation of universal blood and body fluid precautions for all patients eliminates the need for use of the isolation category of "Blood and Body Fluid Precautions" previously recommended by CDC[7] for patients known or suspected to be infected with blood-borne pathogens. Isolation precautions (e.g. enteric, "AFB") should be used as necessary if associated conditions, such as infectious diarrhea or tuberculosis, are diagnosed or suspected.

Precautions for Invasive Procedures

In his document, an invasive procedure is defined as surgical entry into tissues, cavities, or organs or repair of major traumatic injuries:

1. In an operating or delivery room, emergency department, or outpatient setting, including both physicians' and dentists' offices;

2. Cardiac catheterization and angiographic procedures;
3. A vaginal or cesarean delivery or other invasive obstetric procedure during which bleeding may occur; or
4. The manipulation, cutting, or removal of any oral or perioral tissues, including tooth structure, during which bleeding occurs or the potential for bleeding exists. The universal blood and body fluid precautions listed here, should be the minimum precautions for all such invasive procedures
   i. All healthcare workers who participate in invasive procedures must routinely use appropriate barrier precautions to prevent skin and mucous membrane contact with blood and other body fluids of all patients. Gloves and surgical masks must be worn for all invasive procedures. Protective eyewear or face shields should be worn for procedures that commonly result in the generation of droplets, splashing of blood or other body fluids, or the generation of bone chips. Gowns or aprons made of materials that provide an effective barrier should be worn during invasive procedures that are likely to result in the splashing of blood or other body fluids. All healthcare workers who perform or assist in vaginal or cesarean deliveries should wear gloves and gowns when handling the placenta or the infant until blood and amniotic fluid have been removed from the infant's skin and should wear gloves during postdelivery care of the umbilical cord.
   ii. If a glove is torn or a needlestick or other injury occurs, the glove should be removed and a new glove used as promptly as patient safety permits; the needle or instrument involved in the incident should also be removed from the sterile field.

Precautions for Dentistry**

Blood, saliva, and gingival fluid from all dental patients should be considered infective. Special emphasis should be placed on the following precautions for preventing transmission of blood-borne pathogens in dental practice in both institutional and noninstitutional settings.
1. In addition to wearing gloves for contact with oral mucous membranes of all patients, all dental workers should wear surgical masks and protective eyewear or chin-length plastic face shields during dental procedures in which splashing or spattering of blood, saliva, or gingival fluids is likely. Rubber dams, high-speed evacuation, and proper patient positioning, when appropriate, should be utilized to minimize generation of droplets and spatter.
2. Handpieces should be sterilized after use with each patient, since blood, saliva, or gingival fluid of patients may be aspirated into the handpiece or waterline. Handpieces that cannot be sterilized should at least be flushed, the outside surface cleaned and wiped with a suitable chemical germicide, and then rinsed. Handpieces should be flushed at the beginning of the, day and after use with each patient. Munufacturers' recommendations should be followed for use and maintenance of waterlines and check valves and for flushing of handpieces. The same precautions should be used for ultrasonic scalers and air/water syringes.
3. Blood and saliva should be thoroughly and carefully cleaned from material that has been used in the mouth (e.g. impression materials, bite registration), especially before polishing and grinding intraoral devices. Contaminated materials, impressions, and intraoral devices should be cleaned and disinfected before being handled in the dental laboratory and before they are placed in the patient's mouth. Because of the increasing variety of dental materials used intraorally, dental workers should consult with manufacturers as to the stability of specific materials when using disinfection procedures.
4. Dental equipment and surfaces that are difficult to disinfect (e.g. light handles or X-ray unit heads) and that may become contaminated should be wrapped with impervious-backed paper, aluminum foil, or clear plastic wrap. The coverings should be removed and discarded, and clean coverings should be put in place after use with each patient.

Precautions for Autopsies or Morticians' Services

In addition to the universal blood and body fluid precautions listed above, the following precautions should be used by persons performing postmortem procedures:
1. All persons performing or assisting in postmortem procedures should wear gloves, masks, protective eyewear, gowns, and waterproof aprons.

**General infection control precautions are more specifically addressed in previous recommendations for infection control practices for dentistry.[8]

2. Instruments and surfaces contaminated during post-mortem procedures should be decontaminated with an appropriate chemical germicide.

Precautions for Dialysis

Patients with end-stage renal disease who are undergoing maintenance dialysis and who have HIV infection can be dialyzed in hospital-based or free standing dialysis units using conventional infection control precautions.[21] Universal blood and body fluid precautions should be used when dialyzing all patients.

Strategies for disinfecting the dialysis fluid pathways of the hemodialysis machine are targeted to control bacterial contamination and generally consist of using 500–750 parts per million (ppm) of sodium hypochlorite (household bleach) for 30–40 minutes or 1.5–2.0% formaldehyde overnight. In addition, several chemical germicides formulated to disinfect dialysis machines are commercially available. None of these protocols or procedures need to be changed for dialyzing patients infected with HIV.

Patients infected with HIV can be dialyzed by either hemodialysis or peritoneal dialysis and do not need to be isolated from other patients. The type of dialysis treatment (i.e. hemodialysis or peritoneal dialysis) should be based on the need of the patient. The dialyzer may be discarded after each use. Alternatively, centers that reuse dialyzers, i.e. a specific single-use dialyzer is issued to a specific patient, removed, cleaned, disinfected and reused several times on the same patient only—may include HIV-infected patients in the dialyzer-reuse program. An individual dialyzer must never be used on more than one patient.

Precautions for Laboratories***

Blood and other body fluids from all patients should be considered infective. To supplement the universal blood and body fluid precautions listed above, the following precautions are recommended for healthcare workers in clinical laboratories.
1. All specimens of blood and body fluids should be put in a well-constructed container with secure lid to prevent leaking during transport. Care should be taken when collecting each specimen to avoid contaminating the outside of the container and of the laboratory from accompanying specimen.
2. All persons processing blood and body fluid specimens (e.g. removing tops from vacuum tubes) should wear gloves. Masks and protective eyewear should be worn if mucous membrane contact with blood or body fluids is anticipated. Gloves should be changed and hands washed after completion of specimen processing
3. For routine procedures, such as histologic and pathologic studies or microbiologic culturing, a biological safety cabinet is not necessary. However, biological safety cabinets (Class 1 or II) should be used whenever procedures are conducted that have high potential for generating droplets. These include activities such as blending, sonicating and vigorous mixing.
4. Mechanical pipetting devices should be used for manipulating all liquids in the laboratory. Mouth pipetting must not be done.
5. Use of needles and syringes should be limited to situations in which there is no alternative, and the recommendations for preventing injuries with needles outlined under universal precautions should be followed.
6. Laboratory work surfaces should be decontaminated with an appropriate chemical germicide after a spill of blood or other body fluids and when work activities are completed.
7. Contaminated materials used in laboratory tests should be decontaminated before reprocessing or be placed in bags and disposed of in accordance with institutional policies for disposal of infective waste.[24]
8. Scientific equipment that has been contaminated with blood or other body fluids should be decontaminated and cleaned before being repaired in the laboratory or transported to the manufacturer.
9. All persons should wash their hands after completing laboratory activities and should remove protective clothing before leaving the laboratory.

Implementation of universal blood and body fluid precautions for all patients eliminates the need for warning labels on specimens since blood and other body fluids from all patients should be considered infective.

***Additional precautions for research and industrial laboratories are addressed elsewhere.[22,23]

ENVIRONMENTAL CONSIDERATIONS FOR HIV TRANSMISSION

No environmentally mediated mode of HIV transmission has been documented. Nevertheless, the precautions described here should be taken routinely in the care of all patients.

Sterilization and Disinfection

Standard sterilization and disinfection procedures for patient care equipment currently recommended for use[25,26] in a variety of healthcare clinics and offices, hemodialysis centers, emergency care facilities, and long-term nursing care facilities are adequate to sterilize or disinfect instruments, devices, or other items contaminated with blood or other body fluids from persons infected with blood-borne pathogens including HIV.[21,23]

Instruments or devices that enter sterile tissue or the vascular system of any patient or through which blood flows should be sterilized before reuse. Devices or items that contact intact mucous membranes should be sterilized or receive high-level disinfection, a procedure that kills vegetative organisms and viruses but not necessarily large numbers of bacterial spores. Chemical germicides that are registered with the US Environmental Protection Agency (EPA) as "sterilants" may be used either for sterilization or for high-level disinfection depending on contact time.

Contact lenses used in trial fittings should be disinfected after each fitting by using a hydrogen peroxide contact lens disinfecting system or, if compatible, with heat 78–80°C (172.4–176.0°F) for 10 minutes.

Medical devices or instruments that require sterilization or disinfection should be thoroughly cleaned before being exposed to the germicide, and the manufacturer's instructions for the use of the germicide should be followed. Further, it is important that the manufacturer's specifications for compatibility of the medical device with chemical germicides be closely followed. Information on specific label claims of commercial germicides can be obtained by writing to the Disinfectants Branch, Office of Pesticides, Environmental Protection Agency, 401 M Street, SW, Washington, DC 20460.

Studies have shown that HIV is inactivated rapidly after being exposed to commonly used chemical germicides at concentrations that are much lower than used in practice.[27-30] Embalming fluids are similar to the types of chemical germicides that have been tested and found to completely inactivate HIV. In addition to commercially available chemical germicides, a solution of sodium hypochlorite (household bleach) prepared daily is an inexpensive and effective germicide. Concentrations ranging from approximately 500 ppm (1:100 dilution of household bleach) sodium hypochlorite to 5,000 ppm (1:10 dilution of household bleach) are effective depending on the amount of organic material (e.g. blood, mucus) present on the surface to be cleaned and disinfected. Commercially available chemical germicides may be more compatible with certain medical devices that might be corroded by repeated exposure to sodium hypochlorite, especially to the 1:10 dilution.

Survival of HIV in the Environment

The most extensive study on the survival of HIV after drying involved greatly concentrated HIV samples, i.e. 10 million tissue culture infectious doses per milliliter.[31] This concentration is at least 100,000 times greater than that typically found in the blood or serum of patients with HIV infection. HIV was detectable by tissue-culture techniques 1–3 days after drying, but the rate of inactivation was rapid. Studies performed at CDC have also shown that drying HIV causes a rapid (within several hours) 1-2 log (90–99%) reduction in HIV concentration. In tissue culture fluid, cell-free HIV could be detected up to 15 days at room temperature, up to 11 days at 37°C (98.6°F), and up to 1 day if the HIV was cell associated.

When considered in the context of environmental conditions in healthcare facilities, these results do not require any changes in currently recommended sterilization, disinfection, or housekeeping strategies. When medical devices are contaminated with blood or other body fluids, existing recommendations include the cleaning of these instruments, followed by disinfection or sterilization, depending on the type of medical device.

These protocols assume "worst-case" conditions of extreme virologic and microbiologic contamination, and whether viruses have been inactivated after drying plays no role in formulating these strategies. Consequently, no changes in published procedures for cleaning, disinfecting, or sterilizing need to be made.

Housekeeping

Environmental surfaces such as walls, floors, and other surfaces are not associated with transmission of infections to patients or healthcare workers. Therefore, extraordinary attempts to disinfect or sterilize these environmental surfaces are not necessary. However, cleaning and removal of soil should be done routinely.

Cleaning schedules and methods vary according to the area of the hospital or institution, type of surface to be cleaned, and the amount and type of soil present. Horizontal surfaces (e.g. bedside tables and hard-surfaced flooring) in patient care areas are usually cleaned on a regular basis, when soiling or spills occur, and when a patient is discharged. Cleaning of walls, blinds, and curtains is recommended only if they are visibly soiled. Disinfectant fogging is an unsatisfactory method of decontaminating air and surfaces and is not recommended.

Disinfectant-detergent formulations registered by EPA can be used for cleaning environmental surfaces, but the actual physical removal of microorganisms by scrubbing is probably at least as important as any antimicrobial effect of the cleaning agent used. Therefore, cost, safety, and acceptability by housekeepers can be the main criteria for selecting any such registered agent. The manufacturers' instructions for appropriate use should be followed.

Cleaning and Decontaminating Spills of Blood or Other Body Fluids

Chemical germicides that are approved for use as "hospital disinfectant" and are tuberculocidal when used at recommended dilutions can be used to decontaminate spills of blood and other body fluids. Strategies for decontaminating spills of blood and other body fluids in a patient care setting are different than for spills of cultures or other materials in clinical, public health, or research laboratories. In patient care areas, visible material should first be removed and then the area should be decontaminated. With large spills of cultured or concentrated infectious agents in the laboratory, the contaminated area should be flooded with a liquid germicide before cleaning, then decontaminated with fresh germicidal chemical. In both settings, gloves should be worn during the cleaning and decontaminating procedures.

Laundry

Although soiled linen has been identified as a source of large numbers of certain pathogenic microorganisms, the risk of actual disease transmission is negligible. Rather than rigid procedures and specifications, hygienic and common sense storage and processing of clean and soiled linen are recommended.[26] Soiled linen should be handled as little as possible and with minimum agitation to prevent gross microbial contamination of the air and of persons handling the linen. All soiled linen should be bagged at the location where it was used; it should not be sorted or rinsed in patient care areas. Linen soiled with blood or body fluids should be placed and transported in bags that prevent leakage. If hot water is used, linen should be washed with detergent in water at least 71°C (160°F) for 25 minutes. If low temperature [<700°C (158°F)] laundry cycles are used, chemicals suitable for low-temperature washing at proper use concentration should be used.

Infective Waste

There is no epidemiologic evidence to suggest that most hospital waste is any more infective than residential waste. Moreover, there is no epidemiologic evidence that hospital waste has caused disease in the community as a result of improper disposal. Therefore, identifying wastes for which special precautions are indicated is largely a matter of judgment about the relative risk of disease transmission. The most practical approach to the management of infective waste is to identify those wastes with the potential for causing infection during handling and disposal and for which some special precautions appear prudent. Hospital wastes for which special precautions appear prudent include microbiology laboratory waste, pathology waste, and blood specimens or blood products. While any item that has had contact with blood, exudates, or secretions may be potentially infective, it is not usually considered practical or necessary to treat all such waste as infective.[23,26] Infective waste, in general, should either be incinerated or should be autoclaved before disposal in a sanitary landfill. Bulk blood, suctioned fluids, excretions, and secretions may be carefully poured down a drain connected to a sanitary sewer. Sanitary sewers may also be used to dispose of other infectious wastes capable of being ground and flushed into the sewer.

IMPLEMENTATION OF RECOMMENDED PRECAUTIONS

Employers of healthcare workers should ensure that policies exist for:
1. Initial orientation and continuing education and training of all healthcare workers—including students and trainees—on the epidemiology, modes of transmission,

and prevention of HIV and other blood-borne infections and the need for routine use of universal blood and body fluid precautions for all patients.
2. Provision of equipment and supplies necessary to minimize the risk of infection with HIV and other blood-borne pathogens.
3. Monitoring adherence to recommended protective measures. When monitoring reveals a failure to follow recommended precautions, counseling, education, and/or retraining should be provided, and, if necessary, appropriate disciplinary action should be considered.

Professional associations and labor organizations, through continuing education efforts, should emphasize the need for healthcare workers to follow recommended precautions.

SEROLOGIC TESTING FOR HIV INFECTION

Background

A person is identified as infected with HIV when a sequence of tests, starting with repeated enzyme immunoassay (EIA) and including a Western blot or similar, more specific assay, are repeatedly reactive. Persons infected with HIV usually develop antibody against the virus within 6–12 weeks after infection.

The sensitivity of the currently licensed EIA tests is at least 99% when they are performed under optimal laboratory conditions on serum specimens from persons infected for greater than 12 weeks. Optimal laboratory conditions include the use of reliable reagents, provision of continuing education of personnel, quality control of procedures, and participation in performance evaluation programs. Given this performance, the probability of a false-negative test is remote except during the first several weeks after infection, before detectable antibody is present. The proportion of infected persons with a false-negative test attributed to absence of antibody in the early stages of infection of HIV infection in a population (Table 28.1).

The specificity of the currently licensed EIA tests is approximately 99% when repeatedly reactive tests are considered. Repeat testing of initially reactive specimens by EIA is required to reduce the likelihood of laboratory error. To increase further the specificity of serologic tests, laboratories must use a supplemental test, most often the Western blot, to validate repeatedly reactive EIA results. Under optimal laboratory conditions, the sensitivity of the Western blot is highly specific when strict criteria are used to interpret the test results. The testing sequence of a repeatedly reactive EIA and positive Western blot test is highly predictive of HIV infection, even in a population with a low prevalence of infection (Table 28.2). If the Western blot test result is indeterminant, the testing sequence is considered equivocal for HIV infection.

When this occurs, the Western blot test should be repeated on the same serum sample, and, if still indeterminant, the testing sequence should be repeated on a sample collected 3–6 months later. Use of other supplemental tests may aid in interpreting of results on samples that are persistently indeterminate by Western blot.

Table 28.1: Estimate annual number of patients infected with human immunodeficiency virus (HIV) not detected by HIV-antibody testing in a hypothetical hospital with 10,000 admissions/year*.

Beginning prevalence of HIV infection (%)	Annual incidence of HIV infection (%)	Approximate number of HIV-infected patients	Approximate number of HIV-infected patients not detected
5.0	1.0	550	17–18
5.0	0.5	525	11–12
1.0	0.2	110	3–4
1.0	0.1	105	2–3
0.1	0.02	11	0–1
0.1	0.01	11	0–1

*The estimates are based on the following assumptions: (1) The sensitivity of the screening test is 99% (i.e. 99% of HIV-infected persons with antibody will be detected). (2) Persons infected with HIV will not develop detectable antibody (seroconvert) until 6 weeks (1.5 months) after infection. (3) New infections occur at an equal rate throughout the year. (4) Calculations of the number of HIV-infected persons in the patient population are based on the mid-year prevalence, which is the beginning prevalence plus half the annual incidence of infections.

Table 28.2: Predictive value of positive HIV-antibody tests in hypothetical populations with different prevalences of infection.

	Prevalence of infection (%)	Predictive value of positive test* (%)
Repeatedly reactive enzyme immunoassay (EIA)†	0.2	28.41
	2.0	80.16
	20.0	98.02
Repeatedly reactive EIA followed by positive Western blot (WB)††	0.2	99.75
	2.0	99.97
	20.0	99.99

*Proportion of persons with positive test results who are actually infected with HIV.
†Assumes EIA sensitivity of 99.0% and specificity of 99.5%.
††Assumes WB sensitivity of 99.0% and specificity of 99.9%.

Testing of Patients

Previous CDC recommendations have emphasized the value of HIV serologic testing of patients for:
1. Management of parenteral or mucous membrane exposures of healthcare workers.
2. Patient diagnosis and management.
3. Counseling and serologic testing to prevent and control HIV transmission in the community. In addition, more recent recommendations have stated that hospitals, in conjunction with state and local health departments, should periodically determine the prevalence of HIV infection among patients from age groups at highest risk of infection.[32]

Adherence to universal blood and body fluid precautions recommended for the care of all patients will minimize the risk of transmission of HIV and other blood-borne pathogens from patients to healthcare workers. The utility of routine HIV serologic testing of patients as an adjunct to universal precautions is unknown. Results of such testing may not be available in emergency or outpatient settings. In addition, some recently infected patients will not have detectable antibody of HIV (Table 28.1).

Personnel in some hospitals have advocated serologic testing of patients in settings in which exposure of healthcare workers to large amounts of patients, blood may be anticipated. Specific patients for whom serologic testing has been advocated include those undergoing major operative procedures and those undergoing treatment in critical care units, especially if they have conditions involving uncontrolled bleeding. Decisions regarding the need to establish testing programs for patients should be made by physicians or individual institutions. In addition, when deemed appropriate, testing of individual patients may be performed on agreement between the patient and the physician providing care.

In addition to the universal precautions recommended for all patients, certain additional precautions for the care of HIV-infected patients undergoing major surgical operations have been proposed by personnel in some hospitals. For example, surgical procedures on an HIV-infected patient might be altered so that hand-to-hand passing of sharp instruments would be eliminated; stapling instruments rather than hand suturing equipment might be used to perform tissue approximation; electrocautery devices rather than scalpels might be used as cutting instruments; and, even though uncomfortable, gowns that totally prevent seepage of blood onto the skin of members of the operative team might be worn. While such modifications might further minimize the risk of HIV infection for members of the operative team, some of these techniques could result in prolongation of operation time and could potentially have an adverse effect on the patient.

Testing programs, if developed, should include the following principles:
- Obtaining consent for testing
- Informing patients of test results, and providing counseling for seropositive patients by properly trained persons
- Assuring that confidentiality safeguards are in place to limit knowledge of test results to those directly involved in the care of infected patients or as required by law
- Assuring that identification of infected patients will not result in denial of needed care or provision of suboptimal care

- Evaluating prospectively:
  - The efficacy of the program in reducing the incidence of parenteral, mucous membrane, or significant cutaneous exposures of healthcare workers to the blood or other body fluids of HIV-infected patients
  - The effect of modified procedures on patients.

Testing of Healthcare Workers

Although transmission of HIV from infected healthcare workers to patients has not been reported, transmission during invasive procedures remains a possibility. Transmission of hepatitis B virus (HBV)—a blood-borne agent with a considerably greater potential for nosocomial spread—from healthcare workers to patients has been documented. Such transmission has occurred in situations (e.g. oral gynecologic surgery) in which healthcare workers, when tested, had very high concentrations of HBV in their blood (at least 100 million infectious virus particles per milliliter, a concentration much higher than occurs with HIV infection), and the healthcare workers sustained a puncture wound while performing invasive procedures or had exudative or weeping lesions or microlacerations that allowed virus to contaminate instruments or open wounds of patients.[33,34]

The hepatitis B experience indicates that only those healthcare workers who perform certain types of invasive procedures have transmitted HBV to patients. Adherence to recommendations in this document will minimize the risk of transmission of HIV and other blood-borne pathogens from healthcare workers to patients during invasive procedures. Since transmission of HIV from infected healthcare workers performing invasive procedures to their patients has not been reported and would be expected to occur only very rarely, if at all, the utility of routine testing of such healthcare workers to prevent transmission of HIV cannot be assessed. If consideration is given to developing a serologic testing program for healthcare workers who perform invasive procedures, the frequency of testing, as well as the issues of consent, confidentiality, and consequences of test results—as previously outlined for testing programs for patients—must be addressed.

MANAGEMENT OF INFECTED HEALTHCARE WORKERS

Healthcare workers with impaired immune systems resulting from HIV infection or other causes are at increased risk of acquiring or experiencing serious complications of infectious disease. Of particular concern is the risk of severe infection following exposure to patients with infectious diseases that are easily transmitted if appropriate precautions are not taken (e.g. measles, varicella). Any healthcare worker with an impaired immune system should be counseled about the potential risk associated with taking care of patients with any transmissible infection and should continue to follow existing recommendations for infection control to minimize risk of exposure to other infectious agents.[7,35] Recommendations of the Advisory Committee on Immunization Practices (ACIP) and institutional policies concerning requirements for vaccinating healthcare workers with live virus vaccines (e.g. measles, rubella) should also be considered.

The question of whether workers infected with HIV—especially those who perform invasive procedures—can adequately and safely be allowed to perform patient care duties or whether their work assignments should be changed must be determined on an individual basis. These decisions should be made by the healthcare worker's personal physician(s) in conjunction with the medical directors and personnel health service staff of the employing institution or hospital.

MANAGEMENT OF EXPOSURES

If a healthcare worker has a parenteral (e.g. needlestick or cut) or mucous membrane (e.g. splash to the eye or mouth) exposure to blood or other body fluids or has a cutaneous exposure involving large amounts of blood or prolonged contact with blood—especially when the exposed skin is chapped, abraded, or afflicted with dermatitis—the source patient should be informed of the incident and tested for serologic evidence of HIV infection after consent is obtained. Policies should be developed for testing source patients in situations in which consent cannot be obtained (e.g. an unconscious patient).

If the source patient has AIDS, is positive for HIV antibody, or refuses the test, the healthcare workers should be counseled regarding the risk of infection and evaluated clinically and serologically for evidence of HIV infection as soon as possible after the exposure. The healthcare worker should be advised to report and seek medical evaluation for any acute febrile illness that occurs within 12 weeks after the exposure. Such an illness—particularly one characterized by fever, rash, or lymphadenopathy—may be indicative of recent HIV infection. Seronegative healthcare workers should be retested 6 weeks postexposure and on a periodic basis thereafter (e.g. 12 weeks and 6 months after exposure) to determine whether transmission has occurred. During this follow-up period—especially the first 6–12 weeks after exposure, when most infected persons are expected to seroconvert—exposed healthcare workers should follow US Public Health Service (PHS) recommendations for preventing transmission of HIV.[36,37]

No further follow-up of a healthcare worker exposed to infection as described above is necessary if the source patient is seronegative unless the source patient is at high risk of HIV infection. In the latter case, a subsequent specimen (e.g. 12 weeks following exposure) may be obtained from the healthcare workers for antibody testing. If the source patient cannot be identified, decisions regarding appropriate follow-up should be individualized. Serologic testing should be available to all healthcare workers who are concerned that they may have been infected with HIV.

If a patient has a parenteral or mucous membrane exposure to blood or other body fluid of a healthcare worker, the patient should be informed of the incident, and the same procedure outlined above for management of exposures should be followed for both the source healthcare worker and the exposed patient.

REFERENCES

1. Centers for Disease Control (CDC). Acquired immune deficiency syndrome (AIDS): precautions for clinical and laboratory staffs. MMWR Morb Mortal Wkly Rep. 1982; 31(43):577-80.
2. Centers for Disease Control (CDC). Acquired immunodeficiency syndrome (AIDS): precautions for health-care workers and allied professionals. MMWR Morb Mortal Wkly Rep. 1983;32(34):450-1.
3. Centers for Disease Control (CDC). Recommendations for preventing transmission of infection with human T-lymphotropic virus type III/lymphadenopathy-associated virus in the workplace. MMWR Morb Mortal Wkly Rep. 1985;34:681-6, 691-5.
4. Centers for Disease Control (CDC). Recommendations for preventing transmission of infection with human T-lymphotropic virus type III/lymphadenopathy-associated virus during invasive procedures. MMWR Morb Mortal Wkly Rep. 1986;35:221-3.
5. Centers for Disease Control (CDC). Recommendations for preventing possible transmission of human T-lymphotropic virus type III/lymphadenopathy-associated virus from tears. MMWR Morb Mortal Wkly Rep. 1985;34:533-4.
6. Centers for Disease Control (CDC). Recommendations for providing dialysis treatment to patients infected with human T-lymphotropic virus type III/lymphadenopathy-associated virus infection. MMWR Morb Mortal Wkly Rep. 1986;35:376-83.
7. Garner JS, Simmons BP. Guideline for isolation precautions in hospitals. Infect Control. 1983;4(4 Suppl):245-325.
8. Centers for Disease Control (CDC). Recommended infection control practices for dentistry. MMWR Morb Mortal Wkly Rep. 1986;35:237-42.
9. McCray E. Occupational risk of the acquired immunodeficiency syndrome among health care workers. N Engl J Med. 1986;314:1127-32.
10. Henderson DK, Saah AJ, Zak BJ, et al. Risk of nosocomial infection with human T-cell lymphotropic virus type III/lymphadenopathy-associated virus in a large cohort of intensively exposed health care workers. Ann Intern Med. 1986;104:644-7.
11. Gerberding JL, Bryant-LeBlanc CE, Nelson K, et al. Risk of transmitting the human immunodeficiency virus, cytomegalovirus, and hepatitis B virus to health care workers exposed to patients with AIDS and AIDS-related conditions. J Infect Dis. 1987;156:1-8.
12. McEvoy M, Porter K, Mortimer P, et al. Prospective study of clinical, laboratory, and ancillary staff with accidental exposures to blood or other body fluids from patients infected with HIV. Br Med J (Clin Res Ed). 1987;294:1597-7.
13. Needlestick transmission of HTLV-III from a patient infected in Africa. Lancet. 1984;2:1376-7.
14. Oksenhendler E, Harzic M, Le Roux JM, et al. HIV infection with seroconversion after a superficial needlestick injury to the finger. N Engl J Med. 1986;315:582.
15. Neisson-Vernant C, Arfi S, Mathez D, et al. Needlestick HIV seroconversion in a nurse. Lancet. 1986;2:814.
16. Grint P, McEvoy M. Two associated cases of the acquired immune deficiency syndrome (AIDS). PHLS Commun Dis Rep. 1985;42:4.
17. Centers for Disease Control (CDC). Apparent transmission of human T-lymphotropic virus type III/lymphadenopathy-associated virus from a child to a mother providing health care. MMWR Morb Mortal Wkly Rep. 1986;35:76-9.
18. Centers for Disease Control (CDC). Update: human immunodeficiency virus infections in health care workers exposed to blood of infected patients. MMWR Morb Mortal Wkly Rep. 1987;36:285-9.
19. Kline RS, Phelan J, Friedland GH, et al. Low occupational risk for HIV infection for dental professionals. In: Abstracts from the III International Conference on AIDS, 1-5 June 1985. Washington, DC: 155.
20. Baker JL, Kelen GD, Sivertson KT, et al. Unsuspected human immunodeficiency virus in critically ill emergency patients. JAMA. 1987;257:2609-11.
21. Favero MS. Dialysis-associated diseases and their control. In: Bennett JV, Brachman PS (Eds). Hospital Infections. Boston: Little, Brown and Company; 1985. pp. 267-84.
22. Richardson JH, Barkley WE. Biosafety in Microbiological and Biomedical Laboratories. Washington, DC: US Department of Health and Human Services, Public Health Service. HHS publication no. (CDC) 84-8395, 1984.

23. Centers for Disease Control (CDC). Human T-lymphotropic virus type III/lymphadenopathy-associated virus: agent summary statement. MMWR Morb Mortal Wkly Rep. 1986;35:540-2, 547-9.
24. US Environmental Protection Agency. EPA Guide for Infectious Waste Management. Washington, DC: US Environmental Protection Agency (Publication no. EPA/530-SW-86-014), 1986.
25. Favero MS. Sterilization, disinfection, and antisepsis in the hospital. In: Lennette EH, Balows A, Hausler WJ, Shadomy HJ (Eds). Manual of Clinical Microbiology, 4th edition. Washington, DC: American Society for Microbiology; 1985. pp. 129-37.
26. Garner JS, Favero MS. Guideline for Handwashing and Hospital Environmental Control. Atlanta: Public Health Service, Centers for Disease Control. HHS publication no. 99-1117, 1985.
27. Spire B, Montagnier L, Barre-Sinoussi F, et al. Inactivation of lymphadenopathy associated virus by chemical disinfectants. Lancet. 1984;2:899-901.
28. Martin LS, McDougal JS, Loskoski SL. Disinfection and inactivation of the human T-lymphotropic virus type III/lymphadenopathy-associated virus. J Infect Dis. 1985;152:400-3.
29. McDougal JS, Martin LS, Cort SP, et al. Thermal inactivation of the acquired immunodeficiency syndrome virus, human T lymphotropic virus-III/lymphadenopathy-associated virus, with special reference to antihemophilic factor. J Clin Invest. 1985;76:875-7.
30. Spire B, Barre-Sinoussi F, Dormont D, et al. Inactivation of lymphadenopathy-associated virus by heat, gamma rays, and ultraviolet light. Lancet. 1985;1:188-9.
31. Resnick L, Veren K, Salahuddin SZ, et al. Stability and inactivation of HTLV-III/LAV under clinical and laboratory environments. JAMA. 1986;255:1887-91.
32. Centers for Disease Control (CDC). Public Health Service (PHS) guidelines for counseling and antibody testing to prevent HIV infection and AIDS. MMWR Morb Mortal Wkly Rep. 1987;36:509-15.
33. Kane MA, Lettau LA. Transmission of HBV from dental personnel to patients. J Am Dent Assoc. 1985;110:634-6.
34. Lettau LA, Smith JD, Williams D, et al. Transmission of hepatitis B with resultant restriction of surgical practice. JAMA. 1986;255:934-7.
35. Williams WW. Guideline for infection control in hospital personnel. Infect Control. 1983;4(4 Suppl):326-49.
36. Centers for Disease Control (CDC). Prevention of acquired immune deficiency syndrome (AIDS): report of inter-agency recommendations. MMWR Morb Mortal Wkly Rep. 1983;32:101-3.
37. Centers for Disease Control (CDC). Provisional Public Health Service inter-agency recommendations for screening donated blood and plasma for antibody to the virus causing acquired immunodeficiency syndrome. MMWR Morb Mortal Wkly Rep. 1985;34:1-5.

Chapter 29

Mobile Embalming Unit for the Preparation of Specimens for Anatomical Studies*

Andre Bisaillon, Richard Bourassa

The embalming unit (Fig. 29.1), which is mounted on four rubber wheels, is made of 2-cm thick plywood and provided with two sliding Plexiglass doors at the front. The cabinet is divided into two halves by a 2-cm-thick shelf; the bottom half is subdivided into two equal compartments. The external dimensions of the unit are 90 cm in width, 80 cm in height, and 60 cm in depth. The top of the trolley has three holes of about 2 cm in diameter to allow plastic tubing to reach two graduated polyethylene tanks. One length of tubing goes to the upper tank, and the other two reach the bottom container by passing through two rigid plastic pipes. The two polyethylene containers are connected together by a pipe, equipped with a valve. Each tank has a capacity of 45 L with the following external dimensions 30 cm in width, 30 cm in height, and 45 cm in depth. A commercial peristaltic pump is placed on top of the cabinet.

The concentrated formaldehyde solution and the other chemicals used in the preparation of the embalming fluid are transferred through the peristaltic pump from the commercial containers directly to the upper polyethylene tank (Fig. 29.1A). By opening the valve (Fig. 29.1B), the desired quantity of concentrated solution is transferred to the bottom container (Fig. 29.1C). To complete the concentrated embalming solution, the glycerine is poured into the bottom polyethylene container through one of the two rigid plastic pipes. The proper quantity of water necessary for the dilution is added to the concentrated embalming solution in the bottom tank with a length of plastic tubing directly from the tap. By adding the tap water to the solution, a thorough mixing of the embalming components is achieved. However, if a too great quantity of embalming fluid is stored in the bottom tank, the glycerine has a tendency to precipitate. Only one peristaltic pump is used either for the preparation of the embalming fluid or for the embalming of the specimen. For the injection of the embalming solution, one end of the plastic tubing is placed in the bottom tank, and the other end, mounted with a needle of appropriate size, is introduced into the carotid or the femoral artery. Because the pumping system is not equipped with a pressure-gauge, the embalming procedure is controlled by using the rate of flow. This rate of flow varies according to the size of the animals. The pump is set at a rate of 200–250 mL/min for dogs, 500 mL/min for pigs, 600 mL/min for small horses, and 900 mL/min for cows.

The use of this embalming unit enables one to minimize manipulations by the technician during the preparation of the embalming fluid. Pumping the concentrated formaldehyde, or any other product, directly from the commercial container to the polyethylene tank and, after dilution, pumping the diluted fluid directly into the specimen, allows one to work in a closed circuit system and virtually eliminates direct exposure to the chemicals. Unpleasant irritation of the skin, eyes, nose, and throat caused by the formaldehyde during normal embalming procedures is thus greatly reduced.

By using the peristaltic pump, the rate of flow of the embalming fluid for injection purposes is easily controlled and the efficiency and the quality of the embalming are

---

*The Anatomical Record 208: New York: John Willey and Sons Inc.;1984. pp. 147-8.

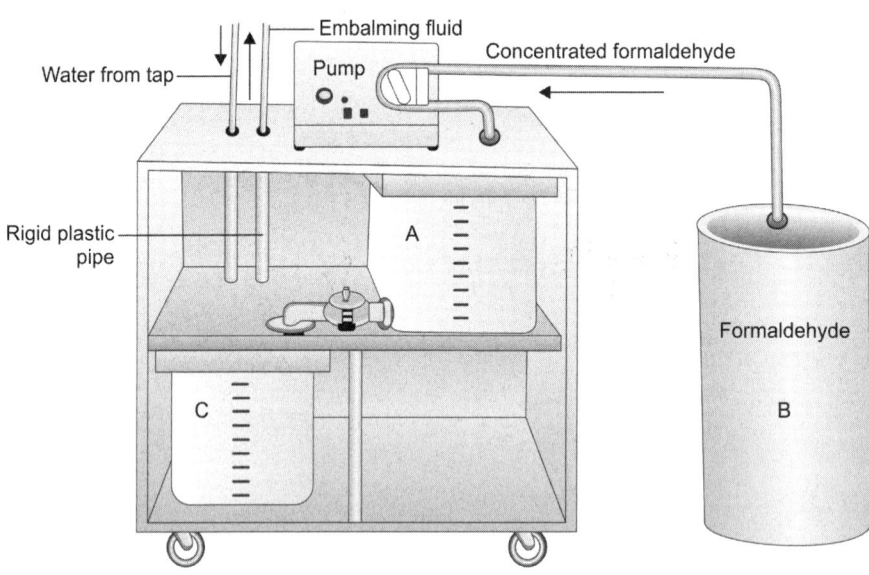

Fig. 29.1: Embalming unit showing transfer of concentrate formaldehyde.

greatly improved. In our laboratory the usual gravity method of embalming was replaced 6 years ago by our present technique. Since that time, the loss of specimens, especially large animals like cows and horses, because of unsuccessful embalming has been practically eliminated. The embalming solution utilized in our department for large animals consists of 10% formaldehyde, 5% isopropyl alcohol, 1% methyl salicylate, 2% glycerine, 2% phenol, and 80% water. With the present embalming cabinet, a large amount of embalming fluid can be injected within a very short time, reducing significantly the work load of the technical staff.

Apart from peristaltic pump, which is a relatively expensive item, the total cost of materials necessary for the building of the embalming cabinet is quite reasonable with a figure of about Canadian $250.

The present embalming unit offers additional advantages for the gross anatomy laboratory. Animals of all sizes can be effectively embalmed, and the cabinet can be easily carried and stored in a small area.

Chapter 30

Exposure to Formaldehyde in Anatomy: An Occupational Health Hazard*

Reinhard Pabst

INTRODUCTION

The adverse effects of formaldehyde have been discussed very emotionally in public. Anatomists, technicians in histology and embalming laboratories, as well as medical students during their dissection course are all exposed to formaldehyde, which in many situations crosses the threshold for irritation of the eyes and upper respiratory tract. There is no doubt about the acute toxic effects and the occurrence of contact dermatitis caused by formaldehyde. Studies in rats and mice using high concentrations over an extremely long period (which would not be tolerated by humans) resulted in squamous carcinoma of the nose. Epidemiologic studies on the mortality of medical personnel exposed to formaldehyde do not provide sufficient evidence of cancerogenicity. A number of recommendations will be given for defining the exact concentration in a dissecting room or laboratory and for ways of reducing formaldehyde concentrations and thus minimizing adverse health hazards. These data could initiate a discussion among anatomists, and with technicians and students, based on a sound scientific background rather than on emotion.

In many countries the dangers of exposure to formaldehyde are periodically discussed in the media, and this reached a peak when it was reported that nasal cancers can be induced in experimental animals. Numerous adverse effects have been attributed to formaldehyde recently, and it has been documented that the publicity "caused" an increase in symptoms, which Norman (1986) called "media-induced symptoms." There is hardly any professional group more exposed to formaldehyde than anatomists-technicians embalming bodies and even medical students during their dissection course are also exposed. Many reports in the lay press are far from objective and not based on hard data. The results of scientific studies, however, are mostly published in journals of toxicology, occupational medicine and mutation and cancer research (Gibson, 1983; Federal Panel on Formaldehyde, 1982), none of which are usually read by anatomists. The aim of the present paper is therefore to summarize the real health hazards of formaldehyde, such as toxic and allergic effects, and to discuss the animal studies and epidemiological surveys on the cancerogenicity of formaldehyde. The properties and origin of formaldehyde will be briefly mentioned, the health hazards will be described, and some recommendations will be given as to how to minimize formaldehyde's adverse effects. These data should enable anatomists to discuss the potential health hazards with technicians and students less emotionally and more scientifically.

PROPERTIES OF FORMALDEHYDE

Formaldehyde (HCHO) is colorless, flammable gas, extremely soluble in water; the aqueous solution about 37% formaldehyde is called formalin. Formaldehyde in an aqueous solution tends to polymerize to paraformaldehyde. A well-known feature is the pungent odor of formaldehyde. The concentration of formaldehyde is usually expressed as ppm (parts per million): 1 ppm = 1.248 mg/m^3.

---

*The Anatomical Record 219. New York: John Willey and sons, Inc.; 1987;109-12.

Formaldehyde is a normal metabolite. Regardless of endogenous production or absorption after inhalation it is rapidly metabolized to formic acid (t½ = 1.5 minutes) (Bernstein et al., 1984). Formaldehyde is present in a variety of foods including many fruits and coffee, so it is commonly introduced via the gastrointestinal tract. No significant increases over average endogenous levels occurred in the nasal mucosa or blood of rats exposed to carcinogenic levels of formaldehyde gas (Bernstein et al., 1984).

Formaldehyde is widely used, e.g. in the chemical, adhesive, paint, plastic, construction, textile, paper, and cosmetic industries (Bernstein et al., 1984). Only a small portion of the amounts produced are used in medicine as disinfectant and for fixation of tissue samples or embalming. It has to be remembered that formaldehyde is ubiquitous in our environment. Formaldehyde is produced by cars and released by all fires, such as those in wood-or coal-burning stoves. Cigarette smoke has been reported to contain more than 20 ppm formaldehyde, and about 0.38 mg of formaldehyde is inhaled per pack of cigarettes in mainstream smoke (Bernstein et al., 1984; Imbus, 1985).

FORMALDEHYDE CONCENTRATION IN ANATOMY LABORATORIES AND DISSECTION ROOMS

The concentration of formaldehyde can be measured relatively easily by calibrated sampling pumps (Bernstein et al., 1984). There are major differences depending on whether air concentrations are measured above the floor or in the breathing zone. Several studies have reported doses ranging from 0.3 to 0.6 ppm (Triebig et al., 1980), 0.3 to 2.63 ppm (Skisak, 1983), 0.9 to 4.5 ppm (Thomsor et al., 1984) up to 20 mg/m^3 (Stofft et al., 1971), 0.2 to 2.35 ppm (Rader, 1974), 1.5 mg/m^3 (Yager et al., 1986), and 0.31 to 6.77 ppm (Perkins and Kimbrough, 1985). This wider range of concentrations can be explained by different types of embalming solutions and fluids in spray bottles used to wet cadaver tissues during class, the size of the room, number of students, temperature, and most important, by the ventilation from windows or active general or local exhaust ventilation. The data mentioned above prove that in most studies concentrations of formaldehyde have been found which are beyond acceptable levels and will produce symptoms in anyone exposed to them. In our medical school we use an embalming fluid consisting of 86.5% ethanol, 8.1% formalin, 2.7% glycerol, and 2.7% phenol and the bodies are stored for at least 3 months in 70% ethanol. Under these circumstances the formaldehyde concentration has never even reached 0.2 ppm in our dissection room.

In the US, the permissible limits for occupational exposure to formaldehyde are 3 ppm for an 8-hour time weight average breathing zone, a ceiling concentration of 5 ppm, and acceptable maximum peak of 10 ppm for no longer than 30 minutes during a 1-day shift (quoted by Bernstein et al., 1984). In West Germany, 1 ppm is the average limit for an 8-hour shift. There is no doubt that such levels are reached and exceeded in laboratories where bodies are embalmed or even in histology laboratories.

Irritation of the Eyes and Respiratory Tract Mucosa

The toxic effects of exposure to formaldehyde can be classified as follows: irritation of mucous membranes, contact dermatitis, and mutagenicity or cancerogenicity. Irritation of the eyes and upper respiratory tract mucosa and contact dermatitis are generally accepted and well documented.

Irritation of the eyes has been documented at as low a concentration as 0.24 ppm but no true dose-response relationship has been found until 0.8 ppm (Imbus, 1985). The thresholds for the irritation effects of acute formaldehyde exposure are summarized in Table 30.1. The irritation at 6 ppm and higher becomes so serious that it is unlikely that anyone would stay in an environment with such levels voluntarily. Normally the lower respiratory tract will hardly be reached by formaldehyde. Two aspects of great practical importance are as follows:

- There is a wide variation as to when and to what extent individuals realized symptoms of irritation.
- Accommodation of the odor threshold and also irritation of the conjunctivae are common (Clark, 1983).

Thus, the warning effect of the odor is lost on some people after a short period, and technicians or students complaining about symptoms at low levels might have a lower threshold and are not necessarily exaggerating the symptoms.

Contact Dermatitis and Asthma-like Symptoms

Many cases of dermatitis due to formaldehyde have been described (Fisher, 1973; Clark, 1983; Imbus 1985, Bernstein et al., 1984). The clinical evaluation of people under

Table 30.1: Adverse effects of inhaling formaldehyde at increasing concentrations.	
Formaldehyde concentration (ppm)	Adverse effects on health
0.05–1.0	Odor threshold
0.05–2.0	Eye irritation, neurophysiologic effects
0.10–25	Irritation of nose and throat
5–20	Maximal tears within a few minutes, lower airway and pulmonary effects (dyspnea, coughing, burning of nose, eyes, and pharynx)
>20	Pulmonary edema and pneumonia

Source:
National Institute for Occupational Safety and Health. NIOSH Criteria Documents: Criteria for a recommended standard: occupational exposure to formaldehyde DHHS (NIOSH) Publication No. 77-126. Washington DC: US Government Printing Office; 1976. pp. 32-59.
Bernstein RS, Styner LT, Elliott LJ, et al. Inhalation exposure to formaldehyde: An overview of its toxicology epidemiology, monitoring and control. Am Ind Hyg Assoc J. 1984;45:778-85.
Imbus HR. Clinical evaluation of patients with complains related to formaldehyde exposure. J Allergy Clin Immunol. 1985;76:831-40.
Triebig G, Valentin H. Gesundheitsrisiken durch formaldehyde. Eine arbeitsmedizinische Bestandsaufnahme. Pathologe. 1985;6:64-70.

suspicion of formaldehyde dermatitis has been described by Imbus (1985). As a precaution gloves should be worn to avoid direct contact. Asthma has also been described in association with formaldehyde exposure (Imbus, 1985). A recent study of bronchial provocation in 15 workers occupationally exposed to formaldehyde showed that in six patients the symptoms were due to a direct irritant effect and three workers had classical occupational asthma (Burge et al., 1985). Despite the widespread use of formaldehyde, it is an extremely rare cause of occupational asthma.

Far fewer studies have been performed on the neurobehavioral effects of formaldehyde exposure. Kilburn et al. (1985) tested women working in histology laboratories with exposure to formaldehyde, xylene, and toluene and compared them to clerical workers of comparable age and smoking habits. The formaldehyde exposure correlated better with neurobehavioral symptoms such as memory, mood equilibrium, and sleep than exposure to xylene and toluene. More studies with controlled exposures are needed to substantiate these data.

Mutagenicity of Formaldehyde

Formaldehyde has been known for some time to be mutagenic to Drosophila, bacteria, and lymphoid cells in vitro (Clark, 1983; Kerns et al., 1983). It was speculated that inhaled or ingested formaldehyde might be toxic at distant sites. In a recent study, Heck et al. (1985) exposed rats to 14.4 + 2.4 ppm formaldehyde for 2 hours and six human volunteers to 1.9 + 0.1 ppm for 40 minutes. In neither experiment could a statistically significant effect of the exposure to the formaldehyde concentrations be found in the blood. The rapid metabolism seems to prevent an increase above the average endogenous level. Thomson et al. (1984) looked at chromosome aberration and the frequency of sister chromatid exchanges in lymphocytes in a small number of pathology workers occupationally exposed to formaldehyde. There was no detectable difference compared to unexposed controls. No mutagens were found in the urine of autopsy service workers exposed to formaldehyde (Connor et al., 1985). When the sister chromatid exchanges were measured in peripheral lymphocytes in medical students before and after a 10-week dissection course, a small increase was noted (Yager et al., 1986). These students were exposed to a mean breathing zone concentration of formaldehyde of 1.2 ppm. Other possible reasons for these sister-chromatid exchanges have to be studied in more detail, using larger groups of students.

Despite the in vitro mutagenic effects of formaldehyde, it is difficult to explain how mutagenic effects could take place at distant sites from the exposure, because of the rapid metabolism. So far there is no convincing evidence of mutagenicity of formaldehyde in occupationally exposed people.

Carcinogenicity of Formaldehyde in Experimental Animals

The basis for the major concern about formaldehyde exposure is studies in which squamous cell carcinomas were induced in Fisher—344 rats by formaldehyde (Kerns et al., 1983). These studies must be quoted in more detail.

Adult rats and mice were exposed to 0, 2.0, 5.6, and 14.3 ppm of formaldehyde gas 6 hours per day, 5 days per week for 24 months. This includes concentrations hardly acceptable to man for short periods and exposure times which make up two-thirds of the rodent's life span. Squamous cell carcinomas were observed in the nasal cavity in about 50% of rats exposed to the concentration of 14.3 ppm and two out of 235 rats at 5.6 ppm, but in only less than 1% of mice at 14.3 ppm. The tumors in rats showed a typical localization on the anterior portion of the lateral aspect of the nasoturbinate and adjacent lateral wall (Morgan et al., 1986). A different group reported similar cancers in rats (Selakumar et al., 1985), while in monkeys, rats, and hamsters exposed to 2.95 ppm for 22 hours per day, 7 days per week for 26 weeks, only monkeys and rats but no hamsters showed squamous metaplasia. The different types of breathing and turbulences in the nose might explain such species differences (Chang et al., 1983).

It is important to stress that in man exposure to such high concentrations is so extremely unpleasant that it would result in a behavioral response of avoidance. The dose relative and absolute length of exposure, and the difficulty in differentiating between toxic and cancerogenic effects in these animal studies prevent an extrapolation to the situation in man, as discussed in detail by Squire and Cameron (1984).

EPIDEMIOLOGICAL STUDIES ON THE TUMOR INCIDENCE IN MEDICAL PERSONNEL EXPOSED TO FORMALDEHYDE

The animal studies on the cancerogenicity of high concentrations of formaldehyde initiated more epidemiological studies. The proportional mortality was analyzed in workers exposed to formaldehyde in the chemical industry. Marsh (1982) could not find any statistically significant excesses or deficits, and no deaths of sinonasal cancer were observed among the chemical workers studied. A comparable study on a cohort of 7,680 men in British factories producing formaldehyde also revealed no excess mortality for cancers at any sites previously reported (Acheson et al., 1984). Hayes et al. (1986), however, recommended further research after having documented a minor increase in the risk of nasal cancers in a retrospective study on workers in whom formaldehyde exposure was thought possible.

Mortality studies of medical personnel are of more interest for anatomists. Based on the Danish Cancer Registry since 1943, neither nasal cancers nor lung cancer cases could be found in physicians specialized in pathology, forensic medicine, or anatomy (Moller Jensen, 1980; Moller Jensen and Kruger Andersen, 1982). The mortality of undertakers in Ontario (Levine et al., 1984) and of embalmers licensed in New York between 1902 and 1980 (Walrath and Fraumeni, 1983) was studied in detail and no increased risk of nasal cancer was found. However, other diseases, such as liver cirrhosis and chronic rheumatic heart disease (Levine et al., 1984), and mortality of cancer of the skin and colon (Walrath and Fraumeni, 1983), were elevated. The latter diseases could have been caused by several factors other than formaldehyde. Mortality studies on pathologists and medical laboratory technicians (Harrington and Skhanon, 1975; Harrington and Oakes, 1984; Brunner and Warich, 1985; Stroup et al., 1986) once again lack any evidence of an increased incidence of nasal cancers.

All these epidemiological studies can be criticized, e.g. because they are retrospective studies and because the exact length of exposure to formaldehyde and its concentration were not known in most cases. A potential carcinogenicity of formaldehyde cannot completely be excluded by the studies, but so far it is very unlikely that long-term formaldehyde exposure in man carries a significant risk of nasal cancer (Squire and Cameron, 1984).

CONCLUSIONS AND RECOMMENDATIONS FOR ANATOMY DEPARTMENTS

The acute toxic effect of formaldehyde and its ability to induce contact dermatitis are beyond any doubt. Animal experiments and epidemiological studies do not provide persuasive evidence for the cancerogenicity of formaldehyde in man, but it cannot be totally excluded. These well-documented and probable health hazards from formaldehyde are so grave that a number of precautions are recommended to reduce occupational formaldehyde exposure to the lowest feasible level (Clark, 1983; Bernstein et al., 1984; Smalky and Schor, 1984; Triebig and Valentin, 1985).

Determine the Concentration

Determine the concentration of formaldehyde in the laboratory where bodies are embalmed, in the dissecting room, and in histology laboratories. Several methods, some relatively easy, are available (for review see Bernstein et al., 1984). It is important to take the air samples in the breathing zone, which can be about five times higher than room air samples (Yager et al., 1986). Blood and urine formaldehyde and formate levels cannot be utilized for monitoring inhalation exposure to formaldehyde. On the basis of exact measurements in the individual laboratory, further steps can be initiated and technicians and students can be informed about the actual data.

Room Ventilation

Effective ventilation using active general or local exhaust ventilation is essential in reducing the concentration of formaldehyde. The ventilation system should be checked under real working conditions, e.g. with all the students in dissecting room and at the beginning and end of the course and working hours. Clark (1983) gives details of how formaldehyde concentrations can be reduced using fume cupboards for handling large volumes of formaldehyde and for mixing embalming solutions.

Look for Alternative Embalming Solutions

Look for alternative embalming solutions to reduce the amount of formaldehyde to hardly detectable levels, as in our department. However, one has to be aware of the health hazards of other chemicals in embalming solutions, such as phenol. This has a low vapor pressure but is absorbed dermally (Morimoto and Wolff, 1980; Yager et al., 1986).

Avoidance of Contact

Technicians and students should be informed about how to avoid unnecessary high concentrations of formaldehyde and about wearing gloves to reduce the likelihood of developing contact dermatitis. Especially technicians should know that acclimatization or tolerance to the irritant effects can occur, thus removing the warning effect of toxic concentrations. Acute symptoms vary largely from one individual to another.

Discussion with the Staff

Detailed discussions with all technicians and with students should take place before starting the dissection course, with the aim of achieving a more critical, balanced attitude toward the health hazards of formaldehyde in anatomy in relation to formaldehyde concentrations in other environments, e.g. cigarette smoke.

BIBLIOGRAPHY

1. Acheson ED, Barnes HR, Gardner MJ, et al. Formaldehyde in the British chemical industry: An occupational cohort study. Lancet. 1984;1:611-6.
2. Bernstein RS, Styner LT, Elliott LJ, et al. Inhalation exposure to formaldehyde: An overview of its toxicology epidemiology, monitoring and control. Am Ind Hyg Assoc J. 1984;45:778-85.
3. Brunner, P, Warich U. Todesursachen bei Pathologen-Zum moglichen EinfluB des Formaldehyds. Pathologe. 1985; 6:43-5.
4. Burge PS, Harries MG, Lam WK, et al. Occupational asthma due to formaldehyde. Thorax. 1985;40:255-60.
5. Chang JC, Gross EA, Swenberg JA, et al. Nasal cavity deposition, histopathology, and cell proliferation after single or repeated formaldehyde exposures in B6C3Fl mice and F-344 rats. Toxicol Appl Pharmacol. 1983;68:161-76.
6. Clark RP. Formaldehyde in pathology departments. J Clin Pathol. 1983;36:839-46.
7. Connor TH, Ward JB Jr, Legator MS. Absence of mutagenicity in the urine of autopsy service workers exposed to formaldehyde: factors influencing mutagenicity testing of urine. Int Arch Occup Environ Health. 1985;56:225-37.
8. Fisher AA. Contact Dermatitis, 2nd edition. Philadelphia: Lea and Febiger; 1973.
9. Gibson JE. Formaldehyde Toxicity. New York: Hemisphere Publishing Corporation; 1983.
10. Harrington JM, Oakes D. Mortality study of British pathologists 1974-1980. Br J Ind Med. 1984;41:188-91.
11. Harrington JM, Shannon HS. Mortality study of pathologists and medical laboratory technicians. Br Med J. 1975;4: 329-32.
12. Hayes RB, Raatgever JW, de Bruyn A, et al. Cancer of the nasal cavity and paranasal sinuses and formaldehyde exposure. Int J Cancer. 1986;37:487-92.
13. Heck HD, Casanova-Schmitz M, Dodd PB, et al. Formaldehyde (CH_2O) concentrations in the blood of humans and Fischer-314 rats exposed to CH_2O under controlled conditions. Am Ind Hyg Assoc J. 1985;46:1-3.
14. Homson EJ, Shackleton S, Harrington JM. Chromosome aberrations and sister-chromatid exchange frequencies in pathology staff occupationally exposed to formaldehyde. Mutat Res. 1984;141:89-93.
15. Imbus HR. Clinical evaluation of patients with complains related to formaldehyde exposure. J Allergy Clin Immunol. 1985;76:831-40.
16. Jensen OM, Andersen SK. Lung cancer risk from formaldehyde. Lancet. 1982;1:913.
17. Jensen OM. Cancer risk from formaldehyde. Lancet. 1980; 2:480-81.

18. Kerns WD, Pavkov KL, Donofrio DJ, et al. Carcinogenicity of formaldehyde in rats and mice after long-term inhalation exposure. Cancer Res. 1983;43:4382-92.
19. Kilburn KH, Seidman BC, Warshaw R. Neurobehavioral and respiratory symptoms of formaldehyde and xylene exposure in histology technicians. Arch Environ Health. 1985;40:229-33.
20. Levine RJ, Andjelkovich DA, Shaw LK. The mortality of Ontario undertakers and review of formaldehyde-related mortality studies. J Occup Med. 1984;26:740-6.
21. Marsh GM. Proportional mortality patterns among chemical plant workers exposed to formaldehyde. Br J Ind Med. 1982;39:313-22.
22. Morgan KT, Jiang XZ, Starr TB, et al. More precise localization of nasal tumors associated with chronic exposure of F-344 rats to formaldehyde gas. Toxicol Appl Pharmacol. 1986;82:264-71.
23. Morimoto K, Wolff S. Increase of sister chromatid exchanges and perturbations of cell division kinetics in human lymphocytes by benzene metabolites. Cancer Res. 1980;40:1189-93.
24. National Institute for Occupational Safety and Health. NIOSH Criteria Documents: Criteria for a recommended standard: occupational exposure to formaldehyde DHHS (NIOSH) Publication No. 77-126. Washington DC: US Government Printing Office; 1976. pp. 32-59.
25. Norman GR. Science, public policy and media disease. Can Med Assoc J. 1986;134:719-20.
26. Perkins JL, Kimbrough JD. Formaldehyde exposure in a gross anatomy laboratory. J Occup Med. 1985;27:813-15.
27. Rader J. Reizwirkungen von Formaldehyde in Prapariersalen: Analytische und experimentelle Untersuchungen, Doctoral Thesis, Faculty of Medicine. Germany: University of Wurzburg; 1974.
28. Report of the Federal Panel on Formaldehyde. Environ Health Perspect. 1982;43:139-68.
29. Sellakumar AR, Snyder CA, Solomon JJ, et al. Carcinogenicity of formaldehyde and hydrogen chloride in rats. Toxicol Appl Pharmacol. 1985;81:401-406.
30. Skisak CM. Formaldehyde vapor exposures in anatomy laboratories. Am Ind Hyg Assoc J. 1983;44:948-50.
31. Smalky K, Schor E. Environmental hazard: Gross anatomy. N Engl J Med. 1984;310:531-2.
32. Squire RA, Cameron LL. An analysis of potential carcinogenic risk from formaldehyde. Regul Toxicol Pharmacol. 1984;4:107-29.
33. Stoff E, Nitsche I, Mayet A. Formaldehyd gehalt in der Luft der Prapariersale. Zbl Bakt Hyg I Abt Orig B. 1971;155:131-41.
34. Sttoup NE, Balair A, Erikson GE. Brain cancer and other causes of death in anatomists. Natl Cancer Inst. 1986; 17:1217-24.
35. Triebig G, Trautner P, Lutjen-Drecoll E. Untersuchungen zur Abschatzung einer Fonnaldehyde-Einwirkung im Anatomischen Prapariersaal. Arbeitsmed. Sozialmed. Pravtntivmed. 1980;11: 264-66.
36. Triebig G, Valentin H. Gesundheitsrisiken durch formaldehyde. Eine arbeitsmedizinische Bestandsaufnahme. Pathologe. 1985;6:64-70.
37. Walrath J, Fraumeni JF. Mortality patterns among embalmers. Int J Cancer. 1983;31:407-11.
38. Yager JW, Cohn KL, Spear RC, et al. Sister-chromatid exchanges in lymphocytes of anatomy students exposed to formaldehyde-embalming solution. Mutat Res. 1986; 174:135 39.

Chapter 31

Phenoxyethanol as a Nontoxic Substitute for Formaldehyde in Long-term Preservation of Human Anatomical Specimens for Dissection and Demonstration Purposes*

KW Frolich, LM Andersen, Arne Knutsen, Per R Flood

INTRODUCTION

Formaldehyde has recently been declared a potential carcinogen. Occupational health authorities throughout the world are therefore likely to put stricter regulations to its use also within anatomical disciplines.

We have been able to reduce the atmospheric concentration of formaldehyde in our dissection rooms to below the detection limit of a conventional Drager tube multigas analyzer (i.e. below 0.5 ppm or 0.6 mg formaldehyde/m^3 air), by extracting previously formaldehyde-fixed material for more than 3 months in 1% phenoxyethanol in tap water.

In this fluid, our material has remained soft and flexible with a consistency and color retention suitable for dissection and demonstration purposes for up to 10 years. Fungal attacks are rare and we have been unable to raise bacteria from such specimens. Even the microscopic structure of most tissues remains satisfactory after 5 years in 1% phenoxyethanol.

The unpleasant and irritating smell traditionally felt in dissection rooms is almost absent in our facilities, but some of our students still mention slight odor, headache, drowsiness, and mild eye, nose, and throat irritation during their dissection practice periods.

From a theoretical point of view, one should distinguish between initial fixation and long-term preservation of animal tissue for dissection or exhibition purposes. The primary aim of the initial fixation is to arrest the tissue structures in a life-resembling fashion or to largely inactivate autolytic enzymes. The long-term preservation, on the other hand, should primarily prevent microbial overgrowth and tissue maceration.[1]

Today there is no reason, beyond saving of labor, to maintain that the same chemicals are the most satisfactory ones for both purposes. On the contrary, there are overwhelmingly strong reasons to exclude our most widely used fixatives, like formaldehyde and phenol, from long-term preservation fluids.

Both substances have prominent toxic, pungent, and unpleasant properties.[2-6] In addition, the evidence for carcinogenic properties of formaldehyde is rapidly growing.

Formaldehyde has been shown to cause mutation in various primitive organisms[7-10] and in cultured mammalian cells.[11-14]

Furthermore, inhaled formaldehyde caused nasal carcinoma in rats and mice[15,16] and subcutaneously injected formaldehyde caused sarcoma in rats.[17] Recent epidemiological surveys among embalmers and industrial workers exposed to formaldehyde[18,19] may indicate an increased cancer risk even to humans.[20,21]

Occupational health authorities throughout the world, accordingly, are likely to put strict regulations on the use of formaldehyde in the near future. In several countries

---

*KW Frølich, LM Andersen, A Knutsen, et al. The Anatomical Record, volume 208. New York: John Willey and Sons, Inc.; 1984. pp. 271-8.

(including Denmark, Norway, Sweden, and West Germany) a ceiling concentration of 1 ppm formaldehyde in the working environment (equivalent to 1.2 mg formaldehyde/ m³ air) has been practiced for some years. Only Russia has set a lower limit (0.4 ppm), whereas other countries still practice more liberal regulations 2 ppm in the United States.[22] It has, however, been proposed that the ceiling concentration should be set as low as 0.03–0.3 ppm.[23]

Fixing tissues in 4% formaldehyde easily results in atmospheric formaldehyde concentration of 5–7 ppm.[24,25] Accordingly, it is evident that the restrictions mentioned above will force many laboratories throughout the world to change their procedures of tissue preservation drastically.

Some laboratories have already found ways of abandoning the use of formaldehyde and phenol for long-term preservation of specimens for dissection and museum purposes. Most widely used among such methods is the immersion of previously formaldehyde and phenol-fixed specimens in alcohol solutions ranging in concentration up to 75%.[26] This principle has recently been reinvestigated by Bjorkman and Christensen (1982) who found the atmospheric formaldehyde concentration was lowered to below 0.5 ppm when the specimens had been extracted for about 3 months in 20–50%. However, ethanol in high concentrations is expensive, flammable, and evaporates rapidly. In addition, most tissues are subject to excessive hardening and loss of natural colors. In lower concentrations, the antimicrobial action of ethanol may be unsatisfactory.

Neumann (1974) reported good results by the use of Merfentincture (a phenylmercury compound with excellent properties as a disinfectant even in concentrations below 0.5 promille). Whole human limbs previously fixed in a solution containing 40% isopropanol, 3% glycerin, 0.64% formol, and 0.5% Merfen compound kept well for several months without fungal growth or decay in one part "Hydro-Merfen" and nine parts water.

A third alternative was described by Owen and Steedman (1956 and 1958).[27,28] They found various zoological specimens, previously fixed by any desirable method, to be well-preserved for years in a solution of 1% propylene phenoxetol (1-phenoxy-propan-2-ol) alone or in combination with 0.2% "Nipa" esters ("Nipastat" or mixture of alkyl esters of 4-hydroxybenzoic acid). This technique was recommended for general use by Spence (1967) and Steinmann et al. (1975) reported good results on veterinary medical and zoological specimens.[26,29] As far as we know, it has never been reported used on human material.

In our institute, we have used a modification of the technique of Owen and Steedman (1956 and 1958) on all our human dissection material for medical and dental students since 1973. As this technique gives very suitable results and satisfy the strictest regulations regarding formaldehyde concentration in working rooms, we will report on our procedure and experience here.

MATERIALS AND METHODS

Since 1973, a total number of 59 human cadavers have been received by our Institute for use in medical research and education. The corpses belonged to persons of both sexes, and were aged between 45 years and 92 years.

Embalming was started between 8 hours and 48 hours postmortem (18 hours average) by the injection of 12 liters of fixative in the femoral artery. Up to September 1979 (30 corpses), the following fixative was used (concentrations given for final mixture are given in Table 31.1).

Later we have used the "new Basler solution" recommended by Kurz (1976).[30] This consists of formaldehyde, Lysoformin, glycerol, chloral hydrate, sodium chloride, and calcium chloride (final concentrations of these are given in Table 31.2).

After the initial vascular injection fixation, the cadavers were observed for a few days and supplementary injections of the same fixative made locally, wherever the initial injection proved unsatisfactory. The cadavers were then transferred to stainless steel containers filled by 600 liters of 4% formaldehyde in tap water. Two corpses were

Table 31.1: Composition of fixative solutions.

Formaldehyde	2%
Phenol	0.25%
Glycerol	13%
Ethanol	11%
Potassium nitrate	5%

Table 31.2: Composition of Basler solution.

Formaldehyde	2.2%
Lysoformin[15]	4.5%
Glycerol	20%
Chloral hydrate	5%
Sodium chloride	4%
Calcium chloride (anhydrous)	1%

allowed in each container and rested there for a period ranging between 2 months and 4 months.

The cadavers were then transferred to similar containers filled by 600 liters of 1% Phenoxetol in tap water and rested there for a period of at least 3 months. Usually, four corpses were kept in the same tray for about 6 months. The phenoxyethanol was renewed at about 3-month intervals or when the solution was discolored by exudates from the cadavers to a significant degree. Most corpses were thus treated in two successive baths of 1% phenoxyethanol to remove most of the remaining free aldehydes left by the fixative solutions.

The active ingredients of Lysoformin are, according to the manufacturer, 16.8 g formaldehyde solution and 3.8 g glutaraldehyde solution (40%) per 100 g Lysoformin.[15] The concentration of formaldehyde solution is not mentioned, but is probably about 40%. In addition; the Lysoformin solution seems to contain a detergent and perfume.

During the dissection practices, the corpses remained on stainless steel tables for up to 4 week covered with plastic foil and blankets soaked in tap water or 1% phenoxyethanol. Between dissections of distinct body parts the corpses were reimmersed in 1% Phenoxetol. According to the integrated preclinical training curriculum used by us, our medical students complete their dissection practices during five to six courses of 3-4 weeks duration spread out through 1½ year. Dissected specimens kept for demonstration purposes were likewise stored in 1% phenoxyethanol. Dissected specimens for permanent exhibition were mounted in Perspex jars filled with 1% Phenoxetol in tap water.

Samples of tissue treated as mentioned above and left in 1% phenoxyethanol in tap water for more than 5 years were dehydrated by ethanol, embedded in paraffin, sectioned, and stained by hematoxylin and eosin according to standard procedures. Similar samples were postfixed in osmium tetroxide, dehydrated in acetone, embedded in Epon plastic, and examined in the light microscope as 1 μm thick sections stained by toluidine blue, and in the transmission electron microscope as 50 nm thick sections stained by uranyl acetate and lead citrate.

Eleven tissue samples (mucosa and content of colon transversum, pulmonary exudate, urethral swabs, and intercostal muscles) from two cadavers subjected to their first dissection were taken by sterile means and submitted to a microbiological laboratory for cultivation of bacteria and fungi by aerobic and anaerobic techniques.

A Drager-tube multigas analyzer with tubes sensitive to formaldehyde vapors in the concentration range 0.5–5 ppm, supplied by Dragerwerk AG, Lubeck, was used to test the aldehyde concentration at various sites in our dissection rooms. In addition, our local Labor Inspection Authority made three measurements of the formaldehyde concentration in our dissection rooms based on the colorimetric analysis of formaldehyde accumulated in 0.1 M hydrogen sulfite through which a certain amount of air had been forced to bubble.[31] The sensitivity of this method varies according to the volume of air that is analyzed and was between 0.1 ppm and 0.3 ppm for the present samples.

At the end of 4 weeks dissection courses, all participating students (240 in total) were asked to give their opinion about certain aspects of the working environment in the dissection rooms and its influence on their health condition. Questionnaires with specified questions and predetermined reply alternatives, mainly concerning known effects of formaldehyde fumes, were used for this purpose (Table 31.3).

RESULTS

For dissection purposes, we find the preservation in 1% phenoxyethanol is very satisfactory. Much of the rigidity of the tissues caused by the initial aldehyde fixation disappears after some weeks in Phenoxetol and all tissues gain a flexible, partly elastic, consistency not unlike the consistency of fresh unfixed tissue, and well suited for dissection and demonstration purposes.

Although we now use a primary fixative specially designed to maintain or restore life like tissue colors,[1] we are of the opinion that 1% phenoxyethanol enhances these colors rather than disturbing them. These colors are stable for years although we have noted a slight fading in some of our exhibition samples subject to much daylight. The tissue samples processed for routine histology and plastic embedding after more than 5 years in 1% phenoxyethanol revealed a tissue preservation (Figs. 31.1 and 31.2) fully comparable to that of tissue stored in more traditional ways. Even at the ultrastructural level, some cell constituents appeared fairly well-preserved (Figs. 31.3 and 31.4).

We saw no sign of microbial activity in any of our histological sections and bacteria or fungi could not be grown from 11 samples submitted to a bacteriological laboratory. However, in about 1 out of 10 cadavers, we found minor fungal attacks on body parts ranging above

Table 31.3: Students' evaluation of working environment in dissection rooms.

No.	Question During/after the dissection I have noticed/suffered from	Reply alternatives 0^a	1^b	2^c	3^d	4^e	Total number replies	Positive replies as % of total	Average numerical score^f
1.	Unpleasant smell	29^g	43	35	6	—	113	74	1.16
2.	Respiratory distress	107	5	1	—	—	113	5	0.06
3.	Dry or sore nose	98	13	2	—	—	113	13	0.15
4.	Running or congested nose	99	11	2	1	—	113	12	0.16
5.	Dry or sore throat	92	16	3	2	—	113	19	0.25
6.	Unusual thirst	100	9	3	1	—	113	12	0.16
7.	Itching or sore eyes	76	19	12	6	—	113	33	0.54
8.	Red eyes (conjunctivitis)	95	12	2	3	—	112	15	0.22
9.	Excessive lacrimation	99	9	3	1	—	112	12	0.16
10.	Disturbance of sight	107	3	—	2	—	112	4	0.06
11.	Disturbed nocturnal sleep	109	1	2	—	—	112	3	0.04
12.	Unusual tiredness or dizziness	73	23	15	1	—	112	35	0.50
13.	Headache	82	19	9	2	1	113	27	0.42
14.	Nausea	103	4	5	1	—	113	9	0.15
15.	Gastrointestinal disturbances	110	7	4	1	—	113	11	0.17
16.	Itching or sore skin on hands	63	1	1	—	—	65	3	0.05
17.	Skin eruptions on face or neck	60	4	1	—	—	65	8	0.09
18.	How often do you use gloves during the dissection?	Always	Usually	Now and then never	—	—	—	—	—
		88	18	7	—	—	113	22	0.28
19.	What is your average consumption of tobacco?	None	<3	3–10	10–20	>20	—	—	—
	(Number of cigarettes per day)	101	9	—	—	—	110	8	0.08
20.	Do you suffer from any kind of allergy?	Number 82	Yes 19	—	—	—	101	19	—

Note:
- ^{a}Not at all, not recognizable
- ^{b}Faint, barely recognizable
- ^{c}Medium unpleasant
- ^{d}Strong, prominent, and irritating
- ^{e}Intolerable
- ^{f}The average numerical score equals the sum of numerical values given to individual answers divided by the total number of answers
- ^{g}Data represent number of replies given to each reply alternative.

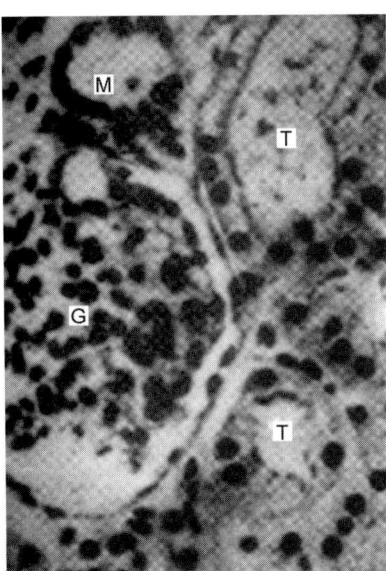

Fig. 31.1: Light micrograft of 10%-thick paraffin section of human kidney stained by hematoxylin and eosin. The tissue, including glomeruli (G) and convoluted tubules (T) seems fairly well-preserved. Magnification, ×500. (M: macula densa).

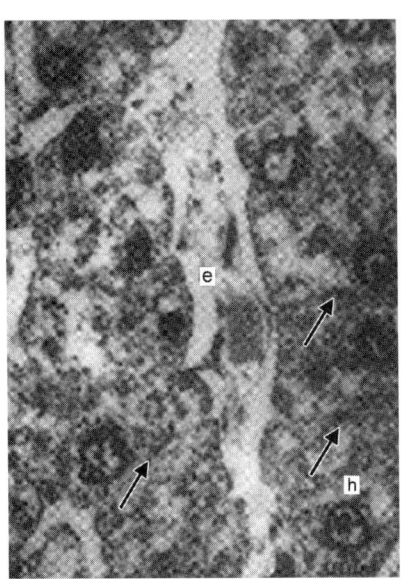

Fig. 31.2: 1 μm thick plastic section of human liver stained by toluidine. Hepatocytes with cytosomes (h), gall capillaries (arrows), and the endothelium of blood sinusoid (e) seem well-preserved.

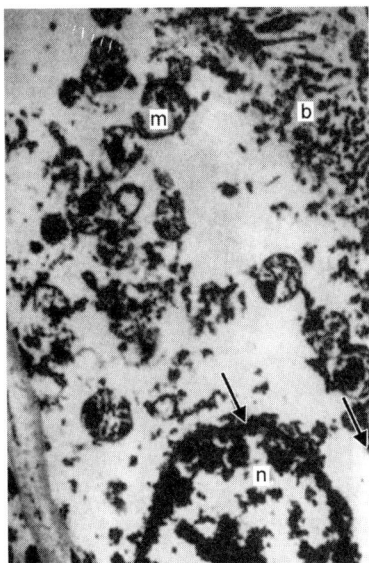

Fig. 31.3: Transmission electron micrograph of ultrathin plastic section of human kidney stained by uranyl and lead. The apical brush border (B), some mitochondria (M), a nucleus (N), and the basement membrane (arrows) are seen fairly well-preserved, magnification, K 7,260.

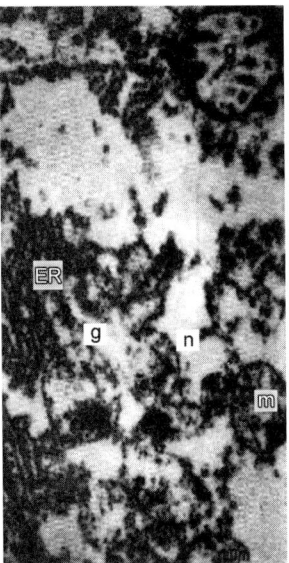

Fig. 31.4: Transmission electron micrograph of ultrathin section of human liver stained by uranyl and lead. The nucleus (n), granulated endoplasmic reticulum (ER), a mitochondrion (m), and gall capillaries (g) are easily identifiable, magnification, K 18,600.

the level of phenoxyethanol solution in our containers, or on cadavers left on the dissection table for several weeks and moistened by towels soaked in tap water only. Such attacks were easily arrested by local application of concentrated Lysoformin solution or reimmersion in 1% phenoxyethanol, and have never been seen on our samples after we moistened towels in 1% phenoxyethanol rather than in tap water.

The unpleasant and irritating formaldehyde and phenol smell traditionally found in dissection rooms is strongly reduced in our premises and we have been unable to detect any formaldehyde vapor by the multigas analyzer at our disposal (detection limit 0.5 ppm) even when the ventilation system was left out of operation for several days. Normally, 20–40 students dissect upon six to eight cadavers in rooms containing 280 m^3 air. A total of 30 measurements were made about 160 cm above floor *level or ca.* 50 cm above the cadavers to be dissected upon, at various times during the daily dissection courses throughout a 2-month period when the room temperature ranged between 17°C and 23°C and the relative humidity between 68% and 80%. When we analyzed the gas accumulated overnight inside the plastic wrapping of a cadaver, a positive reading of 3 ppm formaldehyde was obtained. The three measurements of atmospheric formaldehyde in the dissection room performed by our local Labor Inspection Authority, using a more sensitive method, gave as results 0.15, 0.2, and less than 0.3 ppm.

In spite of these promising measurements, 26 out of 66 (40%) students replied to our first and preliminary questionnaire that they felt barely recognizable to strong eye irritation during the dissection practices. Other specified symptoms like sore skin and rash, sore nose and throat, abnormal thirst, respiratory distress, sleep disturbances, and gastrointestinal symptoms were far less frequently mentioned and were only stated by 2–12% of the students, and as being barely recognizable to medium in strength. On the other hand, 11 out of 66 students (17%) mentioned tiredness and drowsiness as a problem without being confronted with this as a specified question.

In a second questionnaire (circulated to 240 students, with replies received from 113) unusual tiredness and drowsiness was mentioned by 35% of the students, but were mostly classified as being barely recognizable or mild in strength. In this second test questionnaire, unpleasant smell, sore throat, eye irritation, and headache were also mentioned by slightly more students than the remaining symptoms (Table 31.3).

The students were also asked about their use of gloves during the dissection, their smoking habits, and about allergies. It turned out that only 78% of the students used gloves regularly. Less than 10% smoked occasionally or regularly, and about 20% of them suffered from known allergies (Table 31.3).

There seemed to be no correlation between use of gloves and skin problems, between smoking and respiratory symptoms, or between allergies and mucosal irritations.

DISCUSSION

Phenoxyethanol (Phenoxetol, ethylene glycol monophenyl ether, 1-hydroxy-2-phenoxy, ethane, or phenyl cellosolve) is an oily liquid with a density of about 1.1 g/mL and freezing point near 14°C. It has faint aromatic (rose-like) odor and is slightly soluble in water (2.67 g/100 mL).[32] When used in a watery solution, it has fairly good antiseptic properties.[33] It was tried early in local treatment of burns and wounds, especially against *Pseudomonas aeruginosa* or Pyocyanea infections, as it proved to show little skin or tissue irritation on local application as a solution or ointment and low toxicity when injected subcutaneously, intraperitoneally, or intravenously in various laboratory animals.[34] Based on these properties, phenoxyethanol alone or in combination with other bactericides, e.g. quaternary ammonium compounds, has found practical medical use in topical antiseptic solutions and creams. In addition, it is used as a fixative for cosmetics and as insect repellant.[32]

Phenoxyethanol is chemically related to propylene phenoxyethanol, which was used by Owen and Steedman (1956 and 1958) as a preservative for zoological specimens. Both substances have much the same antibacterial activity, whereas propylene phenoxyethanol acts more strongly against molds and yeast (NIPA) information booklet on phenoxetol. Accordingly, propylene phenoxyethanol should in principle be preferred for preservation purposes. However, this substance is more expensive than phenoxyethanol and our experience indicates that phenoxyethanol gives fully satisfactory results. Also, when compared with more conventional preservative techniques[35-40] our method seemed satisfactory from a microbiological point of view.

In fact, from the point of view of preservation, we see no major drawbacks to the use of phenoxyethanol for long-term storage of human corpses for dissection purposes. Our results are thus in good accordance with those reported by Owen and Steedman (1956 and 1958) on zoological samples and by Steinmann et al. (1975) on veterinary and zoological samples. It should, however, be stressed that phenoxyethanol or propylene phenoxyethanol cannot be used for initial fixation purposes. It has no ability to arrest autolysis, and unless other proper fixatives are used, the tissues will decompose rapidly.

From an anatomical point of view, phenoxyethanol gives superior results to those of most other preservatives. The color retention is good[41] and the tissue consistency softer and more flexible than that achieved by ethanol preservation.

The most important advantage of phenoxyethanol preservation still seems to be its low toxicity, as mentioned above. Skin contact, which should be avoided using the phenylmercury compound recommended by Neumann (1974), seems to present no problem with phenoxyethanol. On the contrary, phenoxyethanol is recommended as an antiseptic ingredient in medical creams and ointments.[32]

According to the opinions expressed by our students, the preservative fluid we use causes little skin irritation. This is, however, a prominent and well-known effect of formaldehyde and phenol.[2-5]

The unpleasant or irritating smell and mucosal irritation mentioned by many of our students (questions 3-9, Table 31.3) may partly be due to remnants of formaldehyde still present in our dissection material. The smell was characterized by the students as being sweet or nauseating (8 replies), pungent (3), moldy (2), and as "formalin-smell" (12). Smell and mucosal irritation may be suspected at formaldehyde concentrations as low as 0.15 ppm.[23,42]

Phenoxyethanol fumes are unlikely to cause such irritation, as 2% phenoxyethanol solution applied to the conjunctival sacs of rabbits caused no observable mucosal irritation (Toxicology Report no. 2/70/D 192 of Huntingdon Research Center with permission of NIPA Laboratories, Ltd.)

The slight drowsiness or tiredness reported by 35% of our students probably may be ascribed to the timing of most of our dissection practices between 3 PM and 7 PM, which is certainly not the most ideal time of day. It seems rather unlikely that skin contact or inhalation of trace amounts of phenoxyethanol should cause drowsiness in humans in spite of the fact that this substance, in dilute aqueous solutions, is widely used as an anesthetic or narcotic substance in fish hatcheries.[43,44]

Thus far, our effects to improve the working conditions in the dissection rooms will benefit mainly the students and teachers rather than the technical staff in charge of the embalming procedure itself. The prolonged exposure of the latter group to formaldehyde fumes in the preparation of rooms seems equally important to consider. We believe that a reduced exposure of this group to formaldehyde vapors must be sought via the reduction or replacement of formaldehyde in primary fixative[3] and improved ventilation at critical places within the preparation of rooms.[45,46]

REFERENCES

1. Steinmann W. Uber die Fixierung und Konservierung in Flüssigkeit. Der Praparator (Bochum). 1972;18:3-18.
2. Wirth WG, Hecht CG. Toxikologie-Fibel. Stuttgart; Thieme: 1967.
3. Neumannn MG. Untersuchungen uber die Anwendungsmoglichkeit von "Merfen" also. Konservierungsmittel Anatomischer praparate. Der Praparator (Bochum). 1974; 20:30-5.
4. Putz R, Poisel S, Tiefenbrunner F. Problems with preservation fluids in anatomical preparations 1. Acta Anal. 1974;90:394-402.
5. Schoenberg JB, Mitchell CA. Airway disease caused by phenolic (phenol-formaldehyde) resin exposure. Arch Environ Health. 1975;30:574-7.
6. Plunkett ER, Barbela T. Are embalmers at risk? Am Indust Hyg Assoc J. 1977;38:61-2.
7. Kaplan WO. Formaldehyde as a mutagen in Drosophila. Science. 1948;108:3.
8. Slizynska H. Cytological analysis of formaldehyde-induced chromosomal changes in Drosophila melanogaster. Proc R Soc (Edinb). 1957;66:288-304.
9. Nishioka H. Lethal and mutagenic action of formaldehyde in HCR$^+$ and HCR$^-$ strain in Escherichia coli. Muta Res. 1973;17:261-5.
10. Chanet R, Izard C, Moustacchi E. Genetic effects of formaldehyde in yeast. II. Influence of ploidly and of mutations affecting radiosensitivity on its lethal effect. Mutat Res. 1976;35:29-38.
11. Gosser LB, Butterworth BE. Mutagenicity evaluation of formaldehyde in the L5178Y mouse lymphoma assay. Haskell Laboratory Report. Wilmington, Delaware, United States: EI Du Pont de Nemours and Co.; 1977. pp. 580-81.
12. Obe G, Beek B. Mutagenic activity of aldehyde. Drug Alcohol Depend. 1979;4:91-4.
13. Ross WE, Shipley N. Relation between ONA damage and survival in formaldehyde-treated mouse cells. Mutat Res. 1980;79:277-83.
14. Ragan DL, Boreiko CJ. Initiation of C3H/10TT/2 cell transformation by formaldehyde. Cancer Lett. 1981;13: 325-31.
15. Albert RE, Sellakumar AR, Laskin S, et al. Gaseous formaldehyde and hydrogen chloride induction of nasal cancer in the rat. J Natl Cancer Inst. 1982;68:597-602.
16. Kems WO. Long-term inhalation toxicity and carcinogenicity of formaldehyde in rats and mice. Third CUT Conference on Toxicity. Raleigh, NC: (In Press).
17. Watanabe F, Matsunaga T, Soejima T, et al. Study on aldehyde carcinogenicity I. Experimentally induced rat sarcoma by repeated injections of formalin (in Japanese; summary in English.) Gann. 1954;45:451-2.
18. March GM. Proportional mortality among chemical workers exposed to formaldehyde. Third CUT Conference on Toxicology. Raleigh, NC: (In Press).
19. Walrath J, Fraumeni JF. Proportionate mortality among New York embalmers. Third CIIT Conference on Toxicology. Raleigh, NC: (In Press).
20. Robbins A, Bingham E. Formaldehyde: Evidence of carcinogenicity. US Department of Health US Department of Labor, Joint NIOSH/OSHA Current Intelligence Bulletins No. 34. 1980. p. 15.

21. SFT's og AT's faggruppe for identifisering og klassifisering av kreftfremkallende stoffer. Kriterie dokument for formaldehyd, Oslo. (In Norwegian): 1982.
22. American conference on Government and Industrial Hygiene (ACGIH). Documentation of the threshold limit values for substances in workroom air. Formaldehyde, American Conference on Government and industrial Hygiene. Cincinnati, Ohio: ACGIH; 1980. pp. 197-99.
23. Kane LE, Alerie Y. Sensory irritation to formaldehyde and acrolein during single and repeated exposure in mice. Am Ind Hyg Assoc J. 1977;38:509-22.
24. Stofft E, Nitsche I, Mayet A. Formaldehyde content in the air of dissecting rooms. Zentralbl Bakteriol Orig B. 1971;1(155):131-41.
25. Bjorkman N, Christensen KM. Extraction in dilute ethanol of formaldehyde-fixed dissection specimens. An efficient method to reduce health hazards. Acta Anat. 1982;112:1-8.
26. Spence TF. Teaching and display Techniques in Anatomy and Zoology. Oxford: Pergamon Press; 1967.
27. Owen G, Steedman HF. Preservation of animal tissue, with a note on staining solutions. QJ Microsc Sci. 1956;97: 319-21.
28. Owen G, Steedman HF. Preservation of mollusca. Proc Malac Soc (Land). 1958;33:101-3.
29. Steinmann W, Ebeling R, Goepel U. Die Konservierung medizinischer und biologischer Präparate in Phenoxetol. Der Praparalor (Bochum). 1975;21:8-11.
30. Kurz H. Die Entwicklung moderner Konservierungsmethoden. Der Praparator (Bochum). 1978;24:180-7.
31. Skare I, Dahlner B. Bestamning av aldehyder i luft. (Determination of aldehydes in air.) Arbetaog Halsa, No. 6 Stockholm. (In Swedish); 1973.
32. Stetcher PG. The Merck Index. An Encyclopedia of Chemicals and Drugs, 8th edition. Rahway, NJ: Merck & Co.; 1968.
33. Berry H. Antibacterial values of ethylene glycol monophenyl ether (phenoxetol). Lancet. 1944;247:175-6.
34. Gough J, Berry H, Still BM. Phenoxetol in the treatment of pyocyanea infections. Lancet. 1944;247:176-8.
35. Mrugowsky J. Uber dei Einfluss von Desinfektionsflussigkeiten auf Bakterien in Anatomieleichen. Anat Anz. 1935;80:205-17.
36. Meade GM, Steenken W. Viability of tubercle bacilli in embalmed human lung tissue. Am Rev Tuberc. 1949;59: 429-37.
37. Lyle Aw, Baggenstoss AH. The isolation of pathogens from tissues of embalmed human bodies. Am J Clin Pathol. 1951;21:1114-20.
38. Burke PA, Sheffner AL. The antimicrobial activity of embalming chemicals and topical disinfectants on the microbial flora of human remains. Health Lab Sci. 1976;13:267-70.
39. Lischka MF, Wewalka G, Stanek G, et al. Vergleichsuntersuchungen der Desinfektionswirkung verschiedener Konservierungslosungen fur Anatomieleichen. Anat Anz. 1979; 146:295-306.
40. Wewalka G, Uschka MF, Krammer EB, et al. Microbilogische Uberwachung von konser vierten Studienleichen wahrend des anatomischen Praparierkurses. Anat Anz. 1979;146: 285-94.
41. Gough J, Wentworth JE. The use of thin sections of entire organs in morbid anatomical studied. JR Microsc Soc (Land). 1949;69:231-5.
42. Bourne H, Seferian S. Formaldehyde in wrinkle proof apparel processes-tears for milady. Ind Med Surg. 1959; 28:232-3.
43. Bagenal TB. Propylene Phenoxetol as a fish anesthetic. Nature. 1963;197(4873):1222-3.
44. Sehdev HS, McBride JR. UHM Fagerlund, 2-phenoxyethanol as a general anaesthetic for Sockeye salmon. J Fish Res Bd Canada. 1963;20:1435-40.
45. Tutsch H, Stahl G, Morike KO, et al. Aufbewahrung anatomischer Praparate. Der Praparator (Bochum). 1971;17: 89-95.
46. Wong O. An epidemiologic mortality study of a cohort of chemical workers potentially exposed to formaldehyde with discussion on SMR and PMR. Third CUT Conference on Toxicology. Raleigh, NC (In Press).

Chapter 32

Formaldehyde in Pathology Departments*

RP Clark

INTRODUCTION

Toxic effects of formaldehyde in humans are discussed in relation to occupational exposure and tolerance to this agent. Carcinogenic and mutagenic properties of formaldehyde have been reported in animals and this has led to concern about a possible role in human cancer. The current state of affairs is reviewed in the light of a lack of direct evidence linking formaldehyde with cancer in man and in relation to recommended exposure levels. It is important to employ effective means of containment and practical methods for reducing exposure to formaldehyde in pathology departments and postmortem rooms.

Postmortem changes in cells and tissues can be retarded or even prevented by the use of chemical fixatives. Histological technique is built upon the use of these agents in order that fixed tissue should resemble as accurately as possible the form that it held in life. Early histologists made extensive use of ethyl alcohol but around 100 years ago formaldehyde was established as the "classical" fixative and could now be described as the stock-in-trade of all hospital pathology laboratories.

Formaldehyde (HCHO) is the gas produced by the oxidation of methyl alcohol. It is colorless and flammable with a strong pungent odor and may form an explosive mixture with air and oxygen and is most commonly produced by reacting methanol vapor and air over a catalyst. Produced in this way, it contains trace amounts of methanol and formic acid. Formaldehyde is extremely soluble in water and the aqueous solution containing some 37% formaldehyde is called "formalin". Commercially available formalin is generally a solution containing 37% formaldehyde together with some 10–15% methanol to inhibit polymerization. Without this inhibition, the aqueous phase can slowly polymerize to paraformaldehyde, a form in which it is also available.

Besides being widely used in pathology laboratories, formaldehyde is a basic chemical used in many industrial processes including the manufacture of adhesives, deodorants, dyes, explosives, textiles, laminates, pharmaceuticals, etc. In the building industry, urea formaldehyde is widely used in the manufacture of chipboard and hardboard and in cavity wall insulation.

It is difficult to be accurate about the quantity of formaldehyde produced and used in the United Kingdom (UK) and estimates vary between 60,000 tonnes and 145,000 tonnes per year.[1]

OCCUPATIONAL EXPOSURE TO FORMALDEHYDE

During the last few years, there has been concern about both short- and long-term exposure with conflicting opinions as to the possibility that formaldehyde is carcinogenic. Many groups of people are in some way or other exposed to formaldehyde and the United States (US) Department of Health and Human Services lists some 225 occupations where it might be encountered.[2] In this list are included such unlikely occupations as accountants, health administrators, sailors and deck hands and even writers, artists and entertainers.

It has been estimated that iron foundry workers might be exposed to formaldehyde concentrations between 0.02 ppm and 18.3 ppm whilst dye stuff operatives and people working in plywood industries would be exposed to

---

*Clark RP. Formaldehyde in pathology departments. J Clin Pathol. 1983;36:839-46. (BMJ Publishing Group, London).

between 0.1 ppm and 5.9 ppm, and 1.0 ppm and 2.5 ppm, respectively. By comparison, it was thought that hospital necropsy rooms produced concentrations between 2.2 ppm and 7.9 ppm. The present UK threshold limit value for formaldehyde is 2 ppm[3] whereas, for example, it is 1 ppm in Germany whilst the United States of America has a short-term exposure limit of 1 ppm for 30 min.

TOXICITY TO HUMANS

Absorption and Metabolism

The high solubility of formaldehyde in water means that it is readily absorbed in the upper part of the respiratory tract with relatively small amounts of any inhaled gas penetrating to the lungs. Once absorbed, formaldehyde is metabolized to formic acid both in the liver and blood by the enzyme formaldehyde dehydrogenase. Direct oxidation by red blood cells has also been reported and further oxidation may take place in tissues other than liver or blood. Carbon dioxide and water is finally produced by further oxidation of the formic acid.

Ingestion

There have been reports of death from the ingestion of around 100 mL of formalin in adults (much less in the case of children).[4-6] The symptoms are similar to those produced by a strong acid with severe irritation of all mucosal surfaces of the gastrointestinal tract resulting in ulceration, inflammation and tissue necrosis.

Effects on Eyes and Respiratory Tract

The first signs or symptoms associated with exposure to formaldehyde occur in the eyes at concentrations of 0.1–5 ppm with a burning sensation and the production of tears. It is suggested that the threshold for the eyes to respond to formaldehyde is as low as 0.01 ppm. Accidental splashes of aqueous solution of formaldehyde cause severe irritation to the eyes and have, on occasions, resulted in permanent damage even when the eyes were immediately washed with water.[7-9] 4% formaldehyde solution splashed in the eye has been reported to produce a strong irritant effect with visual disturbance persisting for one day after which time the eye returned to normal.

At concentrations around 0.5 ppm, mild throat irritation and tingling sensation occurs. It is generally regarded that formaldehyde in a concentration of some 5 ppm is intolerable in a room and at concentrations approaching 10 ppm (a danger level) a choking sensation occurs. Exposure to 50 ppm (even of short duration) can be expected to cause serious injury.[10,11]

Effects on Skin

Dilute aqueous solutions of formaldehyde and the vapor itself are irritant to the skin. Many cases of dermatitis have been reported amongst persons exposed to formaldehyde in the course of their work. In normal human volunteers, it has been shown that solutions containing less than 2% formaldehyde are unlikely to produce irritant effects. In addition to the reports of allergic contact dermatitis, skin sensitization has also been noted from experimental studies with volunteers.[12]

There are reports of asthma-like symptoms in workers exposed to formaldehyde.[13] In particular, respiratory symptoms have been reported in nurses in hemodialysis units where formalin was used to sterilize the dialysis equipment. In 1982, a follow-up study of two nurses who were shown to develop occupational formaldehyde asthma in 1977 showed that one nurse, who had ceased to be exposed after 1976, had lost all symptoms. She had also lost her asthmatic sensitivity to formaldehyde and lung function studies were almost normal. The second nurse in this study, however, had continued to be exposed to formaldehyde (although at a reduced level) and persistent asthmatic responsiveness could be demonstrated in 1981. In this case, there was no evidence of any progressive chronic airway obstruction.

In spite of the widespread use of formaldehyde, there have only been a few reported cases of respiratory illness due to allergic sensitization.

TOLERANCE TO FORMALDEHYDE

There is some evidence of acclimatization or tolerance to the irritant effects particularly in the action of tear production. This evidence comes from experiments with healthy volunteers exposed to 13.8 ppm for 30 min.[14] There was initially considerable irritation to the eyes and nose but the effects rapidly wore off with no signs of eye irritation being observed after 10 min.

Formaldehyde and Cancer

A known carcinogen, bischloromethylether (BCME) is produced when formaldehyde reacts with hydrogen chloride.[15-18] The reaction of hydrochloric acid with formaldehyde in situations where the two agents are stored together permits the possibility of forming this potential carcinogen. However, the concentrations of both agents would need to be considerably in excess of their respective threshold limit values and in such an atmosphere work would become impossible. The separate storage of these substances and the maintenance of their levels below the threshold limit values are regarded as providing adequate safeguards against carcinogenic risk due to the formation of BCME.[19]

Mutagenicity, or the ability of an agent to cause a change in the genetic material within a cell, is associated with most chemicals known to cause cancer. Tests for mutagenicity can therefore help in determining carcinogenic potential. In this regard, formaldehyde has been known to be mutagenic for some time from laboratory experiments with fruit flies (Drosophila) grasshoppers, flowering plants, fungi and bacteria.[20-22]

There is a recent report that formaldehyde at a level of 4 ppm was found to be mutagenic in diploid human lymphoblasts in culture.[23] In another study, no chromosome abnormalities were found in a group of 15 workers exposed to formaldehyde over a long period (average 28 year).[24]

In March 1979, workers at the University of Birmingham published a report on the possible carcinogenic hazards of formaldehyde.[25] In reviewing human data, they concluded that the Registrar General's occupational mortality tables for 1961-1970 did not show any increased incidence of cancer in two groups of workers, namely chemists, physical and biological scientists. In the study of the causes of death of 131 pathologists, death from some cancers (especially respiratory cancers) were less than expected but there were significantly more deaths from lymphoid tumors (8 were found when 3.3 were expected). There authors concluded that the possibility that this was associated with exposure to formalin should perhaps not be excluded.

They also concluded that "it seems to us that carcinogenicity tests carried out so far would probably have shown if formaldehyde itself had a high degree of carcinogenic activity. It is, however, possible that more thorough tests now being carried out may show up a relatively weak carcinogenic action."

In October 1979, preliminary results from studies in animals showed that when rats were exposed to 15 ppm for 6 hour/day/week for 16 months, three developed squamous cell carcinoma originating in the epithelium of the nasal turbinates.[26] Further, results from this study in 1980 showed that after 24 months of exposure to 15 ppm of formaldehyde, some 93 rats developed squamous cell carcinomas of the nasal turbinates. Two developed respiratory epithelial carcinomas and two rats exposed to 6 ppm and two mice exposed to 15 ppm had also developed squamous cell carcinomas of the nasal turbinates.[27]

In April 1981, the United States National Institute of Occupational Safety and Health (NIOSH), in consideration of these carcinogenic features of formaldehyde, recommended that formaldehyde be handled in the workplace as a potential occupational carcinogen.[2] Since that time, there have been a number of investigations seeking to clarify any relation between occupational exposure to formaldehyde and the incidence of cancer in humans. Concurrently, there have been call to limit the general exposure of workers to this agent and to seek ways of producing containment whereby environmental contamination by formaldehyde is kept at a very low level.

At the time, that US NIOSH issued its recommendations concerning the potential carcinogenicity of formaldehyde, there had been no hard evidence of specific cases of human cancer due to the agent. The prime reason for the recommendation seems embodied in the statement that "although humans and animals may differ in their susceptibility to specific chemical compounds, any substance that produces cancer in experimental animals should be considered a cancer risk to humans." In 1981, the Health and Safety Executive in the UK issued a Toxicity Review about formaldehyde and stated "there is at present no evidence that exposure of formaldehyde has produced cancer in humans". A number of epidemiological studies are in progress to investigate this aspect.

One of the immediate results of the US recommendation was that the American Consumer Product Safety Commission decided to ban the use of urea formaldehyde foam used for insulation in the building industry. This was because of "unreasonable risks to consumers from the irritation, sensitization and possible carcinogenic effects of formaldehyde emitted by this substance". The Commission concluded that at that time no standards, voluntary or mandatory, to reduce the risk, were feasible.

In recent publication, the British Plastics Federation, sought to defend the use of urea formaldehyde foam and to criticize the American Consumer Product Safety Commission for recommending a ban on the substance.[28] In regard to the release of formaldehyde in dwellings it asserts, "there remains no evidence to suggest that formaldehyde can cause anything more than short-term irritation to humans to the levels liable to be experienced in properly insulated dwellings." Further concern for the industrial use of formaldehyde is expressed in a publication from the Chemical Industries Association which says "the acute (short-term) effects of excessive exposure to formaldehyde are mainly transitory and reversible."[29] The long-term effects are summarized as chronic skin disorders and chronic respiratory tract conditions but with very few examples cited in the scientific literature.

Recently, Sir George Young, Under Secretary of State for Environment, in a written answer in Parliament concerning the carcinogenicity of chemicals in food consumer products and the environment, said that an Advisory Committee was looking at research on the effects of formaldehyde and that "in its view there is no evidence that formaldehyde gas causes cancer in man."

From the available literature, there would, therefore, appear to be no evidence to suggest that the concentrations of formaldehyde agent are effectively self-limiting because of the extremely unpleasant effects at relatively low concentrations with the consequent behavioral response of avoidance.

Nevertheless, there do exist problems of formaldehyde toxicity related to asthma, dermatitis, sensitization and irritation where guidelines for exposure reduction are appropriate.

By 1982, it was thought that there might be some pressure from the Health and Safety Executive (HSE) to impose restrictions on the use of formaldehyde but there was some disagreement between this agency and the Health and Safety Commission (the governing body of the HSE) who were less satisfied that such constraints were justified. A number of agencies and organizations were already preparing guidelines and policies in anticipation of new regulation which might result but which in the event did not materialize.

PRACTICAL CONTAINMENT MEASURES

In 1980, the Medical Research Council had indicated that work with formaldehyde should be carried out with the following reasonable precautions:
- Solutions should be made up in a fume cupboard.
- Vessels should be covered as much as possible.
- Work should only be done in well-ventilated rooms.
- Time of exposure should be kept to a minimum.

The reduction exposure should be kept to a minimum. The reduction of operator exposure to splashes and gross contamination by formaldehyde is a matter of laboratory technique together with the use of gloves and eye protection where appropriate. However, the formaldehyde vapor concentration in the air may need to be controlled and this can be achieved in a number of ways.

Room Ventilation

The laboratory may be ventilated in order that any formaldehyde gas released into the atmosphere is purged and the concentration maintained below the threshold limit value. Care must be taken not to produce excessive air change rates; for example, in laboratories some 7 m × 5 m, the minimum air removal rate for comfort conditions would be of the order of 0.2 m^3/s. Greater extract would also increase revenue costs as far as heating of input air is concerned.

Fume Cupboards

To complement the effects of overall ventilation systems, more local extraction of formaldehyde vapor is often appropriate and here there are a number of alternatives. The most obvious is to make use of the laboratory fume cupboard, particularly when handling large volumes of formaldehyde.

In correctly designed cupboards, the vapor will be carried away and diluted before discharge to the atmosphere at high level. In older buildings where multiple fume cupboards may be on one air system, the fume cupboard and its duct work should be proved to be effective and should on no account allow leakage of formaldehyde gas back into other laboratories.

Recently, there has been considerable interest in the use of relatively inexpensive portable fume cupboards which do not require major installation work. These devices incorporate absorption filters to remove gases and vapors from the air before returning it to the laboratory.

Such cupboards initially appear very attractive in terms of capital cost, installation and operating expenses. There are, however, a number of significant problems which should be reviewed in the light of a potential use as far as formaldehyde absorption in the pathology laboratory is concerned.

If a recirculating fume cupboard is to be safe and effective at removing formaldehyde and maintaining the concentration below the correct threshold limit value, it must:
- Achieve adequate containment of fume at the front by an inflow air velocity of at least 0.5 m/s (and not greater than 1.0 m/s).

- In order that the harmful agent is effectively removed by the filter, the contact time with the filter medium must be sufficient for adequate absorption to take place. In addition, because these filters have a finite absorption capacity, there must be some reliable indication of filter saturation. In the case of formaldehyde, it has been suggested that the sense of smell by those within the laboratory would be adequate to determine the end-point of filter life.

The charcoal filters have a wide range of absorption characteristics for different chemical agents. Their effectiveness for particular compound is generally expressed as the proportion of the dean filter weight that can be absorbed. The absorption can be as high as 15–20% for some agents but in the case of formaldehyde, it is very much lower at only around 1–2%. One consequence of this is that for a filter to be effective over a reasonable period of time, it must be fairly large and one manufacturer suggests that filter weight for a practically useful life is some 36 kg.

The use of recirculating fume cupboards is generally regarded as unsatisfactory and only in exceptional and rather specific circumstances where the fume has a nuisance value rather than being toxic could the use of these cupboards be considered.[30]

Postmortem Room

Airborne contaminants can pose problems in the postmortem room. The minimization of the release of potentially pathogenic droplets or tissue aerosols together with the reduction of exposure to formaldehyde at the cut-up bench requires special measures. There is some debate as to the extent of the problem and whether effective precautions can be devised whereby the overall "air quality" in these areas can be guaranteed, and if so do the chances of acquiring infection, particularly tuberculosis, become smaller.

New designs of ventilated necropsy tables in conjunction with overhead canopies producing downflowing air curtains can contain aerosols liberated during the postmortem procedures. Exhaust air from these systems are filtered in order to remove particulates before the air is discharged to outside. Such systems can also purge the postmortem room of noxious vapors including formaldehyde. As gases will not be arrested by filtration, the exhaust should be treated in much the same way as for a fume cupboard. Figures 32.1A and B show a novel ventilated necropsy table using exhaust ports which are adjustable in height and length appropriate to the work area.

Cut-up Benches

Cut-up benches adjacent to the necropsy table require local air extraction of formaldehyde and Figure 32.2 shows such a system incorporated into a postmortem room where there is also a ventilated necropsy table and overhead air curtain.

Besides being suitable for postmortem rooms, the ventilated cut-up bench is also important in preventing a build-up of formaldehyde in the pathology laboratory. Care should be taken that the design is effective for gathering formaldehyde from a reasonably large working volume on the bench and partial enclosures to entrain the contaminated air are generally required as shown in Figure 32.3.

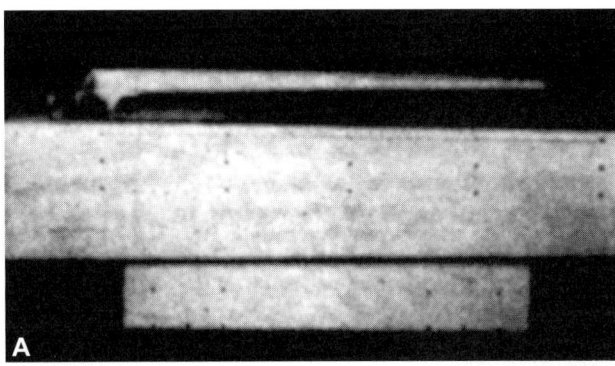
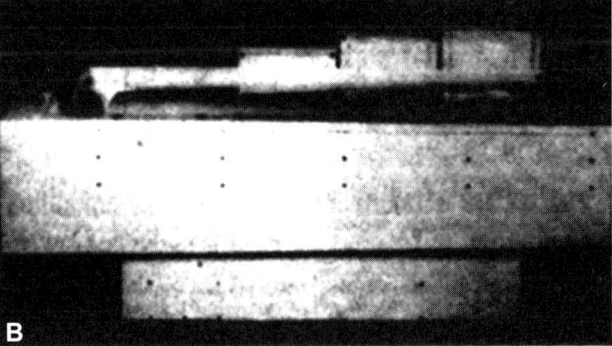

Figs. 32.1A and B: A novel ventilated necropsy table with air exhausted from over the surface of the body by means of adjustable exhaust ports which may be positioned at a height and length appropriate to the work area concerned.
Source: Howorth Air Engineering Ltd.

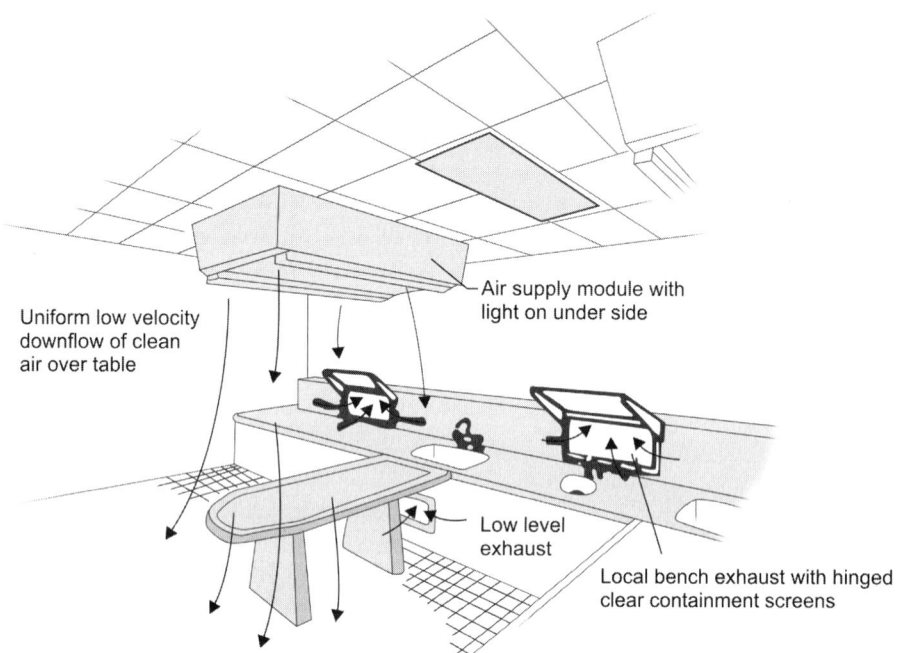

Fig. 32.2: Postmortem room layout incorporating a clean air zone over the table and local exhaust at the cut-up bench.
Source: Medical Air Technology Ltd.

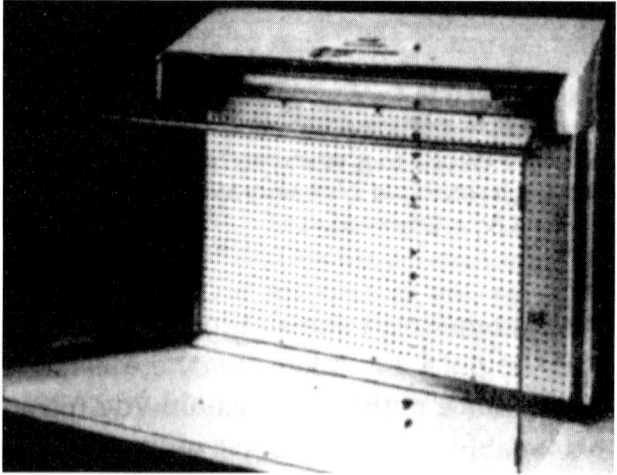

Fig. 32.3: An example of a local fume extraction unit suitable for bench extraction of formaldehyde in the postmortem room or pathology laboratory.
Source: Howorth Air Engineering Ltd.

Fumigation

The widespread use of microbiological safety cabinets and the requirement for routine servicing means that the laboratory staff are frequently called upon to effectively decontaminate these cabinets before maintenance engineers start work. Many contractors now require certification of decontamination procedures and the Health and Safety at Work Act requires that appropriate safety measures are carried out.

The normal method of decontaminating safety cabinets and their filters is by fumigation with formaldehyde gas. It is now also fairly common for complete laboratories to require fumigation, from time to time. This requirement may be extended to postmortem rooms' necropsy tables and air handling systems that are being proposed for new installations. There are several methods of fumigating safety cabinets and rooms with formaldehyde. In the case of a safety cabinet, the front closure should be in place and the exhaust duct blocked off. 25 mL of formalin can be vaporized by being placed in a dish in an electric heater. Alternatively, 25 mL of formalin can be placed in a 500 mL beaker and 10 g of potassium permanganate added. The mixture will react vigorously producing formaldehyde gas. If too much potassium permanganate is used, there is risk of explosion. Once the formaldehyde is produced in the cabinet, it should be introduced into the filter by running the cabinet fan for a few seconds. After this, it should be left overnight. At the end of the fumigation period, cabinet should be run normally to purge the formaldehyde gas. It should be noted that fumigation is only fully effective as long as adequate water vapor is present. Liberation of formaldehyde gas, for example, by subjecting paraformaldehyde to dry hot air is not satisfactory.

When cabinets are not ducted to the outside fumigation produces considerable problems if formaldehyde is not released into the laboratory. These may overcome by, for example, incorporating a damper into the safety cabinet exhaust and using a flexible tube attached to the exhaust duct to take the formaldehyde to a window or fume cupboard at the end of the fumigation period. Most of these decontamination procedures involve larger volumes of formaldehyde than are encountered in general laboratory work and staff should therefore be fully instructed in the appropriate techniques and safety precautions.

When installing new safety cabinets, the provision of external ducting should be reviewed in the light of decontamination procedures which may be required at reasonably frequent intervals and should produce minimum exposure of staff to formaldehyde.

The author is grateful to C Gilchrist of the Safety Section of the Medical Research Council for help in researching much of the literature.

REFERENCES

1. ASTMS. Health and Safety Monitor No. 2. London: The Association of Scientific, Technical & Managerial Staffs; 2014.
2. NIOSH (National Institute for Occupational Safety and Health, US Department of Health and Human Services), Current Intelligence Bulletin 34, Formaldehyde: evidence of carcinogenicity. Washington, DC: NIOSH; 1981.
3. HSE (Health & Safety Executive) Guidance Note EH 15/80. Threshold Limit Values. London: HMSO; 1980.
4. Levison LA. A case of fatal formaldehyde poisoning. JAMA. 1904;42:1492.
5. Rathery F, Piedelieure R, Delarue J. Death by absorption of formalin. Ann Med Leg Criminol Police Sci Toxicol. 1940;20:201-9.
6. Ely F. Formaldehyde poisoning. JAMA. 1910;54:1140-1.
7. Grant WM. Toxicology of the Eye, 2nd edition. Springfield, Illinois: Charles C Thomas; 1974.
8. Kelecom J. Corrosive eye damage with formalin. Arch Ophthalmol. 1962;22:259-62.
9. Sagar DS. The effect of formaldehyde on the cornea. Ophthalmoscope. 1906;4:63-4.
10. Patterson RM. Assessment of formaldehyde as a potential air pollution problem. GCA Report No. TR-75-32G(8). Bedford, Indiana: GCA Corporation; 1975.
11. Fassett DW. Aldehydes and acetals. In: Patty FA, Clayton GD, Clayton FE (Eds). Industrial Hygiene and Toxicology, 2nd edition. New York: Interscience; 1970-2, 1963.
12. Epstein E, Maibach HI. Formaldehyde allergy. Arch Dermatol. 1966;94:186-90.
13. Hendrick DJ, Rando RJ, Lane DJ, et al. Formaldehyde asthma: challenge exposure levels and fate after five years. J Occup Med. 1982;11:893-97.
14. Sim VM, Pattie RE. Effect of possible smog irritants on human subjects. JAMA. 1957;165:1908-13.
15. Kallos GJ, Solomon RA. Investigations of the formation of bis(chloromethyl) ether in simulated hydrogen chloride formaldehyde atmospheric environments. Am Ind Hyg Assoc J. 1973;34:469-73.
16. Van Duuran BL, Katz C, Goldschncidt BM, et al. Carcinogenicity of halo ethers. J Natl Cancer Inst. 1972;48:1431-39.
17. Franket LS, McCallum KS, Collier L. Formation of bis (chloromethyl) ether from formaldehyde and hydrogen chloride. Environ Sci Technol. 1974;8:356-59.
18. Albert RE, Pasternak BS, Shore RE, et al. Mortality patterns among workers exposed to chloromethyl ethers. Environ Health Perspect. 1975;11:209-14.
19. MRC (Medical Research Council). Health Hazard Note NO. 8. MRC; 1978.
20. Fishbein L. Environmental sources of chemical mutagens. In: Flamm WG, Mehlman MA (Eds). Advances in Modern Toxicology. Washington, DC: Hemisphere; 1978. pp. 257-348.
21. Auerbach C. Mutation Research-Problems, Results and Perspective. London: Chapman and Hall; 1976.
22. Auerbach C, Moutschen-Dahmen M, Moutschen J. Genetic and cytogenetical effects of formaldehyde and related compounds. Mutat Res. 1977;39(3-4):317-61.
23. Goldmacher VS. Mutagenic effects of formaldehyde in bacterial and human cells. Proceedings of "Formaldehyde Toxicology 1982 Update". Washington; 1982.
24. Fleig I, Petri N, Stocker WG, et al. Cytogenic analysis of blood lymphocytes of workers exposed to formaldehyde in formaldehyde manufacturing and processing. J Occup Med. 1982;24:1009-12.
25. Searle CE, Teale OJ. Possible carcinogenic hazards of formaldehyde. Department of Cancer studies, The University of Birmingham. Birmingham, United Kingdom; University of Birmingham; 1979.
26. Chemical Industry Institute of Toxicology: Statement concerning research findings, docket number 11109. North Carolina: CIIT; 1979.
27. Kerns WD. Long-term inhalation toxicity and carcinogenicity studies of formaldehyde in rats and mice. Presented at the 3rd CIIT Conference on Toxicology, Raleigh, North Carolina: CIIT; 1980.
28. BPF News. Separating the facts from the confusion. Newspaper of the British Plastics Federation (November/December); 1982.
29. Formaldehyde exposure in industry. London: Chemical Industries Association; 1982.
30. Medical Research Council Health Hazard Note NO. 47. "Recirculating" fume cupboards. London: MRC; 1982.

Chapter 33

Danger of Infection*

Leandro Rendon

INTRODUCTION

The possibility of acquiring disease as the result of handling and caring for human remains is very real and is of concern to funeral licensees. Unfortunately, there are those who do not seem to be aware of the potential risks involved or who do not seem to believe such danger exists or that it is even possible. Such individuals, in and out of funeral service, seem to minimize the existence of disease-producing organisms in dead human remains.

At the Continuing Education Program sponsored April 18, 1980, by the faculty of San Antonio College, San Antonio, Texas, Dr Kendall O Smith, Professor of Microbiology, University of Texas Health Science Center at San Antonio, was one of the participants. He presented information about some of the biological hazards that should be of conern to the funeral licensee. The following discussion is based on some of the information presented by Dr Smith. It is hoped that this discussion serves to further stress the potential dangers of infection that the licensee does encounter in his or her work and the need, therefore, to follow prescribed hygienic practices and certain procedures of disinfection and decontamination to protect himself or herself against infection.

The most often reported infections associated with handling of human remains are tuberculosis and infectious hepatitis. In the survey among funeral licensees made by this department some time ago, of those who sustained one or more infections, about 14% said they had contracted tuberculosis and 12.7% infectious hepatitis. The medical literature makes reference to similar and other incidence of infection.[1]

Causes of death in cancer patients for the year 1970 were studied in New York[2] at a hospital on the basis of clinical and pathology reports of 506 cases. The single major cause of death was infection (36%), which also was contributory factor in an additional 68% of the cases. The organisms causing the infection were mostly Gram-negative and antibiotic-resistant bacteria. Other important causes of death were hemorrhagic and thromboembolic phenomena (18%), which also were contributory factors in an additional 43%.

In a study performed by personnel of the MD Anderson Hospital and Tumor Institute, Houston, Texas,[3] the causes of death in patients with malignant lymphoma were reviewed. The records of some 206 patients over an 8-year period were used for the report.

The most common cause of death in those patients was infection, which accounted for 51% of the deaths. These infections were primarily caused by Gram-negative bacilli.

Toxoplasmosis is a disease caused by infection with the protozoan, *Toxoplasma*. In infants and children, the disease usually is characterized by an encephalomyelitis. In adults, a form clinically resembling a spotted fever has been reported.

Five patients with lethal-disseminated toxoplasmosis were seen within a 2-year period at the Swedish Hospital Medical Center and the University of Washington Hospital.[4] In all patients, there was a severe underlying disease treated with various chemotherapeutic agents, corticosteroids, splenectomy, or irradiation. Although the clinical symptoms were variable and masked by the underlying illness, therapeutic measures, or concomitant infectious processes, or both, the autopsy findings were

---

*Printed from the Expanding Encyclopedia No. 508. Springfield, Ohio: Champion Chemical Company; 1980.

strikingly uniform in that the brain, myocardium, and lungs were invariably affected. Reports in the literature and the experience of the investigators indicate that disseminated toxoplasmosis in compromised hosts is being recognized with increasing frequency.

One episode has been reported[5] in which toxoplasmosis was transmitted during postmortem examination. The occurrence of lymphadenitis in human toxoplasmosis is well recorded. However, the mode of transmission and time course of the disease remains far from clear.

Most of the knoweldge of acquired toxoplasmosis is based on infections in labortory workers and on occasional cases of accidental inoculation. A case is recorded when a pathologist became acutly ill with toxoplasmosis 2 months after the autopsy of a patient who died with Hodgkin's disease and toxoplasmic ventriculitis.

Personnel from the National Institute of Neurological Diseases and Stoke, National Institutes of Health, call attention to another type of potential infection.[6] Precautions are mentioned in conducting biopsies and patients with presenile dementia.

The report mentions that such patients may have Creutzfeldt–Jakob disease, a transmissable disease by a virus likely to be extremely resistant to inactivation. It is recommended:

- That instruments used in any surgical or autopsy procedures on patients with presenile dementia be autoclaved for at least 30 minutes
- That all organs, including those fixed in formalin, be treated as infectious materials
- That floor and other surfaces in contact with tissues from such patients be decontaminated with a solution known to inactivate the scrapie agent, for instance 0.5% NaOCl solution. The fact that the agent is susceptible to sodium hypochlorite but not to the well-known disinfectants tells us something about the newly emerging pathogens that seemingly are highly resistant to the commonly used chemical sterilants!

The literature references many instances of cross-infections among patients in hospitals. The May, 1980 issue (507) of this Encyclopedia alludes to infections of this type among hospitalized populations. A typical situation found in the literature is the following case. Serological evidence of cross-infection in a dialysis unit, hepatitis-B epidemic has been reported.[7]

It is of interest to call this report to the attention of the reader because it points to the ease with which personnel can acquire infections. If this can happen in a hospital, consider the possibility of such occurence in the preparation room while handling the remains of individuals who have been in a dialysis unit.

There were 74 patients and staff who developed HBAg-positive hepatitis during a 28-month surveillance period. 26 of these cases were intimately related to the dialysis unit (21 dialysis/transplant patients and five hospital staff) and 48 were not. Representative sera from each group of cases were further tested for HBAg subtype specificity. 13 of 14 dialysis/transplant patients and subtype ay, whereas 10 of 15 general hospital patients had the alternate phenotype ad.

All four staff invididuals who had probably acquired their infection from dialysis/transplant patients were ay subtype. Eight of the dialysis/transplant patients had never received blood. Transfusion rate in the infected dialysis patients was one-third that of leukemic patients but the hepatitis rate was higher.

The bacteriological procedures are mentioned in detail simply to illustrate the thoroughness of establishing proof of cross-contamination. There is little doubt as to the source of the infection.

An interesting incident is found in the literature[8] that should be of pertinent interest to funeral licenses-tubercular infection.

Inoculation tuberculosis of the skin, occurring in physicians and medical students engaged in performing postmortem examinations, has been referred to by a variety of names among which "prosector's wart" appears to be a particularly appropriate term. A medical student-prosector developed typical primary cutaneous tuberclosis of the hand despite having practiced most currently accepted precautionary methods in performing an autopsy on a patient who had harbored active tuberculosis. The nature of the infection was established by culture as well as by demonstration of acid-fast bacilli in the surgically excised lesion of the hand.

In a study to establish the incidence of tuberculosis among workers in medical laboratories, an investigator[9] at the London School of Hygiene and Tropical Medicine made a survey among personnel of the National Health Service and the Public Health Laboratory Service. There was a larger number of incidence of infection among individuals employed in laboratory and mortuary tasks, which exposed them to the risk of contact with infected pathological material. The incidence was highest in the 2nd and 3rd years of such employment.

Tuberculosis as an occupational disease among workers in pathology institutes is the subject of a report from West Germany.[10] Incidence of tuberculosis among pathologists was found to be 20-fold greater in one study, and 35-fold greater in another than in general population.

Investigators in Europe[11] have shown that *Streptococci* and *Staphylococci* multiply 10–100 times and even more in the blood and tissues of corpses kept at room temperatures. Additional investigations have also shown that there is an increase not only of the number of septicemic agents (*Pasteurella*, the erysipeloid, and bacterium pyocyaneum), but also in their virulence. The virulence of the strains isolated from dead remains held at room temperature rises immediately after death and reaches maximum at the 5th–7th hours for the *Streptococci* after which it may gradually decrease.

The newly emerging pathogens that are frequently arriving on the scene seem to be "unconventional" types. They are difficult to isolate in some cases and present problems in classification. Some seem to be able to change their structure, i.e. mutate, and thereby become resistant to commonly used drugs.

Often infections are acquired and the host is unaware of the infection. The organisms may not indicate their presence for day, weeks, months, and even years. As can be seem from the very brief overview of the literature, there is ample scientific evidence for the need to practice effective measures in the preparation room to reduce as much as possible, the risk factors of such environment.

REFERENCES

1. Proc R Soc Med. 1973;66:25.
2. Ambrus JL, Ambrus CM, Mink IB, et al. Causes of death in cancer patients. J Med. 1975;6:61-4.
3. Feld R, Bodey GP, Rodriguez V, et al. Causes of death in patients with malignant lymphoma. Am J Med Sci. 1974;268(2):97-106.
4. Gleason TH, Hamlin WB. Disseminated toxoplasmosis in the compromised host. A report of five cases. Arch Intern Med. 1974;134:1059-62.
5. Neu HC. Toxoplasmosis transmitted at autopsy. JAMA. 1967;202:284-5.
6. Traub RD, Gadjusek DC, Gibbs CJ. Precautions in conducting biopsies and autopsies on patients with presenile dementia. Technical note. J Neurosurg. 1974;41(2): 394-5.
7. Hamilton JD, Hatch MH, Gutman RA. Serological evidence of cross infection in a dialysis unit hepatitis-B epidemic. Kidney Int. 1974;6(2):118-21.
8. Minkowitz S, Brandt LJ, Rapp Y, et al. "Prosector's wart" (cutaneous tuberculosis) in a medical student. Am J Clin Pathol. 1969;51(2):260-3.
9. Reid DD. Incidence of tuberculosis among workers in medical laboratories. Br Med J. 1957;2(5035):10-4.
10. Purrmann W. Tuberculosis as an Occupational Disease in Workers of Pathological Institutes. Deutsche Gesundheit. 1964;19:2389-90.
11. Dold Bolg Akad Nauk. 1965;18:179-81.

Index

Note: Page numbers followed by *t* indicate tables; numbers followed by *f* indicate figures

A

Abdomen, nine regions of 102*f*, 102*t*
Abdominal
    aorta 77, 112
        aorta bifurcates 71
    cavity 119
        aspiration of 103
        removal of 109
    regions to locate to internal organs 101
    wall 13
        branches, lateral 70
        tributaries from 71
Absinthi 13
Accavederata 13
Acid glutaraldehyde 43
Acids 21
    use of solutions of 17
Acquired immunodeficiency syndrome 41, 128, 131, 165
Actin 56
Adenodiphosphate 56
Adipocere 58
    formation of 54, 58
Aerosols, form of 40*f*
Agonal
    algor 54
    fever 54
    period 54
Air
    handling in preparation room 42
    pressure machine 95
Albert H Worsham 31
Algor mortis 54, 114
Alkali salts 17
Alkalies 21
Alkaline 55
Alkalinized (cidex) glutaraldehyde 43
Aloes 8, 13
Alum 18
Alumina
    acetate of 18
    salts of 21
Ambroise Pare (1510-1590) 13
Aminoglycosides 125
Ammonia 121
Ammonium
    chloride 27
    nitrate 138
Amphetamines 124, 125
Amytal 124
Anatomical considerations 63
Anatomical dissection 13
Anatomical specimens, collection of 14
Anatomists, period of (AD 650-1861) 11
Anatomy departments 182
Ancient
    ethiopians 8
    persians 8
    restorative art 6
Anethi 13
Animals experimental 181
Antibiotic chemotherapy, combination of 122
Anticoagulants 83
    sodium citrate 83
Antihypertensives anticlotting agents 125
Anti-inflammatory drugs 123
Antimicrobial procedures 50*t*
Aorta 67, 70
    arch of 68, 75
    ascending 68, 75, 112
    descending 68
Appendix 102
Aqueous 49
    formalin 51
Army order for embalmers 25
Arsenic 27
Arsenicals 21
Arterial fluid for
    obese subjects, composition of 85*t*
    preparation of 110
    thin subjects, composition of 85
Arterial injection 2, 119
    and cavity treatment 2
    chemicals, rate of flow of 44
    of the blood vessels 33
Arterial route 110
Arteries and veins of upper limb 66*f*
Arteries of
    abdomen 70
    body 75
    head and neck 64, 64*f*
    lower limb 71
    neck 64
        common carotid artery 64
        external carotid artery 64
        internal carotid artery 64
        subclavian artery 64
    thorax and abdomen 68*f*
    upper limbs 66
Arteriosclerosis 117
Artery forceps 148*f*
Artery in autopsied bodies, choice of 93
Artificial cold 2
Ascites 116
Aspergillus 56
Asthma-like symptoms 180
Astonishing 35
Atherosclerosis 117
Atomic bombardment 35
Auguste Renouard's chemical formulas for embalming fluid 28*f*
Auricular artery, posterior 64
Autodigestion of gastric mucosa 56
Autolysis 56
Autopsy
    body 110
    preparation of 109
    gloves 131
    postmortem examination of dead body 109
    precautions for 168
Axilla, contents of 76*f*
Axillary and brachia/arteries 76
Axillary
    artery 66
    vein 67

B

Babylonians 8
Bacteremia 44
Bacterial
    agents 40
    etiology 41

septicemias 47
wound infections 47
Balantidium aerogenes capsulatus 56
Balantidium coli 56
Balantidium proteus 56
Balsami 13
Barbed tracks 35
Barbiturates 124, 125
Bard-Parker solution 43
Baron Leopold Cuvier (1769-1832) 17
Bartholin (1585-1629): developed continuous flow syringe 12
Basler solution, composition of 186
Belly Punchers 33
Benjamin F Lyford 26
Benjoini 13
Benzedrine 124
Bernardino Ramazzini 20
Betadine 49
Bichloride of mercury 21, 27
Biohazard 131
Blood
 circulation of 73
  changes at birth 74
  fetal 73
 cleaning and decontaminating spills of 171
 clots 125
 vascular system 26
 vessels, removed blood 12
 vessels, surface anatomy and exposure of 75
Blow fly 118
Body
 cavities 108
 contusion of 55t
 flesh of 9
 fluid precautions 131
 identification of 134
 orifices 109
 packing polythene bag 108
 preservation of 8, 88
 proteins 92
 size and weight of 110
 system
  circulatory 53
  nervous 53
  respiratory 53
 tissue pH 55
 wash and dry 108
 wrapping bandage soaked in petroleum jelly 108
Boric acid 138
Brachial artery 67

Brachiocephalic
 artery 75
 trunk 68
 vein
  left 69
  right 69
Brain
 adult 58
 removal of 60, 109
British Epidemiology Study 163
British Medical Research Council's Environmental Epidemiology Unit 163
Buccal cavity 163
Buffered and unbuffered, composition of 91
Buffers 82
Burn injuries 109

C

Cadaver storage facilities 90
Cadaveric
 lividity 55
 spasm 56
Cadavers
 drying of 12
 type of 88
Calami aromat 13
Calliphora erythrocephala 118
Camphor 27
 powder of 17
Canadian Funeral Licensees 163
Canary islands 8
Cancer chemotherapeutic agents 123
Cancer chemotherapy 125
Candida 127
Canopic urns 6f
Carbolic acid 82
Carcinogenicity of formaldehyde 181
Carl Lewis Barnes 31
Carotid artery
 common 17, 75, 112
 external 75
 internal 75
Caryophyll 13
Cavity
 closure of 111
 embalming 101
  instruments required for 101
  period for 103
 fluid
  composition of 86, 131
  injection of 103

injection and immersion 2
injector 101
treatment
 advocates 33
 chemicals, use of 46
 need of 101
 techniques 46
Cecum 102
Cedar, cases of 7
Celiac
 artery 77
 trunk 70
Cell
 death 55
 membranes less permeable 125
Cellular death 53
 early changes 54
Cellular material 56
Cellular metabolism 55
Centers for Disease Control 131
Central nervous system 40
Cerebral artery
 anterior 64
 middle 64
Cerebrospinal fluid 40
Cervical artery, superficial 65
Cervical injection 93
Cervical portion of trachea, removal of 109
Chamomile 13
Chemical
 agents and drugs 120
 and ingredients 81
 and physical decontamination, methods of 47
 body defense 39
 constituents of soft embalming 138t
 for embalming and techniques 22
 sterilant 43
 substance, type of 120
Chemotherapeutic agent 122
Chemotherapeutic agents, problems caused 125
Chemotherapy
 case 121
 problems, possible solutions to 126
 treatment of disease 120
Chickenpox 44
Chin rest method 106
Chloride of alumina 18
Chlorine compounds 49
Chlorpropamide (diabinese) 124
Choroidal artery 64
Cidex 49

Cinamoni 13
Cincinnati College of Embalming 30
Circle of Willis 64
Circulation, cessation of 54
Circulatory
    drugs 125
    system 20
Circumflex iliac artery, superficial 71
Cisterna cerebellomedullaris 51
Civil war times 21
Clarence G strub 31
Clean up procedure 132
Clearance from embassy 135
Close eye method 106
Clostridium welchii 55
Cloth fluid 118*t*
    composition of 87*t*
Clotting 107
Cocaine 124, 125
Coffins shaped 7
Coils of small intestine 102
Colic artery
    inferior left 70
    middle 70
    right 70
    superior left 70
Colonel Ellsworth's embalming 22
Communicating artery, posterior 64
Compazine 124
Concurrent disinfection 42
Confirmed studies 39
Consent 134
Contact dermatitis 180
Copper-mercury alum 18
Cornelius stated 26
Coronary artery
    left 68
    right 68
Coroner's physician 22
Corticosteroids 123, 125
Cosmetic
    and presentation 133
    treatment 108
    use of 133
Cosmetology
    ornamental 133
    technical 133
Costocervical trunk 65
Cotton-like circulatory blockages 125
Crane's electrodynamic mummifier 27
Cranial cavity 109, 111
    aspiration of 103
Creosote 26
Creutzfeldt-Jakob disease 88

Criminal abortions 109
Crooked spine 7
Cryptococcus 127
Cut diaphragm 60
Cuticle intact 55
Cut-up benches 197
Cyperi 13
Cytotoxic drugs act 123

D

Daniel H Prunk (1829-1923) 24
Dark ages 12
Dead body, luminescence of 57
Dead methods of disposal 58
Death
    and postmortem changes 53
    baby 109
    biological 53
    brainstem 53
    cause of 110
    cellular 53
    cerebral 53
    clinical 53
    individual cells 53
    molecular 53
    stage of somatic 53
    types of 53
        molecular death 53
        somatic 53
    whole brain 53
Decontamination 42
    embalmer(s) 43
Decubitus ulcers 117
Deep cervical artery 65
Deep external pudendal artery 71
Deep veins 65, 67, 73
    femoral vein 73
    popliteal vein 73
Dehydration 59, 125
Dental tie method 106
Dentistry, precautions for 168
Deodorants 84
Determine concentration 182
Dexedrine 124
Dialysis, precautions for 169
Diaparine chloride 49
Diluents 84
Diodorus siculus 4
Discussion with staff 183
Disinfect body 112
Disinfectant 131
    solution 109
    intermediate-level 49
    low-level 49

Disinfection 170
Disinfection 84
    activity, levels of 49*t*
    and decontamination chemistry 39
    antimicrobial activity 84
    concurrent 48
    disinfectant 84
    germicide 84
    high-level 48
    primary 48
    sterilization 84
    terminal 48
Dissection
    and demonstration purposes 185
    material 191
    rooms, working environment in 188*t*
Domestic flies, types of 118
Doorway 149
Dorsal venous arch 67
Dorsalis pedis artery 78
Dosi-tube readings for formaldehyde
    vapor 91*t*
Double rubber gloves 129
Drainage technique 98
    contents of drainage 98
    drainage sites 99
        femoral vein 99
        inferior vena cava 99
        internal jugular vein 99
        right atrium of the heart 99
    methods of 100
        alternate drainage 100
        concurrent (continuous) drainage 100
        intermittent drainage 100
    purpose of drainage 99
Droplet infection particle 40
Droplet nuclei 40, 51
Dry
    cold 1
    grass 10
    heat 1
Duamutef 6*f*
Dutch physician Peter Forestus (1522-1597) 12
Dyes 83
    eosin 83
    ponceau 83

E

Ears cavity 107
Earthquakes 35
Ecuador 9

Egypt's new Kingdom period 59
Egyptian
　burial site 3f
　embalming practice 7
　law 11
　preparation steps in 5
　　covering with natron 6
　　evisceration 5
　　removal from natron 6
　　removal of brain 5
　　wrapping and spicing 6
Electric
　aspirator 101
　pump 148f
Embalmed cadavers 137
Embalmer 42
　arterial 33
　as sanitarian 40
　legal responsibility 134
　self-manufactured 21
Embalming
　AIDS body, guidelines for 128
　anatomical 117
　and chemical manufacturers association 39
　and subsequent dissection 91t
　art and science of 33
　bodies in state of rigor mortis 114
　body 147
　　exposed to radiation 116
　burnt bodies 116
　certificate of 135
　changing room 148
　chemical continuously 21
　chemicals 81
　completion of 131
　decomposed bodies 115
　delayed 114
　facilities, establishment of 146
　fluids 40, 81f, 84, 88, 130
　　arterial fluid 85
　　cavity fluid 85
　　composition of four different 91t
　　percentage composition of 89
　　preinjection fluid 86
　　to kill microorganisms 82
　hands 108
　history of 18, 20
　human dead bodies, form of application for 134
　human remains, recommended minimum standards for 44
　hypodermic 95
　ideal method of 108
　improvement in 26
　infant procedure 112
　　cavity treatment 113
　　fluid strengths and volume 113
　　pressure 113
　　rate of flow of injection 113
　　selection of blood vessels 112
　knowledge 21
　methods of 95, 129
　　arterial embalming 95, 129
　　cavity embalming 95, 129
　　supplemental methods of 95, 129
　　　hypodermic embalming 130
　　　surface embalming 130
　　variation in 3
　modern 92
　multidisciplinary science of 39
　near battlefield during the civil war 24f
　need of 146
　origin and history of 1
　periods of history 2
　powders 159
　practical 92
　practice of 32
　preparation room 148
　procedure 12, 90, 130
　　arterial embalming 95
　　　electric pump 95
　　　gravity injection 95
　　hypodermic embalming 96
　process and materials 12
　process of 105
　professionalism in 33
　refrigerated bodies 115
　reports concerning arterial injection 32
　room 129, 146, 156
　　equipment and furniture 147
　　preparation 148
　schools
　　establishment of 2
　　increase in 31
　soft 137
　　alternative to thiel 138
　　procedure 137
　　role of various components of 138
　solutions, look for alternative 183
　specific purpose of 14
　surface 95
　surgeons of the civil war 22
　table 35
　techniques, modern 88
　third mode of 4
　unautopsied adult bodies 105
　unit 178f
　waiting room 149
Endogenous
　invasion 40
　microflora 40
Endothelial, surface of pleura 57
Endothelium of blood sinusoid 189f
Endotracheal tubings 128
England's customs and achievements 14
Environment 39
　safety branch 41
Enzyme 121
　action of 56
　immunoassay 172
Eosin 85
Epigastric artery, superficial 71
Equanil 124
Esophagus, removal of 109
Ethyl alcohol 51
Ethylene glycol 138
　monophenyl ether 190
Ethylene oxide gas 51
Europe from the dark ages, emergence of 11
Europe's access to cadavers 17
Evisceration 2
　and drying 2
　and immersion 2
　local incision 2
Exhaust duct against the back wall 43f
Exposure
　and cannulation 94
　effects of 162
External pudendal artery, superficial 71
Eye
　and respiratory tract, effects on 194
　bank story 32
　changes in 54
　irritation of 180
　osiris 61

F

Facemask 129
Facial vein 66
Factory accidents 109
Falcon electric embalmer 35
Falconry 19
Faulty theories 39
Felix Aloysius Sullivan (1843–1931) 30
Femoral artery 17, 71, 77, 107, 112
Femoral triangle 77f
Fetal death 109

Fixative solutions, composition of 186
Flaccidity muscles 55
    primary 55, 114
    secondary 56, 114
Flammable gas 179
Fluid
    for nervous tissue 87
    manufacture 21
    oozes 108
    required, quantity of 86
Forceps 147f
Forensic
    autopsy 109
    expert 109
Forestus embalming 12
Formaldehyde 49, 51, 81, 91, 138, 193
    adverse effects of 179
    alternatives to 89
    and cancer 194
    and paraformaldehyde
        methods and materials 152
        results 152
    chemical structure of 81f
    concentration 152, 158, 163, 159t
        comparison of ventilation systems 153
        dissection rooms 180
        in anatomy laboratories 180
        in funeral homes 153t
    demand 121
    exposure, reported studies on effects of 162
    fumes 34
    in anatomy 179
    in long-term preservation of human anatomical specimens 185
    in Medical Schools in the UK, use of 89
    in pathology departments 193
    levels, experiments to monitor 90
    mutagenicity of 181
    properties of 179
    risks and problems in the use of 88
    safe levels of 88
    safe limit of 157
    study in funeral homes 151
    study in preparation rooms 158
    tolerance to 194
    toxicity 158
    transfer of concentrate 178
    vapor emission study 156
    workers 151
Formalin 34, 85, 87
Foul-smelling gases, liberation of 57

Francois Chaussier (1746–1828) 17
Freezing 1
Frozen cases 105
Frozen solid state 115
Fume cupboards 196
Fume extraction unit 198f
Fumigation 198
Funeral home 153
    personal health policies 44
Fungal infection 117
Fungal infections 44, 47

G

Gabriel clauderus (late 17th century) 14
Galen's teachings and writings on human anatomy 11
Gall capillaries 189f
Gaseous compounds injected 26
Gases, liberation of 57
Gastric juice 56
Gastrointestinal
    tract 40, 119
    ulcerations 123
General guidelines 43
Genicular artery, descending 71
Genitourinary tract 40
Gentiana 13
Germicide protective barrier attire 51
Germicides 82
Germs die with the host 39
Girolamo Segato 19
Gloves 131
Gluing lips 106
Glutaraldehyde 49, 82
    activated 51
Gluteal artery
    inferior 70
    superior 70
Glycerin 85
Glycerol 91
Glycolytic 56
Goatskins 9
Goggles 129
Grave wax 58
Gravity fluid injection 20f
Guanches' method of embalming 9

H

Hair covering 129
Handling sharp instruments 131
Harlan's translation of history of embalming 19f

Hazardous chemical particulates 42
Head and face, injection treatment of 110
Health hazard 149
Healthcare workers
    acquiring HIV in healthcare settings 166
    definition of 165
    management of exposures 174
    testing of 174
    with AIDS 165
Heart 63, 63f
    right side of 102
    surfaces diaphragmatic (inferior) 63
    surfaces left surface 63
    surfaces sternocostal (anterior) 63
Heat
    simple 1
    sterilization 51
Hepatic veins 71
Hepatitis 109
    B virus 174
Hepatocytes with cytosomes 189f
Hinged instruments 50
Histoplasma infections 127
Homicides 109
Host of salts 21
Hot tap water 138
Household bleach 109
Housekeeping 170
Howard S Eckels (1865-1837), manufacturer of embalming chemicals 31
Human immunodeficiency virus 41, 128, 165, 172t
    antibody tests 173t
    in environment, survival of 130, 170
    infection during pregnancy 132
    infection, serologic testing for 172
    precautions to prevent transmission of 167
    testing of patients 173
    transmission in healthcare settings 165
    transmission, environmental considerations for 170
Human
    liver stained 189f
    remains 42
    skeleton 79f
Hydrochloric acid 21
Hydrocyanic acid poisoning 55
Hypodermic
    embalming 115
    needles 50

Hypostasis 55
Hypostasis stain 57

I

Ileocolic artery 70
Iliac artery
    common 70, 77
    external 70, 77, 112
    internal 70
Iliac veins
    external 71
    internal 71
Iliolumbar artery 70
Illness
    contagious 88
    terminal 88
Immersion solution 138
Immunization 43
Incisions, various types of 94, 94f
    combined 94
    longitudinal 94
    transverse 94
    wedge 94
Indian Medical Council 144
Industrial methylated spirit 89, 91
Infected healthcare workers,
    management of 174
Infection
    danger of 200
    prevalence of 172
    risk-handle with care 129
    risks of 46
Infectious
    agent 47
    diseases, refusal on the ground of 136
    hepatitis 47
Infective waste 171
Information, lack of 40
Ingestion 194
Inguinal ligament 71
Inhalation of infectious 42
Inhaling formaldehyde, adverse effects
    of 181t
Injected wax to secure castings 12
Injection
    and drainage 107
    solution 138
    syringe 24f
    techniques 97
        multipoint injection 97
        one-point injection 97
        restricted cervical injection 98
        six-point injection 98
        split injection 97

treatment of
    lower extremities 110
    upper extremities 110
Instruments
    disposal of used 132
    for injection, early 12
Intercostal artery
    posterior 68
    superior 65
Intermittent (restricted) drainage,
    use of 45
Intestine
    large 58, 60, 63
    removal of 60
    small 63
Inventor of the microscope 14
Investigators in Europe 202
Iodophors 49
Iowa state department of health 163
Irosflorent 13
Isopropyl alcohol 51
Isotope 116, 124

J

Jackal's head 6f
Jaundice, conquest of 32
Jean-Nicolas Gannal (1791–1852) 17
Jejunal and ileal arteries 70
John Hunter (1728–1793) 16
John Morgan (Circa 1863) 19
Jugular vein
    anterior 65
    external 65
    internal 64, 65, 116

K

Kidneys, removal of 60
Kodiak archipelago 10
Kodiak Archipelago practiced
    preservation 10

L

Laboratories, precautions for 169
Larynx and trachea 58
Larynx, removal of 109
Laundry 171
Lavendula 13
Law and dead 141
    Indian practice 141
    Western scenerio 141
Legionnaires' disease 44

Lensed instruments 50
Librium 124
Lifespan of less-specialized cells 54t
Lingual
    artery 64
    vein 66
Lipolytic action of enzymes 56
Liquid microbicide 49
Liver
    part of 102
    removal of 60
Living from disease 41
Livor mortis 114
Louis Jacques Thenard (1777–1857) 17
Ludwig De Bils (1624–1671) 14
Lung diseases, treatment of 28
Lungs, removal of 60
Lysosomes 56

M

Macula densa 189f
Maggots 118
    event of 118
Magic bullet 120, 123
Mammary artery, internal 65
Mantoux skin test for tuberculosis 43
Marjoran 13
Massage cream to face 110
Materials and methods 186
Matter insoluble in water 61
Matthew Baillie (1761–1823) 16
Maxillary artery 64
Mechanical pump 90
Medical Schools 90
Medicolegal case 135
Medicolegal examination 109
Mediterranean 11
Meningitis 109
Meprobamate 124, 125
Mercurial compounds organic 49
Mesenteric artery
    inferior 70, 77
    superior 70, 77
Mesenteric vein
    inferior 71
    superior 71
Metal and materials 35
Methanol 82, 85
Methe 13
Mexico's outstanding anthropologist 10
Microbial contamination, controlling 48t
Micrograft 189f
Military religious campaigns 11

Miltown 124
Mission and high commissions 135
Mobile embalming unit 177
Modern period 21
Moisture, lack of 58
Mood-altering drugs 124
Morticians' services, precautions for 168
Mortuary services, practitioners of 41
Mourner's room 149
Mouth gags 128
Multi-site injection and drainage 44
Mummies, wrapped 7
Mummification 54, 58, 59
    procedure 60
    results 60
Mummifier's table 61*t*
Mummiform coffin 8*f*
Musca domestica 118
Muscle
    atrophy 125
    cell life, end of 56
    protein 56
    relaxants 84
    infection 117
Myosin 56
Myrrh 8, 13

N

Narcotics 124
Nasal and oral cavities 110
Nasal cavities 57, 107
National Accreditation of Mortuary
    Schools 32
National Funeral Directors Association 28
National Institute of Neurological
    Diseases and Stroke 201
National Institutes of Health 41, 201
Natron dimensions 61
Natron salt wrapped in linen 61
Neck, side of 75
Needle injector method 106, 106*f*
Neutralizing chemotherapeutic agents
    125
New technique, discovery of 13
New York State Supreme Court 1
New York University Medical College 22
Niter 17
Nitrate of potash 18
No objection certificate from police 135
North American Indians 10
Nostrils 110, 149
Notifiable diseases 136
Novel ventilated necropsy table 197*f*

Nucis moschat 13
Nylon thread 104

O

Obesity 118
Obturator artery 64, 70, 72
Occupational health authorities 185
Occupational health hazard 179
Occupational safety and health
    administration 41
Oil of cedar 4
Omnium quod sut'ficit 13
Operative antemortem epithelial 40
Ophthalmic artery 64
    supplies the eye 64
Opiates 124
Opponents of formalin fluids 34
Oral drugs control 124
Oral-nasal masks 44
Organs, removal of 60
Ormation of alkaline product 55
Orphanages and poorhouses,
    establishment of 11
Oxygen starvation 53

P

Pacemaker 118
Paint mixture 86, 118*t*
    composition of 86
Pancreas 58
    removal of 60
Pancreaticoduodenal artery inferior 70
Paraffin section of human kidney 189*f*
Paraformaldehyde powders 153
Paraformaldehyde study in funeral
    homes 151
Pasteurella 202
Pelvic cavities 46
    removal of 109
Penicillins 125
Performance procedures 46
Perfumes 84
Pericardium 57
Peritoneum 57
Personal health considerations 39
Personal hygiene and safety 41
Personal involvement dealing with the
    embalmer's 39
Peru 9
Petrosal sinus, inferior 66
pH
    buffered 91
    unbuffered 91

Pharyngeal artery, ascending 64
Pharyngeal vein 66
Phenol 82, 85, 91
Phenolic
    compounds 49
    derivatives 82
Phenomenon, internal 57
Phenothiazines 124, 125
Phenoxetol 190
Phenoxyethanol 185, 190, 191
Phrenic veins, inferior 71
Physical examination 43
Physicians and anatomists 19
Pituitary gland 109
Plastic apron 129
Plutarch 5
Poisoning by nitrates 55
Poisoning suspected or evident 109
Poisonous chemicals 34
Polyethylene
    catheters 50
    tubing 50
Popliteal
    artery 72, 77
    fossa 77*f*
Portal circulation 63
Portal of "host" entry 47
Portal veins 71
Portrait of
    Dr Thomas holmes 22*f*
    Henry P Cattell 23*f*
    Jean-Nicolas Gannal of age 4*U* 18*f*
    Joseph Henry Clarke, founder of
        Cincinnati College of
        Embalming 29*f*
Postmortem
    caloricity 55
    changes 54, 114, 193
    delivery of fetus 57
    regurgitation 119
    room layout 198*f*
    staining 55, 55*t*, 57
    suggillation for 55
Potassium
    bicarbonate 55
    chlorate 55
    nitrate 26, 138
Powdered mixture of alum salt 27
Powdered resin 9
Practical containment measures 196
Precautions
    for invasive procedures 167
    implementation of recommended
        171

Pre-embalming
  consideration criteria for selection of vessel 92
  preparations 128
  treatment 119
Pregnant workers 132
Preludin 124
Preservation
  artificial means of 1
  body in peru 9
  natural means of 1
Preservative 81
  agents by drugs, inactivation of 122
  chemicals 82
  concentration of 45
Profunda femoris artery 71
Properties 156
Prophylactic antibodies, administration of 44
Propylene glycol 138
Prosector's wart 201
Protective barrier attire 39
Proteins 120
  chemistry of 120
Proteolytic 56
  enzymes 122
Protozoan 200
Pseudomonas aeruginosa 190
Public and professional acceptance 26
Public health
  areas of 41
  guideline 47
    for risk embalmer "host" 47*t*
    premise 42
    purpose 41
  safety 39
Pudendal artery internal 70
Pulmonary
  circulation 63
  trunk 69, 75
  veins 70
Pulsating devices 35
Purge 119
Putrefaction 56
  and autolysis 54
  factors affecting the rate of 58
  in water 58
  modified 58
Putrefactive changes 57
Pyocyanea infections 190
Pyramids 59

Q

Qebeh-Snewef 6*f*
Quartermaster
  general 21
  officer 21
Quaternary ammonium
  compounds 49
  solutions 51

R

Radial artery 67, 76
Radiation, type of 116*t*, 124
Radioactive isotopes
  effect of 124
  used to treat malignancy 116*t*
Radioisotopes, used to treat malignancies 124*t*
Receptacle jar 101
Receptacles 7
Rectal artery
  middle 70
  superior 70
Rectum 149
Red blood cells, hemolysis of 57
Red tagging 40
Renal veins 71
Reserpine 124
Resin 17
Respiration, cessation of 54
Respiratory
  infections of viral 41
  tract mucosa 180
Reticuloendothelial system 40
Richard Harlan (1796-1843) 18
Richardson's eye process 33
Rigid plastic pipes 177
Rigor mortis 54, 55, 114
  time of onset of 56
Ritalin 124
Road side accidents 109
Rodgers' method of single-entrance 33
Room ventilation 183, 196
Rorismar 13
Royal College of Surgeons 15, 16
Rubber
  tube 101
  tubing rubber catheters 50
Rubella vaccination 43
Ryle's tube 128

S

Sacral artery
  lateral 70
  median 70
Salvia 13
Sanitation survey 47
Santel 13
Saphenous vein
  great 73
  small 73
Saponification 58
Saprophytic bacteria 56
Scalpel 101
Scalpel and blades 147*f*
School of Embalming and Organic Chemistry 29
Scissors 148*f*
Seconal 124
Sedatives drugs 124, 125
Selected microbicides, activity levels of 49*t*
Semiopaque cream 133
Septicemia 44
Serum hepatitis 43
Simmons School of Embalming in Syracuse 32
Skin changes in 54
Skin effects on 194
Smooth muscles 55
Sodium
  bicarbonate 61
  borate 85
  carbonate 61
  chloride 18, 61
  citrate 85
  hypochlorite 51
    solution of 131
  sulfate 61, 138
Soft-embalmed cadavers
  advantages and disadvantages of 139
  surgical procedures performed 139
Soil, nature of 1
Soluble wintergreen 85
Somatic death, immediate 54
Sonacide 43, 49
Specimens for anatomical studies, preparation of 177
Spices grossly powdered 13
Spinal cord, removal of 109
Spleen 63
  removal of 60
Splenic vein 71

Sporicidin 49
Staphylococci 56, 202
Starves 120
Sterilization 170
Sternocleidomastoid muscle 64
Stimulants drugs 125
Stomach 102
    removal of 60
Streptococci 56, 202
Styracis calamita 13
Subclavian
    artery 68, 76
    vein 66
Sugar of lead 21
Suicides 109
Supplemental chemicals, use of 45
Suprarenal vein, right 71
Suprascapular artery 65
Surgical instruments 147
Syrians 8
Syringes 147*f*
Systemic failures
    asphyxia 53
    cases of 109
    coma 53
    syncope 53
Systemic mycoses 41

T

Tank (immersion) fluid 86
Tank (immersion) fluid, composition of 86*t*
Tap water 91
Temporal artery, superficial 64
Terminal
    branches 70
    disinfection 42, 43
Tetrabromofluorescein 83
Tetracyclines 125
Thermometers 50
Thomas Joseph Pettigrew 19
Thomas Marshall 19
Thoracic aorta descending 75
Thoracic cavity
    aspiration of 103
    removal of 109
Thoracic, treatment of 46
Thorazine 124
Threshold limit value 151
Throat
    cavity 107
    cutters 33
Thymi 13

Thymol 85
Thyrocervical trunk 65
Thyroid artery
    superior 64
Thyroid gland, removal of 109
Thyroid vein
    middle 66
    superior 66
Tibial artery
    anterior 72, 78
    posterior 72, 78
Tissue decomposition, order of 58
    firm tissue 58
    hard tissue 58
    soft tissue 58
Tissues, liquefaction of 57
Tofranil 124
Tolbutamide (orinase) 124
Total volume of arterial 45
Toxic gas 151
Toxicity survey 153
Toxicity to humans 194
Toxoplasma 200
Toxoplasmosis 200
Tranquilizers drugs 124, 125
Translations, differences in 5
Transmission electron micrograph 189*f*
Tributaries 66
Tripod of life
    brain 53
    heart 53
    lung 53
Trocar
    guides 103*f*
    insertion of 102
Tuberculosis 47
Tuberculosis incidence of 47
Tumor, incidence 182
Turnip watch 118

U

Ulnar artery 67, 76
Ultrathin section of human liver stained 189*f*
Ultraviolet light illuminator furnished 35
Umbilical artery 70
Undertaker's manual 28*f*, 33
Universal blood 131
Universal precautions 167
Universal work precautions 131
Urea 121
Urethral catheters 128

Uric acid 121
Urinary bladder 103
Uterine artery (in female) 70

V

Vaccination (heptavax B) 43
Vacuum breakers 43
Vaginal
    artery (in female) 70
    orifice 149
Vagus nerve 64
Valium 124
Vascular system 44
Vehicles 84
Veins 71
Veins of
    abdomen 71
    body 78
        external jugular vein 78
        femoral vein 78
        great saphenous vein 78
        inferior vena cava 78
        internal jugular vein 78
        left brachiocephalic vein 78
        portal vein 79
        right brachiocephalic vein 78
        small saphenous vein 78
        subclavian vein 78
        superior vena cava 78
    head and neck 65*f*
    lower limb 72
    neck 65
    thorax 69
    and abdomen 69*f*
    upper limb 67
Veins, superficial 65, 67, 72
    basilic vein 67
    cephalic vein 67
Vena cava, inferior 63, 70, 71, 92, 112
    tributaries of 71
Vena cava, superior 69
Venous
    blood 63
    coagula 107
    drainage, reasons for 108
Ventilation systems 153, 156, 159, 159*t*
Vertebral artery 65
Vesical artery inferior 70
Vessel
    choice artery 92
    choice in infants and children 92
    depth location of 92
    exposure of 93

axillary artery and vein 93
basilic vein 93
brachial artery 93
common carotid artery 93
femoral artery and vein 94
internal jugular vein 93
radial artery 94
proximity of heart 92
selection of 107, 114
size of 92
Viral
encephalitides 41
upper respiratory infections 47
Viscera of body 79, 80
ascending colon 80
cecum 80
descending colon 80
gallbladder 80
heart 79
kidney 80
liver 80
lungs 79
pancreas 80
spleen 79
stomach 79
trachea 79*t*
transverse colon 80
Viscera, preservation of 104
Viscera, treatment of 111
Visceral branches
anterior 70
lateral 70
Visceral tributaries 71

W

Warmth enhances 58
Washing solution 109
Waste materials 121
Water 85
Weight loss 125
Werowance Indian 10
Wescodyne 49
Wetting agents 83
glycerin 83
sodium lauryl sulfate 83
sorbitol 83
William Hunter 15
William J Bunnell 22
William Peter Hohenschuh 31
Women embalmers 32
Wooden anthropoid 8*f*
Wooden coffin 7*f*
World War II, end of 35

Z

Zephiran chloride 49, 82
Zinc chloride 21, 26, 27